AMERICAN JOURNAL of PUBLIC HEALTH
JULY 2025
Issue 7

# AJPH

A PUBLICATION OF THE
AMERICAN PUBLIC HEALTH ASSOCIATION

## THE ENVIRONMENTAL, HEALTH, AND HUMANITARIAN CRISES IN GAZA

Ongoing Environmental Destruction and Degradation of Gaza, p. 1053
Conflict and the Environment, p. 1042
A Maelstrom of Misfortune, p. 1044
Israel and Gaza's Public Health Cooperation, p. 1046
Opportunities for Action, p. 1050

Also in this issue:

AJPH EDITOR-IN-CHIEF
Ten Years at the Helm, p. 975

QUALITY IN SCIENTIFIC PUBLICATION
A Guidance Document, p. 966

Uncovering Racial, Ethnic, and Gender Disparities, p. 1129

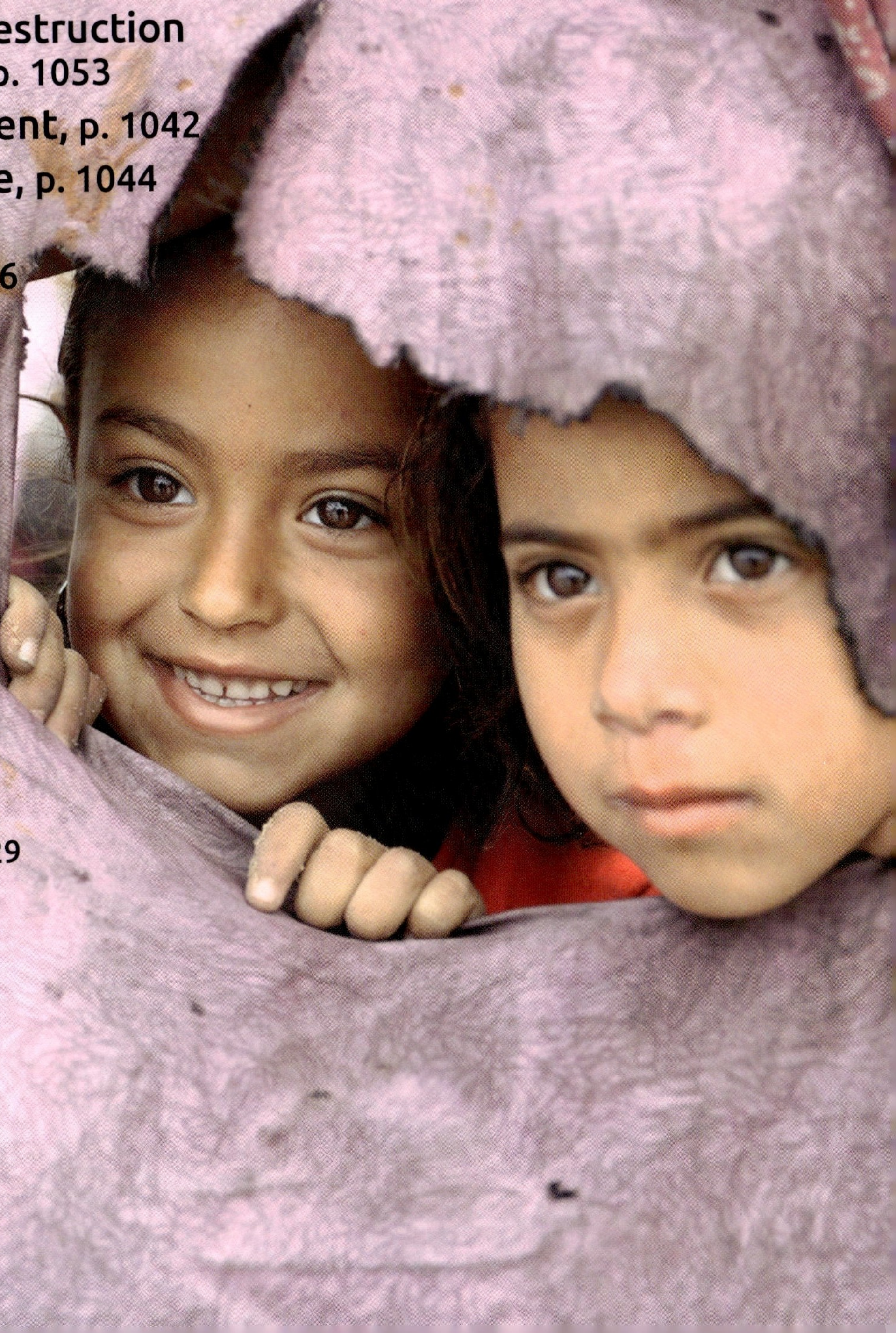

AMERICAN PUBLIC HEALTH ASSOCIATION
*For science. For action. For health.*

*AJPH*®, published monthly, is the official Journal of the American Public Health Association®, 800 I St NW, Washington, DC 20001-3710; (202) 777- APHA; TDD (202) 777-2500. APHA is a nongovernmental professional society founded in 1872, representing all disciplines and specialties in public health.



The *American Journal of Public Health*® (*AJPH*) (print ISSN: 0090-0036; electronic ISSN: 1541- 0048), first published in 1911, is the official journal of the American Public Health Association® (APHA). The oldest and largest organization of public health professionals in the world, APHA represents approximately 30 000 members from more than 50 occupations of public health.

**Submissions:** Visit www.editorialmanager.com/ajph or ajph.edmgr.com for online manuscript preparation and submission guidelines. Contributions of original unpublished research, social science analyses, scholarly essays, critical commentaries, departments, and letters to the editor are welcome. Questions? Write ajph.submissions@apha.org or call APHA at (202) 777-2469.

**Print plus online subscriptions:** Institutional price (print copy with online access for a single institution and all authorized users, regardless of geographic location) varies by size of organization and ranges from \$993–\$1445 for US organizations, and \$1073–\$1526 for international organizations (air delivery); multiple campuses not permitted without special arrangement. Details of the tiered pricing system at https://subscriptionoffice.com/pages/apha-landing-page. To order, write apha.subscriptions@apha.org.

**Online-only subscriptions:** Institutional price for one institution and its authorized users (regardless of geographic location) is \$878–\$1307. To order, write apha.subscriptions@apha.org. For academic consortia or multisite corporate subscriptions, contact apha.subscriptions@apha.org.

**Print-only subscriptions:** Institutional price is US \$701, \$782 international.

**Back print issues:** A limited number of print issues are for sale. Single copies are US \$65, \$75 international (air delivery). Shipping included; prepay only. To order, write apha.subscriptions@apha.org.

**Reprints:** For prices and ordering information on 50 or more reprints, check the Reprints section at www.ajph.org. To order smaller quantities of reprints (rush delivery), use the "Purchase Article" link on the article site itself.

**Electronic access:** Online articles more than 10 years old are available free for personal use at www.ajph.org. Recent articles are available through pay-per-view: single PDF article for \$24, single issue access for 24 hours for \$33, or entire site access for 24 hours for \$38.

**Postal information:** Periodicals postage paid at Washington, DC, and additional mailing offices. Postmaster: Send address changes to American Journal of Public Health, 800 I St NW, Washington, DC 20001-3710.

**Address changes:** Send to AJPH, Membership Department (members) or AJPH Subscriptions (subscribers), APHA, 800 I St NW, Washington, DC 20001-3710. Or write to membership.mail@apha.org (members) or apha.subscriptions@apha.org (subscribers).

**Advertising:** For pricing and other information, see www.ajph.org. Please write to brian.selzer@apha.org or call (202) 777-2470 for other advertising opportunities. Ask about special exhibit packages and sponsorships. Acceptance of advertising by the *Journal* does not imply endorsement of products.



**Indexes:** Publications that index or abstract articles from *AJPH* include the following: Ageline, Assia (Applied Social Science Index and Abstracts), Biological Abstracts, Chemical Abstracts, CINAHL, Criminal Justice Abstracts, EMBASE, EMCare, Environmental Abstracts, e-psyche, ERIC, ETOH (Alcohol and Alcohol Problems Science Database), Excerpta Medica, Food Science and Technology, General Science Index, Grateful Med, Hospital Literature Index, Human Resources Abstracts, International Pharmaceutical Abstracts (IPA), Medline, Physical Education Index, Pollution Abstracts, Psychological Abstracts, PsychINFO, Safety Science Abstracts, Sage Family Studies Abstracts, Sage Human Resources Abstracts, Science Citation Index, SCOPUS, SIIC Data Bases, Social Work Research and Abstracts, and Statistical Reference Index (SRI)/LexisNexis.

Medscape Publishers Circle

# AJPH

A PUBLICATION OF THE
**AMERICAN PUBLIC HEALTH ASSOCIATION**

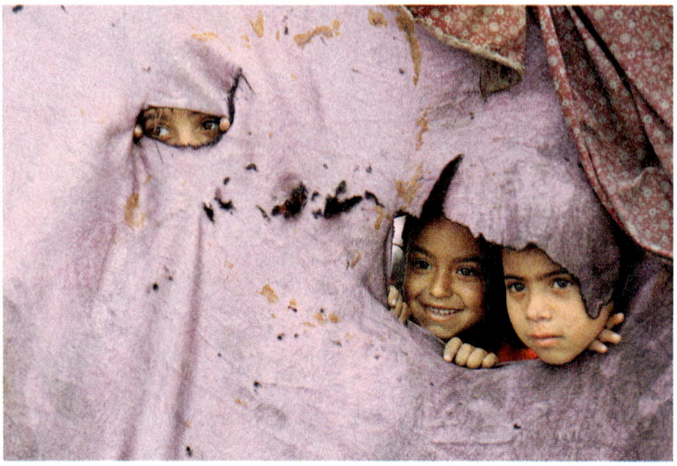

COVER: Palestinian children peek out of holes in their tent at a makeshift displacement camp set up amid building rubble in Gaza City on May 12, 2025. Israeli Prime Minister Benjamin Netanyahu said on May 12 that the release of a US–Israeli hostage announced by Hamas would not lead to a ceasefire in the Gaza Strip or the release of Palestinian detainees.

Cover concept and selection by Aleisha Kropf. Photo by OMAR AL-QATTAA/AFP via Getty Images. Printed with permission.

APHA
AMERICAN PUBLIC HEALTH ASSOCIATION
*For science. For action. For health.*

Promoting public health research, policy, practice, and education is the *AJPH* mission. As we widen our scope to embrace global issues, we also sharpen our focus to support the needs of public health practitioners. We invite contributions of original unpublished research, opinion and commentary, and letters to the editor.

The *Journal* is printed on acid-free recycled paper.

OPEN ACCESS ONLINE ONLY PODCAST DATA SUPPLEMENT AVAILABLE


EDITOR'S CHOICE

966 Ensuring Quality in Scientific Publication Through Inclusivity and Transparency
*M. Loui and A. Morabia*

BOOKS & MEDIA

968 Do Data Still Matter in Gun Rights States? Review of *What We've Become: Living and Dying in a Country of Arms*
*J. L. Pomeranz*

971 An Insider's (Plus Protégés') Take on (North–South) Global Health During Troubled Times
*P. Trivellato and A-E. Birn*

## OPINIONS, IDEAS, & PRACTICE

EDITORIALS

975 Ten Years at the Helm: Reflections From the *AJPH* Editor-in-Chief
*A. Morabia*

979 Minimum Legal Age Restrictions on Cannabis Sales: Just One Important Tool for Prevention
*J. A. Dilley and R. G. Hendrickson*

982 Masking the Health Impacts of Anti-LGBTQ+ Policies by Political Suppression of Data and Informational Erasure
*J. R. Cimpian and M. T. McQuillan*

985 On The Efficacy and Legality of Vaccine Mandates
*J. G. Hodge Jr.*

988 An Effective HIV Response Means HIV Decriminalization
*J. Csete*

990 The Need for Comprehensive and Timely City-Level Fatal and Nonfatal Firearm Injury Surveillance
*A. A. Braga*

993 Equity as a Pragmatic Application of Ethics: Considerations for Scarce Resource Allocation During a Pandemic
*R. Gur-Arie*

PERSPECTIVES

996 Health Inequalities, Disparities, Equity: What's in a Name?
*P. Braveman*

1003 Integrating Reproductive Justice in Public Health Practice, Research, and Advocacy: An Imperative to Advance Health Equity
*M. Velarde and A. Hassan*

1008 Law and Policy Efforts to Dismantle Diversity, Equity, and Inclusion
*D. G. Aaron, F. C. Stanford, and A. E. Emery*

1014 The American Public's Disengagement With Highly Pathogenic Avian Influenza (HPAI): Considerations for Vaccination and Dietary Changes
*R. Piltch-Loeb, K. Wyka, T. M. White, S. G. Gibbs, S. Gorman, A. Joshi, S. Kimball, J. V. Lazarus, J. J. Lowe, K. Rabin, S. C. Ratzan, and A. El-Mohandes*

1019 The Unsettled PREEMIE Reauthorization Act and the Recalcitrant Challenge of Preterm Births
*E. Y. Adashi, D. P. O'Mahony, and I. G. Cohen*

1022 Fluoride, Teeth, and Developing Brains: Dental Health in Tension With Environmental Health, Millions Affected
*H. Hu and L. Birnbaum*

RADICAL HOPE

1025 Yellow Power: Building Asian Student Community Voices Against Gender-Based Violence Through Public Health Research and Art
*E. V. Park*

1027 Disability Dream Work for the Public's Health
*V. Sivamani and S. V. Lu*

1029 Stride by Stride: How Run Clubs Foster Public Health
*L. N. Bui*

EDITORS' CORNER

1032 *AJPH* Project Examines the *Journal*'s Past Representation of Historically Marginalized Populations
*T. M. Brown, M. M. Jones, and C. Roth*

IMAGES OF HEALTH

1034 Point of View: Portraits of Maternal Mental Health
*J. Glance and J. A. Nielson*

NOTES FROM THE FIELD

1037 Beyond Boundaries: Navigating Challenges and Charting the Future of Reproductive Health Care in the Post-*Roe* Landscape
*T. M. H. Hoang, R. DeLuna, E. Albertson, A. Wong, A. Santoyo, and V. Ferrara*

CONFLICT AND THE ENVIRONMENT: THE TRAGIC EXAMPLE OF GAZA

1042 Conflict and the Environment: The Tragic Example of Gaza
*J. M. Samet*

1044 Personal Reflections on the Environmental Destruction and Degradation of Gaza: A Maelstrom of Misfortune
*L. O. Gostin*

1046 Israel and Gaza: Keeping Room for Hope Based on Past Cooperation in Public Health
*T. H. Tulchinsky, A. M. Troen, D. Nitzan, R. Lobel, and G. DeFriese*

1050 Destruction of Public Health and the Environment in Wars in Gaza and Beyond: What Must be Done
*L. Rubenstein*

## RESEARCH & ANALYSIS

CONFLICT AND THE ENVIRONMENT: THE TRAGIC EXAMPLE OF GAZA

1053 The Ongoing Environmental Destruction and Degradation of Gaza: The Resulting Public Health Crisis
*A. Abuawad, M. Griffiths, G. H. Edwards, A. Eftekhari, M. Al-Ebweini, H. Al-Najar, A. Butmeh, R. Abu Dayyeh, M. El-Shewy, and A. Aker*

CLIMATE CHANGE

1062 A Flexible Framework for Urgent Public Health Climate Action
*H. A. Joseph, S. C. Lemon, K. V. Goins, S. A. Aytur, S. Zimmerman, E. Alexander, C. Brown, S. Saha, and P. J. Schramm*

HISTORY

1074 History of Risk Assessments of the Organophosphate Pesticide Chlorpyrifos at the US Environmental Protection Agency, 1980–2024
*C. Sellers, E. Kohl, M. Sullivan, G. Gehrke, J. Varner, M. Chambers, and the Environmental Data and Governance Initiative*

POLICY

1085 Was the Allocation of COVID-19 Vaccines Globally Fair and Equitable?
*E. J. Emanuel and M. Jung*

HEALTH MONITORING

1095 Self-Reported Versus County-Based Rurality of People Who Gave Birth in 6 US States, 2020
*K. B. Kozhimannil, E. C. Sheffield, J. D. Interrante, C. Liu, and J. R. Daw*

1106 State-Level Estimates of Nonfatal Firearm Injury Hospitalizations, 2000–2021
*R. Smart, J. Murphy, T. L. Schell, A. R. Morral, and N. Nicosia*

1115 Sequencing-Based Detection of Measles in Wastewater: Texas, January 2025
*S. Javornik Cregeen, M. J. Tisza, B. Hanson, M. Cook, A. Surathu, R. Schneider, J. Wu, K. Short, K. Domakonda, L. Hopkins, M. C. Ross, J. F. Petrosino, J. Deegan, L. B. Stadler, E. Boerwinkle, and A. Maresso*

OPEN-THEMED RESEARCH

1120 World Trade Center (WTC) Exposures and Cardiometabolic Risk Among WTC Health Program General Responders
*H. Krasnov, K. A. Patel, P. Knobel, H-H. L. Hsu, S. L. Teitelbaum, M. A. McLaughlin, A. C. Just, and M. Y. Sade*

1129 Evaluating Algorithmic Approaches to Uncover Racial, Ethnic, and Gender Disparities in Scientific Authorship
*Y. Song, N. Dasgupta, and M. L. Bell*

1137 Adverse Childhood Experiences Among LGBTQ+ High School Students: National Evidence From the 2023 Youth Risk Behavior Survey
*J. Mittleman*

1146 COVID-19 Vaccine Mandate and Vaccination Rates in the US Military, 2020–2022
*E. J. Dullea, A. A. Eick-Cost, C. H. Olsen, and J. D. Mancuso*

1157 A Decarceral Response to HIV Criminalization in the Black LGBTQIA+ Community
*L. Listerud, S. Meanley, A. Richards, B. Kosciow, and S. Bonett*

1166 Minimum Legal Age of Nonmedical Cannabis Purchase Laws and Cannabis-Related Hospitalizations in Canada, 2015 to 2022
*D. T. Myran, R. Talarico, R. L. Pacula, J. Xiao, D. Manuel, E. Hobin, L. Konikoff, P. Tanuseputro, and M. Taljaard*

**BACKMATTER**

LETTERS & RESPONSES

1175 "Whiteness" and the Opioid Epidemic: A Construct in Need of Elaboration
*A. Pendyal*

# Ensuring Quality in Scientific Publication Through Inclusivity and Transparency

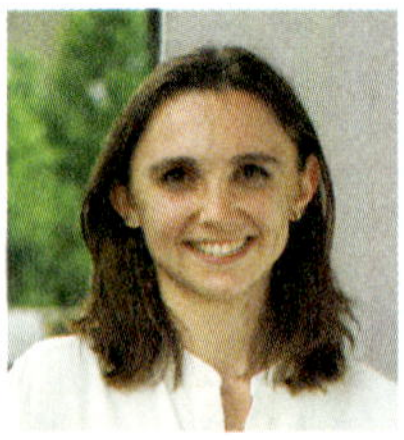
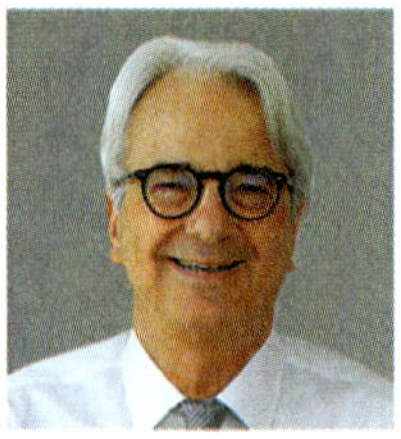

Meredith Loui, MPH
Alfredo Morabia, MD, PhD
Editor-in-Chief, *AJPH*

AJPH July 2025, Vol. 115, No. 7

High-quality scientific publication depends not only on rigorous research but also on equitable editorial practices. This includes ensuring that researchers from all backgrounds have access to the publishing process and that published findings are presented accurately, transparently, and reliably.

A coalition of leading journals—including *American Pediatrics*, *Health Affairs*, *JAMA*, *The Lancet*, and *AJPH*—supported by the Robert Wood Johnson Foundation, formed a working group to develop guidance for improving editorial processes and advancing diversity of thought in scientific publishing.

The *Guidance for Ensuring Quality in Scientific Publication Through Inclusivity and Transparency* (*EQSPI*) outlines key practices that journals can adopt or adapt based on their unique capacities (see the Appendix, available as a supplement to the online version of this article at http://www.ajph.org). Recognizing that journals vary in size, funding, and staffing, *EQSPI* offers flexible implementation approaches—from small-scale actions to more substantial structural reforms.

Below are the eight core strategies included in the guidance:

1. Transparency: Journals are encouraged to openly communicate their editorial standards and decision-making processes. Transparency can be advanced through collecting stakeholder feedback, analyzing review disparities, publishing data on review timelines and acceptance rates, and conducting internal audits aimed at improving the peer review process.
2. Organizational operations: Inclusive practices at the organizational level help create a culture that supports high-quality science. This may include appointing an equity officer, offering targeted training on inclusive publishing, consulting external experts, regularly updating terminology, and encouraging authors to apply a health equity lens.
3. Data collection and reporting: Collecting demographic data from authors, reviewers, and editors is one option for journals to assess their inclusivity. Journals are encouraged to use privacy-conscious methods to share such data, maintain currency, and adapt

Continued on page 967...

## HISTORY CORNER

### 15 YEARS AGO

**Persistent Psychopathology in the Wake of Civil War: Long-Term Posttraumatic Stress Disorder in Nimba County, Liberia**

There is ample evidence that there is a substantial burden of psychopathology among those engaged in war—on combatants and civilians alike. . . . Using data from a population-based representative survey in Nimba County, Liberia, combined with a historical analysis, we showed both that the prevalence of PTSD in Nimba County remains high nearly 2 decades after the end of the principal conflict and that the geographical patterns of traumatic event experiences and of PTSD are consistent with the best available information about the path of the violent civil conflict that Nimba County experienced from 1989 to 1990. . . . [I]nterventions in the postconflict era could fruitfully target areas with a history of conflict and that interventions aimed at rebuilding social and physical infrastructure in these areas may be an inextricable part of mental health treatment in these countries.

From *AJPH*, September 2010, pp. 1745, 1749–1750

collection strategies to meet evolving needs.

4. Diversity of authors: Journals are encouraged to work to ensure that their pool of authors reflects the diversity of the field. Supporting junior investigators, exploring new dissemination formats, and actively engaging underrepresented communities are all ways to broaden participation and enrich the literature.
5. Diversity of editors: A diverse editorial team brings varied perspectives and strengthens decision-making. Strategies include building representation at all levels, offering fellowships, and using inclusive recruitment practices.
6. Diversity of reviewers: A varied reviewer pool strengthens peer review by bringing in different perspectives and reducing potential bias. Journals can track reviewer demographics and ensure that their reviewer community is broad in both background and expertise.
7. Inclusive coverage and perspectives: Journals are encouraged to welcome submissions on underrepresented topics and perspectives. This could involve identifying gaps in the literature, supporting nontraditional topics or formats, and using editorials and public messaging to invite new voices.
8. Inclusive language: Language matters. Journals can help authors use respectful, inclusive, and precise terminology that reflects diverse human experiences. Guidance, editorial oversight, and regular updates are encouraged to help maintain cultural and academic relevance.

By adopting these strategies, journals can uphold scientific integrity, foster trust, and create a more equitable publishing environment.

Looking ahead, *EQSPI* will evolve through feedback and collaboration. A dedicated Web site will host updates, register participating journals, and build a learning community committed to continuous improvement. Together, we can move from intention to transformation—strengthening science through transparency, equity, and inclusion. AJPH

DOI: https://doi.org/10.2105/AJPH.2025.308174

ORCID iD:
Meredith Loui https://orcid.org/0000-0003-3022-3814

## HISTORY CORNER

### 16 YEARS AGO

### Water, Conflict, and Hope

Water has been both a source of conflict and a weapon used in conflicts, and water systems have been targets in conflicts started for a wide range of reasons. Water-related disputes often end before obvious ecological and human health consequences emerge, but not always. . . . In a minority of water-related disputes countries have fired weapons, attacked a dam, or engaged in other military actions. Those disputes that threaten to become violent or become violent are often grounded in preexisting and long-standing animosity over differences in religion, ethnicity, race, or lifestyle. . . . At this time, water in the Middle East, such as the Jordan River Basin, is probably the most threatening to public health, environmental, and economic stability.

From *AJPH*, November 2009, pp. 1928–1930

# Do Data Still Matter in Gun Rights States? Review of *What We've Become: Living and Dying in a Country of Arms*

*Jennifer L. Pomeranz, JD, MPH*

**ABOUT THE AUTHOR**

*Jennifer L. Pomeranz is with the Department of Public Health Policy and Management, College of Global Public Health, New York University, New York.*

AJPH July 2025, Vol. 115, No. 7

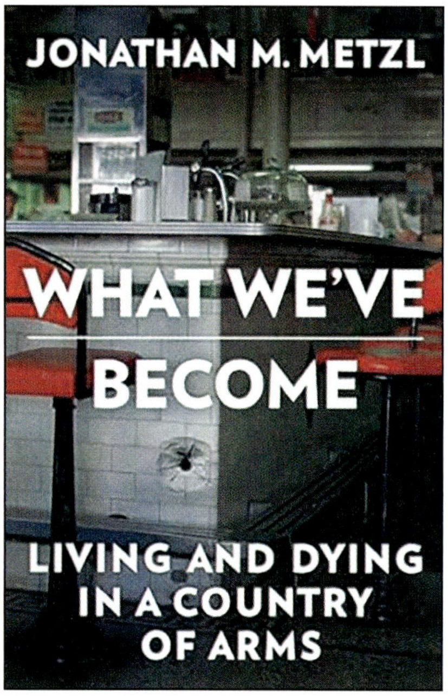


**What We've Become Living and Dying in a Country of Arms**
**By Jonathan M. Metzl**
W. W. Norton & Company, New York, NY; 2024
372 pp; $29.99
ISBN 978-1-324-05025-4

In a piercing examination of the United States itself, Jonathan M. Metzl asks us to reconsider what we think we know about guns, gun policy, and gun culture. Metzl uniquely allows the reader inside his head as he paints a clear and convincing picture of the US "civilian arms race"—which exists not in the shadows but out in the open for all the world to see.

Metzl sets his book apart from others by weaving the life story of the "Waffle House shooter" into a narrative of the modern history of US gun rights. A mostly naked White man, Travis Reinking, opened fire with an AR-15 at a Nashville, Tennessee, Waffle House, targeting and killing Black and Brown youths. What led to this reveals the failure and perhaps inability of institutions, laws, law enforcement, mental health providers, and public health research to prevent mass shootings. Travis was off the grid, home schooled. He was delusional. Taylor Swift was stalking him. His violation of social norms and the law were written off with slaps on the wrist. As Metzl observes about the race-based shooting: "The inevitability of a system that cast armed White men as patriots until proven otherwise has led to this moment" (p. 217). Metzl provides insight into failed gun control efforts in the United States and seeks a new way forward.

Part One of *What We've Become* provides a detailed look at the pivotal moment that sealed the fate of a guilty verdict at Travis Reinking's trial through the testimony of Sharita Henderson. The story is heart-wrenching. Travis is found guilty on all 16 counts. Metzl delves into why Travis was not also brought up on a weapons charge for unlawful possession of a firearm—which would be a 17th count—when he used a semiautomatic rifle he unlawfully possessed. As Metzl explains, the 17th count would have charged him with a crime "before he pulled the trigger." In a gun rights state,[1] this 17th count could be disastrous for the prosecution because it would place gun control laws on trial alongside Travis. The conservative media was quick to blame Waffle House for the shooting because of the restaurant's policy of not allowing guns inside. The book starts to reveal itself as an incisive look into political and social aspects of the United States today. It is US culture that turned a race-based shooting into a conservative political statement about armed gun owners' role in protecting Americans; perhaps, the reader must consider, they really mean protecting White Americans.

Part Two delves into the "insanity of the system" by documenting various interests in preventing gun violence from mental health, public health, and legal perspectives. Importantly for Metzl, this part begins to highlight the limitation of the public health approach and perspective. Not everyone puts health first. People's concepts of safety and safe spaces differ. What makes someone feel safe (arming themselves) may be different than what public health data tell us about their actual safety.

The chapters expose nonenforcement of gun safety laws in blue states (in this case a red flag law), the absence of gun safety laws in red states, handshake deals, White male privilege, and lack of familial interventions when doing so would conflict with conservative values.[2] If Travis was Black, wouldn't he have been arrested for trying to break into Trump's White House? Indeed, there were multiple missed touchpoints to reach Travis: family, friends, law enforcement, his YouTube channel, and the list goes on—where he should have gotten help or lost access to his firearm license and his firearms—but that did not happen. Instead, Travis received a slap on the wrist and a handshake deal to transfer his firearms to his father.

Acknowledging Travis's mental illness, Metzl sets forth data on alternative risk factors for firearm violence in the United States. People with mental illness tend to be less violent, more likely to use firearms for suicide, and anyway the term is too broad to be meaningful.[3] Metzl posits that examining gun violence as a mental health issue stems from the public health framework, but there is evidence that the National Rifle Association (NRA) blamed mental health as a method to distract from firearm's role in morbidity and mortality in the United States.[3,4] Regardless, this part compels the reader to question policing in the United States and law enforcement's special treatment of White men who commit crimes. It requires thinking about how to get mental health treatment to people outside the system. It asks why public health research on firearm violence is not enough to sway voters and gun owners to seek more protective laws—as public health defines it.

We then discover that Travis's father gave him back his guns.

Part Three provides a play-by-play account of the Waffle House shooting. Wearing only a green bomber jacket, Travis targeted and shot eight Black and Brown youths, killing four of them. Travis was tackled while trying to reload his Bushmaster AR-15 to continue his shooting spree. We know Travis was found guilty, but Metzl quickly unsettles the reader that "justice" from the trial will be short-lived.

Indeed, Part Four examines the aftermath. After such a shooting, those of us in public health think this is the impetus "they" need for stronger gun laws. But we are wrong. After the shooting, we discover, the NRA is stronger than ever in Tennessee and funded the winning electoral campaign of a far-right candidate for governor. Governor William Byron Lee went on to pass a sweeping deregulatory law—permitless carry—and defund regulatory safety agencies. Deregulation coupled with defunding is now an all too familiar conservative strategy playing out across the United States.

This part reveals Citizens United at work.[5] The 2010 US Supreme Court decision in *Citizens United v FEC* ushered in modern campaign rules that allow big money entities (e.g., corporations, the NRA) to fund political campaigns with no limit.[6] Indeed, the NRA is credited with securing Donald Trump's first presidency in 2016.[7] And President Trump did not speak out against the race-based Waffle House shooting.

In Part Four, Metzl seeks a new way forward. He finds the prevention-based model ill-equipped to address firearms in the United States. Metzl calls for deep discussions between public health researchers and gun owners, most notably in the South. He recommends that we reassess ideas of safety in public spaces and policing that goes along with that and find common ground on conceptions of safe public spaces. Clearly, in places with permitless carry laws, citizens' idea of safety is different from what the public health data bear out; Metzl calls on us to understand these values. He also recommends a health in all policies approach[8] for community to invest in structural solutions. Metzl suggests that a new strategy to change minds, culture, and policy in the South is necessary, as is the building of global networks. Metzl asks us to consider how Americans can create a unifying framework.

The epilogue delves into the 2022 case, *N.Y. State Rifle & Pistol Association v Bruen*, in which the Supreme Court struck down New York State's public carry licensing law, extending the right to self-defense from inside the home to public places.[9] The court adopted a new test for reviewing firearm laws. Public health research is no longer relevant, as courts were admonished against weighing the government's interest in controlling firearm violence.[9] Now "the government must affirmatively prove that its firearms regulation is part of the historical tradition that delimits the outer bounds of the right to keep and bear arms."[9]

The epilogue portends the outcome of the 2024 presidential election. It asks a poignant and crucial question: what if nationalizing "disastrous" Southern policies that have "caused immeasurable suffering in red states" (p. 301) is the goal? These policies allowed Republican values to consolidate judicial power and resulted in the reelection of

Donald J. Trump. Metzl asks us to consider if perhaps the overall objective is to destabilize the North? After all, the North has better health outcomes and more civil rights and social services than the South. We must ask ourselves if the North can survive the next four years intact.

This book is directed to all who live in the United States. It highlights our lack of shared values. Public health seeks to use data to reduce morbidity and mortality. But this goal is not necessarily the most important to all citizens where freedom and fear of other resound. Metzl's critique of public health should be seen as exposing the inherent limitations of a field that is underfunded and undervalued and prioritizes data. There is only so much that data can do. The important lesson is Metzl's point that perhaps no level of data will ever matter in gun rights states. Indeed, public health data are no longer relevant in court after *Bruen*. How can we in public health adapt to the new raw realities of the United States' "civilian arms race"? AJPH

## CORRESPONDENCE

Correspondence should be sent to Jennifer L. Pomeranz, School of Global Public Health, New York University, 708 Broadway, 7th Floor, New York, NY 10003 (e-mail: jlp284@nyu.edu). Reprints can be ordered at https://www.ajph.org by clicking the "Reprints" link.

## PUBLICATION INFORMATION

Full Citation: Pomeranz JL. Do data still matter in gun rights states? Review of *What We've Become: Living and Dying in a Country of Arms*. *Am J Public Health*. 2025;115(7):968–970.

Acceptance Date: April 16, 2025.

DOI: https://doi.org/10.2105/AJPH.2025.308169

## CONFLICTS OF INTEREST

The author has no conflicts of interest to disclose.

## REFERENCES

1. Pomeranz JL, Silver D, Lieff SA. State gun-control, gun-rights, and preemptive firearm-related laws across 50 US states for 2009–2018. *Am J Public Health*. 2021;111(7):1273–1280. https://doi.org/10.2105/AJPH.2021.306287
2. Berens N. Father of convicted Waffle House shooter to serve time in prison for providing gun. *News Channel 5 Nashville*. March 6, 2023. Available at: https://www.newschannel5.com/news/father-of-convicted-waffle-house-shooter-to-serve-time-in-prison-for-providing-gun. Accessed May 1, 2025.
3. Swanson JW, McGinty EE, Fazel S, Mays VM. Mental illness and reduction of gun violence and suicide: bringing epidemiologic research to policy. *Ann Epidemiol*. 2015;25(5):366–376. https://doi.org/10.1016/j.annepidem.2014.03.004
4. Lexington. Why the NRA keeps talking about mental illness, rather than guns. *The Economist*. March 13, 2013. Available at: https://www.economist.com/lexingtons-notebook/2013/03/13/why-the-nra-keeps-talking-about-mental-illness-rather-than-guns. Accessed May 1, 2025.
5. Weiner DI, Lau T. Citizens United explained. January 29, 2025. Available at: https://www.brennancenter.org/our-work/research-reports/citizens-united-explained. Accessed May 1, 2025.
6. *Citizens United v FEC*, 558 US 310 (2010).
7. Spies M, Balcerzak A. The NRA placed big bets on the 2016 election, and won almost all of them. November 9, 2016. Available at: https://www.opensecrets.org/news/2016/11/the-nra-placed-big-bets-on-the-2016-election-and-won-almost-all-of-them. Accessed May 1, 2025.
8. American Public Health Association. Health in all policies. Available at: https://www.apha.org/topics-and-issues/health-in-all-policies. Accessed May 1, 2025.
9. *N.Y. State Rifle & Pistol Association v Bruen*, 597 US 1 (2022).

# An Insider's (Plus Protégés') Take on (North–South) Global Health During Troubled Times

Paulo Trivellato, MSc, and Anne-Emanuelle Birn, ScD, MA

**ABOUT THE AUTHORS**

*Paulo Trivellato is with the School of Public Health, University of São Paulo, Brazil. Anne-Emanuelle Birn is with the Department of Global Development Studies and the Dalla Lana School of Public Health, University of Toronto, Canada.*

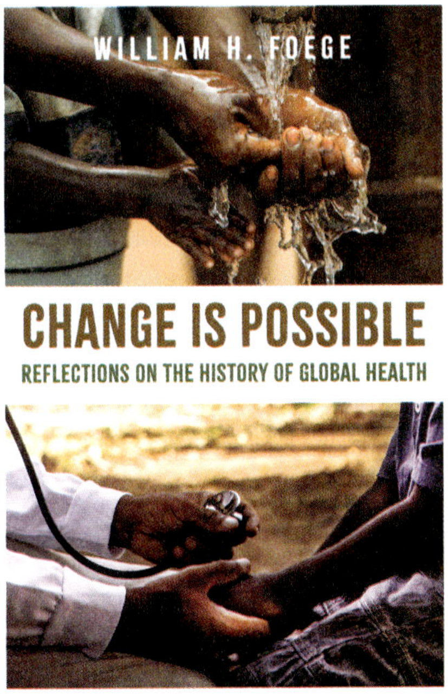


**Change Is Possible: Reflections on the History of Global Health**
**by William H. Foege, Paul Elish, Alison T. Hoover, Madison Gabriella Lee, Deborah Chen Tseng, and Kiera Chan**
Baltimore, Maryland
Johns Hopkins University Press; 2024
paperback; 321 pp; $34.95.
ISBN 978-1-4214-5042-1

Published two months before the start of the second Trump administration, the latest book by eminent public health physician William "Bill" Foege, *Change Is Possible: Reflections on the History of Global Health*, finds its "speaking place"[1] at a pivotal crossroads.[2,3]

In the context of the contentious debates sparked by the slew of global health–related edicts of early 2025,[4–6] the volume's reflections on the range of actors involved in global health, intertwined with snippets from Foege's own trajectory, take on an up-to-the-moment urgency. This resonance goes from personal anecdotes regarding the tensions between (and possibilities of) international health priorities and military and foreign policy interests (pp. 66, 110) to Foege's championing of the global diffusion of technological innovations, and his thoughts on the first Trump administration.

In sharing a decidedly US perspective on global health, the book is representative of, if lacking great analytical pretensions about, the ethical and political dilemmas presently facing the field.

## A HYBRID APPROACH TO HISTORY

Through the mentored collaboration of five public health graduate students from Emory University, whom he invited to join him as coauthors in 2020, Foege blends the memoir style of his autobiographical trilogy[7–9] with chapters covering many different categories of actors and several overarching global health themes. As such, the book complements Foege's prior volumes with a patina of impartiality.

Not unexpectedly, highlights from Foege's storied global health career, spanning the World Health Organization's (WHO's) smallpox eradication campaign, child survival programs, and "neglected" disease initiatives, are peppered throughout the volume. For example, chapters on "Militaries and Global Health" and "Bilateral Programs," written, respectively, by Paul Elish and Alison T. Hoover, return to an episode Foege previously proudly recounted, regarding the refusal of David Sencer, then director of the Centers for Disease Control and Prevention, to give the Central Intelligence Agency permission to interview Foege while he was working on relief efforts during the Nigeria–Biafra War (1967–1970).

Atop his acolytes' retelling of various memorable biographical events, Foege has a hand in virtually all of the book's 15 chapters, directly authoring one third and inserting a reflective or evaluative epilogue to the others. For instance, his brief chapter on "Hybrid Organizations"—a euphemism for corporate-driven entities (p. 4)—revisits Foege's most recent book, focused on his experience cofounding and leading the Task Force for Child Survival, a multi-UN agency–Rockefeller Foundation collaboration formed in 1984 to

AJPH July 2025, Vol. 115, No. 7

raise childhood immunization rates. Two more of his chapters, "Politics and Global Health" and "Pharmaco-Philanthropy and Global Health," spotlight the achievements of the Carter Center, which Foege directed from 1986 to 1992.

Additionally, in his "Personal View of Philanthropy" section of a chapter on "The New Philanthropy," penned by Kiera Chan, Foege briefly recounts his time on the boards of six foundations. As noted in the preface, the title of this book, as suggested by Foege's trainees, coincides with the motto of one of these foundations, the Marguerite Casey Foundation (p. ix).

Given Foege's deep personal engagement with so many of the events and approaches covered here, the book almost serves as a summary installment of his multitome biography.

Nonetheless, drawing from the students' research synthesizing some of the field's best known English-language bibliography, combined with his own approach to history, editor–author Foege aspires to a more objective style. In particular, he provides the book with a leitmotif through "an attempt to identify some triumphs and tragedies in a concluding paragraph for each chapter" (p. 4).

This personal–professional evaluative approach is based on Foege's own admittedly simplistic abbreviation of global health as "any activity that promotes 'global health equity'" (p. xii). His reflections at the end of each chapter show how his normative definition combines with a descriptive one, that of the global health field as "an amalgamation of ingredients and historical developments over the centuries" (p. 3).

Global health thus emerges as a journey whose destination—"equity"—is propelled by "the skills and knowledge garnered in rich countries for the benefit of low-income areas" (p. 19). To elaborate further, for Foege and coauthors, the epic arc of global health is predetermined, with progress almost entirely dependent on the motivation and know-how of—and financial support for—the actors involved.

With this teleological and political will-driven understanding, the authors assess the putative costs and benefits, as well as the impetus, they associate with each theme and category of actors. In the conclusion to Elish's chapter on "The Legacy of Colonialism in Global Health," for example, Foege highlights "globalism" as "one of the lasting contributions" of colonialism even as he condemns "power and greed" as its driving forces. Amplifying this contradictory stance, Foege's condemnation that ". . . the avarice of strong countries leads them to impose their will on weak areas of the world" (p. 46) comes just 25 pages after having lauded global health's North–South generosity.

The book returns repeatedly and uncritically to the notion of shared benefits of the contemporary (what many call the neoliberal capitalist)[10] era of global health. Referencing the possibilities of Big Pharma's unidirectional technology transfer, without citing the aforementioned avarice regarding global health's colonial legacy, Foege argues that "Pharmaceuticals provide a positive case for globalism. Remoteness no longer precludes benefiting from cutting-edge science" (p. 258).

Perhaps most problematically, Foege underscores the US military's unsung involvement in health as propitiously linking military medicine, tropical medicine, and "the current concept of global health," enabling the field's extension more broadly "to health problems in tropical countries, such as malnutrition, measles, pneumonia and maternal mortality" (p. 66).

## INTERROGATING GLOBAL HEALTH AS POSITIVE CHANGE

Foege sees "the current concept of global health [as] inclusive in a way that international health could never be" (p. 66). Yet a chapter by Alison T. Hoover and Madison Gabriella Lee extolling "Multilateral Organizations" puzzlingly evaluates the WHO only as an example of multilateralism's "potential dark side." This is in direct contrast to the way that public–private partnerships such as the Global Fund and Gavi are celebrated (p. 147).

In their message of "Promoting Positive Change," the authors appear reluctant to embrace intergovernmental cooperation as a means of rescuing global health, in contrast to the resounding "gratitude" accorded to military medicine and philanthropy (pp. 66, 216–217) and a triad of actors. This triad comprises professional politicians, "the prime example" being Jimmy Carter and his postpresidential performance (pp. 8, 20); nongovernmental organizations (NGOs), which Foege argues "may be second only to political engagement in their potential to improve global health" (p. 184); and hybrid programs (i.e., public–private partnerships) themselves.

Confusingly presented as overlapping multilateral and NGO programs, these "latest major participants in global health" will, Foege holds, ultimately "becom[e] more powerful and more effective in delivering global health improvements," likely "mapping the future of global health" (pp. 185, 189).

In sum, despite having admirably afforded a unique opportunity to Foege's mentees to explore the past and present challenges of global health, the book comes off mostly as a vindication of Foege's own professional legacy. He rationalizes this as upholding an ethos, but it also serves to defend the agendas of the actors with whom Foege built his career.

## BRINGING POWER AND POLITICS BACK IN

Regrettably, this volume is a departure from Foege's previous, more direct style of recalling the highs and lows of his notable career. In posing a kind of global health history that turns out to be largely allegorical, the volume detracts from—rather than contributing to—the overall credibility of this proposed evaluation exercise; alas, the approach instills little confidence in the "transparency and feedback" of what the book calls the "best" philanthropic foundations (p. 217).

The point here is not to question the authors' motivations, but rather to reveal the limitations generated by their way of understanding history.[11] In addition, in watering down politics to a question of good management motored by a strong evidence basis, the book adheres to a dominant scientific triumphalism that offensively reduces the Global South to a passive object of salvation. Drawing on our own backgrounds—an emerging global health and international relations scholar from Brazil and a Canadian global health historian who has decades of research and collaborative work with colleagues and comrades in Latin America—we found the near absence of "Southern" protagonism to be shocking, if not surprising.[12] From the more than half-century of Cuban medical internationalism, to Brazil's leadership in horizontal global health cooperation, to countless health innovations, to the solidarity engagement of the People's Health Movement, global health in, across, and from the South surely warrants attention as *a*, if not *the*, transformational hope of the field.[13–16]

Perhaps the book's silence on this perspective is to be expected in view of the background and provenance of the lead author, yet it also shows a remarkable lack of learning from the many initiatives in which he has been involved on the front lines. This is especially troubling given the current political context of US global health's apparent demise. Indeed, Foege's comments on the first Trump administration, in the book's opening chapter on "The Triumph and Tragedy of Global Health," are illustrative. His assessment of the paradox of that administration's COVID-19 policy seems incredulous:

> How could the same political group that thwarted a reasonable public health response have supported this [vaccine] breakthrough in science and technology? . . . How did we get to this point of combining chaos and scientific excellence? . . . But it is no exception: triumph and tragedy have been factors in every step of the global health journey (pp. 2–3).

Judging the Trump administration's appalling pandemic policies (and, by extension, those of other countries) as a form of "human incompetence" boils it down to something that seems easy to understand and even dismiss. Ultimately, the book blames social media for the overall context: "What it has done to civilized discourse is cause for great concern" (p. 271).

This vague hypothesis regarding what has become not only a serious threat, but a growing reality, of de-democratization across growing swathes of the world is symptomatic of the book's naive and uncritical stance. Understanding where and how power resides in global health and the world order writ large is fundamental to recognizing and resisting tyranny[17]; the call for properly managing (global health) technology is but a sideshow to the struggles and challenges at hand.

Notwithstanding this critique, the book leaves readers with a tantalizing set of questions and conundrums at this particular historical conjuncture: Will philanthropic and pharmaceutical (or hybrid organizations') interest in global health continue despite the US government's withdrawal from this arena? How will these actors respond to WHO's move to sustain its funding by creating its own foundation? Will these private players help offset Trump's budget cuts, smelling opportunity? Will they seek to unilaterally set the global health agenda?[18] Or will there be a renewal and democratization of multilateralism toward a postimperial[19] and ethical counterpoint to growing autocracy, with the hope, if pie-in-the-sky, that public sector–civil society Global South alliances will replace and potentially transform the global health field? AJPH

## CORRESPONDENCE

Correspondence should be sent to Paulo Trivellato, Faculdade de Saúde Pública, Universidade de São Paulo, Av. Arnaldo, 715, São Paulo - SP, Brasil CEP 01246-904 (e-mail: paulo.trivellato@usp.br).


## PUBLICATION INFORMATION

Full Citation: Trivellato P, Birn AE. An insider's (plus protégés') take on (North–South) global health during troubled times. *Am J Public Health*. 2025;115(7):971–974.

Acceptance Date: March 1, 2025.

DOI: https://doi.org/10.2105/AJPH.2025.308104

ORCID iDs:
Paulo Trivellato https://orcid.org/0000-0002-3372-2494

Anne-Emanuelle Birn https://orcid.org/0000-0002-0314-5913

## CONTRIBUTORS

The authors jointly discussed the content of the article and prepared an outline. P. Trivellato wrote the first draft. A.-E. Birn reviewed and edited the draft. Both authors approved the final draft.

## ACKNOWLEDGMENTS

P. Trivellato acknowledges the support from the São Paulo Research Foundation (FAPESP; grant no. 2024/01644-3).

## CONFLICTS OF INTEREST

The authors have no conflicts of interest to declare.

## REFERENCES

1. Ribeiro D. *Where We Stand.* Viswanathan P, trans. New Haven, CT: Yale University Press; 2024.
2. Fletcher E. From Mpox to influenza—USAID collapse and CDC blackout upend WHO response to deadly outbreaks. *Health Policy Watch.* February 12, 2025. Available at: https://healthpolicy-watch.news/from-mpox-to-influenza-usaid-collapse-and-cdc-blackout-upend-who-response-to-deadly-outbreaks. Accessed February 16, 2025.
3. Stobbe M, Johnson C. HHS is losing thousands of workers under Trump administration probationary job cuts. *AP News.* February 14, 2025. Available at: https://apnews.com/article/trump-job-cuts-health-cdc-0d002fd6f528a7b91ced79628bf68196?s=08. Accessed February 16, 2025.
4. Ntusi N. US aid cuts are an opportunity to reimagine global health. *Nat Med.* 2025;31(3):719. https://doi.org/10.1038/d41591-025-00009-9
5. Torres I, López-Cevallos D. A vision for PAHO/WHO from and for Latin America. *Latinoamérica21.* February 10, 2025. Available at: https://latinoamerica21.com/en/a-vision-for-paho-who-from-and-for-latin-america. Accessed February 16, 2025.
6. Gostin L, Friedman A, Wetter S. Dismantling US global health aid. *Health Affairs.* February 14, 2025. Available at: https://www.healthaffairs.org/content/forefront/dismantling-us-global-health-aid?s=08. Accessed February 16, 2025.
7. Foege W. *House on Fire: The Fight to Eradicate Smallpox.* Berkeley, CA: University of California Press/Milbank Memorial Fund; 2011.
8. Foege W. *The Fears of the Rich, The Needs of the Poor: My Years at the CDC.* Baltimore, MD: Johns Hopkins University Press; 2018. https://doi.org/10.1353/book.88357
9. Foege W. *The Task Force for Child Survival: Secrets of Successful Coalitions.* Baltimore, MD: Johns Hopkins University Press; 2018. https://doi.org/10.56021/9781421425603
10. Baru R, Mohan M. Globalisation and neoliberalism as structural drivers of health inequities. *Health Res Policy Syst.* 2018;16(suppl 1):91. https://doi.org/10.1186/s12961-018-0365-2
11. Parisi V, Sivaramakrishnan K. The limits of linearity: recasting histories of epidemics in the Global South. *Isis.* 2023;114(S1):S247–S287. https://doi.org/10.1086/726987
12. Perez-Brumer A, Hill D, Parker R. Latin America at the margins? Implications of the geographic and epistemic narrowing of "global" health. *Glob Public Health.* 2023;19(1):2295443. https://doi.org/10.1080/17441692.2023.2295443
13. Ventura D, Martins J, Leme A, Pereira P, Trivellato P, Viegas L. Brazil should use its G20 leadership to support public health systems and promote decolonisation of global health. *BMJ.* 2024;386:e080209. https://doi.org/10.1136/bmj-2024-080209
14. People's Health Movement. 2025. Available at: https://phmovement.org. Accessed February 19, 2025.
15. Birn A-E, Necochea López R, eds. *Peripheral Nerve: Health and Medicine in Cold War Latin America.* Durham, NC: Duke University Press; 2020. https://doi.org/10.1215/9781478012221
16. Yaffe H. Cuban medical internationalism: a paradigm for South–South cooperation. *Int J Cuban Stud.* 2023;15(2):203–234. https://doi.org/10.13169/intejcubastud.15.2.0203
17. García Márquez G. *El otoño del patriarca.* Buenos Aires, Argentina: Editorial Sudamericana; 1975.
18. Puyvallée A, Harman S, Rushton S, Storeng K. Global health partnerships for a post-2030 agenda. *Lancet.* 2025;405(10477):514–516. https://doi.org/10.1016/S0140-6736(24)02816-2
19. Montenegro C, Fonseca S. "Stop looking north, look to the world." Can we imagine global health without the USA at its centre? *Speaking of Medicine and Health.* February 14, 2025. Available at: https://speakingofmedicine.plos.org/2025/02/14/stop-looking-north-look-to-the-world-can-we-imagine-global-health-without-the-usa-at-its-centre. Accessed February 18, 2025.

# Ten Years at the Helm: Reflections From the *AJPH* Editor-in-Chief

*Alfredo Morabia, MD, PhD*

**ABOUT THE AUTHOR**

*Alfredo Morabia is* AJPH *editor-in-chief (2015–2025) and is with the Barry Commoner Center for Health and the Environment, Queens College, City University of New York, and the Department of Epidemiology, Mailman School of Public Health, Columbia University.*

As I conclude my decade-long tenure as editor-in-chief of the *American Journal of Public Health* (*AJPH*), I do so with deep pride, gratitude, and a sense of urgency. These are difficult times for public health. Yet I leave *AJPH* strong—in its science, its financial footing, and its unwavering commitment to diversity, equity, and inclusion (DEI). I am particularly proud that the *Journal* has stood firm in defending the integrity of science against obscurantist attacks and political pressure. It has served as a sanctuary for rigorous, timely, and courageous public health scholarship.

When I began in 2015, *AJPH* was already a cornerstone of public health publishing.[1] I sought to build on that foundation by streamlining the editorial process, amplifying marginalized voices, promoting a dialogue in the public health community beyond the partisan divide, broadening the *Journal*'s reach, and reinforcing the essential link between research and public health practice. The past 10 years have reaffirmed my belief in the power of scientific publishing to influence not only professional norms but also the nature of the public discourse on health.

## ADVANCING THE SCIENCE

*AJPH* is indisputably the premier journal in public health. Its scientific standing is evident in its citation footprint, which grew from 32 270 citations in 2015 to 43 414 in 2023 (Table 1). The *Journal*'s impact factor rose from 4.1 to a peak of 12.7 in 2022 before recalibration under new Clarivate indexing criteria in 2023. In that year, *AJPH* ranked in the 97th percentile for both the Science Citation Index Expanded and the Social Sciences Citation Index categories of "Public, Environmental & Occupational Health."

*AJPH* receives between 3000 and 3500 submissions annually, excluding the exceptional COVID-19 spike to 5500 in 2020. The senior deputy editor Michael C. Costanza and I have triaged 36 630 submissions in 10 years. Of these, 90% were peer-reviewed submissions, but only about 5% ultimately reached publication. Our commitment to quality requires a rigorous but transparent process: approximately 80% of submissions are desk-rejected during the initial triage, with the remainder undergoing an in-depth review by associate editors, statistical evaluation, and assessment of tables and figures.

Speed and responsiveness have also improved. In 2015, the time from submission to publication for peer-reviewed articles averaged 6 months. In 2025, that figure is 2.5 months, allowing *AJPH* to more swiftly support evidence-informed policy and practice.

We also launched new article formats, including Notes From the Field and Qualitative Notes From the Field, to bring local and grassroots interventions and local innovations into scholarly view.[2] *AJPH* Open Access supplements act as a repository, as well as a bank of best public health practices, featuring the experience of thousands of public health professionals and community activists.[3]

## EDITORIAL INNOVATION AND EXPERIMENTATION

*AJPH* has not shied away from experimentation. With support from the Robert Wood Johnson Foundation, we conducted a two-year workshop on DEI in scientific publishing, culminating in two landmark documents: a scoping review (in press) and the Ensuring Quality in Scientific Publications Through Inclusivity and Transparency (EQSPI) platform (Loui and Morabia, p. 966 of this issue). These provide a foundation for future equity-driven editorial practices.

In another major innovation, *AJPH* has conducted a randomized controlled trial comparing double-blind and triple-blind peer review. The results will soon be made public, and I hope they will inform broader reforms in scholarly communication.

*AJPH* also maintained its independence in the face of political pressure. We refused requests to alter the content of accepted articles[4] and created

AJPH July 2025, Vol. 115, No. 7

**TABLE 1— Key Performance Metrics of *AJPH* in "Public, Environmental & Occupational Health": 2015–2025**

| Metric | 2015 | 2019 | 2022 | 2023 | 2025 |
|---|---|---|---|---|---|
| Total citations (Clarivate), no. | 32 270 | ... | ... | 43 414 | ... |
| JIF | 4.1 | ... | 12.7 | 9.7[a] | ... |
| JIF percentile (SCIE/SSCI) | 91/97 | ... | ... | 97/97 | ... |
| Influence score | ... | 2.6 | ... | 4.7 | ... |
| Average time from submission[b] to publication, mo | 6 | ... | ... | ... | 2.5 |

*Note.* JIF = journal impact factor; SCIE = Science Citation Index Expanded; SSCI = Social Sciences Citation Index.
[a]The 2023 JIF was calculated on a merged scale owing to the unification of SCIE and SSCI categories by Clarivate.
[b]Only peer-reviewed research articles and analytic essays.

the Public Health Interventions: Rapid Reports section to quickly publish high-priority findings—beginning with the inaugural report by Cregreen et al. featured in this issue (p. 1115). *AJPH* has been the refuge for many articles that other journals can no longer publish freely.

## CULTIVATING THE NEXT GENERATION

A fulfilling part of my tenure was building the next generation of public health editors and thinkers. In 2016, we launched the Student Think Tank and a student editor fellowship. Over the years, we welcomed 60 Think Tank members from across the United States and trained 5 student editors in a hands-on, two-year mentorship. These students helped guide *Journal* priorities and even led initiatives such as social media engagement and new communication formats.

## COMMUNICATION, PODCASTS, AND THE STATE OF THE UNION

Science is only powerful if it is heard. Since 2015, the *AJPH Podcast* has grown from short bilingual summaries to in-depth audio and video interviews. It has had 184 000 plays on SoundCloud alone and is widely accessible across platforms, including YouTube. In 2022, we launched the State of the Public Health Union—an annual address modeled on the US presidential tradition (https://www.youtube.com/live/PizfB9pv1dA?si=QcIA6o8CV8-EzLCj). It gave grassroots public health organizations a national stage. Each event drew more than 1 000 live viewers and helped reconnect research with community voice.

The weekly *AJPH* newsletter now reaches more than 100 000 subscribers, a vibrant, engaged audience that represents the breadth of our field.

## RELATIONSHIP WITH THE AMERICAN PUBLIC HEALTH ASSOCIATION

*AJPH*'s close but independent relationship with the American Public Health Association (APHA) has been one of mutual benefit. As outlined in our bylaws, the *Journal* enjoys complete editorial independence, and that autonomy has been essential. Still, the relationship with APHA leadership, particularly through monthly meetings with the executive director, Dr. Georges Benjamin, and the advisory role of the APHA Editorial Board, have been mutually enriching. In October 2024, *AJPH*, through its editor-in-chief, received the APHA Impact Award (Figure 1).

Through APHA, *AJPH* had direct access to the entire ecosystem of public health: from the surgeon general and leaders of the US Department of Health and Human Services, the Centers for Disease Control and Prevention, the National Institutes of Health, the Occupational Safety and Health Administration, and the US Food and Drug Administration to state and local health departments and academic institutions. My office at APHA headquarters enabled regular collaboration with the production and communications teams, grounding the *Journal* in the daily life of the APHA.

## FINANCIAL STEWARDSHIP

For many decades, APHA has supported *AJPH* financially. During my tenure, I prioritized achieving financial stability through diversified revenue streams, including grants and sales. Ensuring *AJPH*'s sustainability is essential not only for its survival but also for safeguarding its editorial independence.

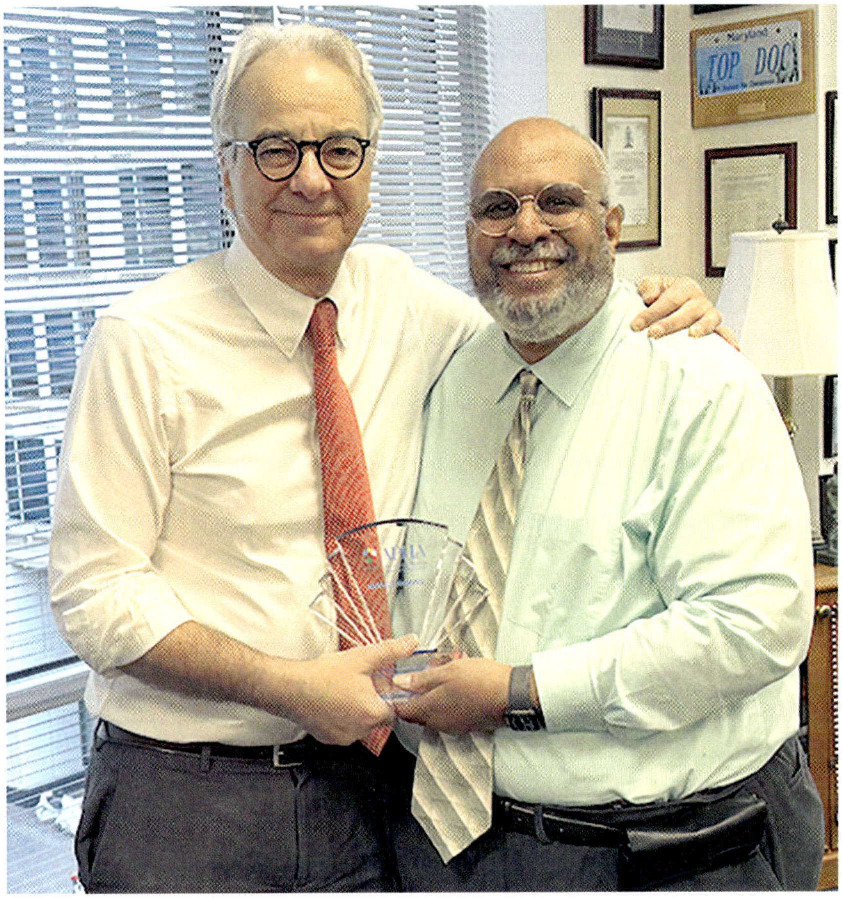


**FIGURE 1—** Dr. Georges Benjamin, Executive Director of American Public Health Association (APHA; Right) and Alfredo Morabia, Holding the APHA Impact Award Awarded to Alfredo Morabia for His Achievements as Editor-in-Chief of *AJPH* at the Opening General Session of the APHA Meeting in Minneapolis, MN, on October 27, 2024

## A PERSONAL NOTE ON AMERICAN PUBLIC HEALTH

Although I was initially hired with the idea that my European background would bring a global touch to *AJPH*, I learned quickly that understanding US public health—its strengths, contradictions, and histories—is indispensable to leading this *Journal*.

Over the years, I visited 44 US states, thanks to the hospitality of health departments and universities. I was advised by a bipartisan group of former state health officials, who met with me regularly, wrote for the *Journal*, and sharpened my understanding of the public health landscape. Their guidance was invaluable.

## GRATITUDE

No editor works alone. I was blessed to work alongside an extraordinary editorial and production team, including Brian Selzer, now APHA director of publications, whose partnership over the past decade was instrumental to the *Journal*'s success. To the editors (see Appendix Table A, available as a supplement to the online version of this article at http://www.ajph.org), student editors (see Appendix Table B), Think Tank members, reviewers, and authors—you shaped the voice and vision of this *Journal*. I thank you.

To the APHA staff, the executive board, the editorial board, and the public health professionals who make up this field—your work inspired the pages of every issue. I am also deeply grateful to the readers who challenged us, corrected us, and stood by us.

## REGRETS AND WARNINGS

I regret that my warnings about rising authoritarianism[5] and the threats posed by the current US presidential administration[6] were not more seriously heard. This is a dangerous administration for public health—but also troubling is the capitulation by many institutions, including universities, and scholars, who met shameful demands with silence.

## FAREWELL AND THE ROAD AHEAD

Ten years is a small chapter in *AJPH*'s 115-year history, but these have been transformative years. The coming era will be difficult. The bipartisan consensus that public health was a public good is eroding. The conservative revolution under way threatens decades of achievements—and there will be no returning to the pre-2024 world.

But in crisis lies opportunity. Public health can be reimagined—perhaps, finally, as a system centered on prevention rather than reactive medical care. *AJPH* will have a critical role to play in this transformation. Safeguarding its independence will be essential to preserving its science, its equity, and its pride.

It is a great time to become *AJPH*'s next editor-in-chief. AJPH

### CORRESPONDENCE

Correspondence should be sent to Alfredo Morabia, Professor of Epidemiology, Queens College, Barry Commoner Center, 65-30 Kissena Blvd, Remsen #311, Flushing, NY 11367 (e-mail: am52@cumc.columbia.edu). Reprints can be ordered at http://www.ajph.org by clicking the "Reprints" link.



### PUBLICATION INFORMATION

Full Citation: Morabia A. Ten years at the helm: reflections from the *AJPH* editor-in-chief. *Am J Public Health*. 2025;115(7):975–978.

Acceptance Date: April 16, 2025.

DOI: https://doi.org/10.2105/AJPH.2025.308173


### CONFLICTS OF INTEREST

The author has no conflicts of interest to report.

### REFERENCES


1. Morabia A. *AJPH! Am J Public Health*. 2016;106(1):7. https://doi.org/10.2105/AJPH.2015.302983
2. Morabia A. Notes from the field: a repository of best practices. *Am J Public Health*. 2022;112(8):1079. https://doi.org/10.2105/AJPH.2022.306957
3. Morabia A. A repository of public health best practices from the heart of the pandemic. *Am J Public Health*. 2024;114(4):357–358. https://doi.org/10.2105/AJPH.2024.307614
4. Morabia A. *AJPH* and the threat of political interference in scientific publishing. *Am J Public Health*. 2025;115(5):626–627. https://doi.org/10.2105/AJPH.2025.308100
5. Morabia A. The fascist threat. *Am J Public Health*. 2021;111(4):538–539. https://doi.org/10.2105/AJPH.2021.306169
6. Morabia A. The US presidential election of 2024 is a public health emergency. *Am J Public Health*. 2024;114(8):757–759. https://doi.org/10.2105/AJPH.2024.307737

# Minimum Legal Age Restrictions on Cannabis Sales: Just One Important Tool for Prevention

Julia A. Dilley, PhD, MES, and Robert G. Hendrickson, MD

**ABOUT THE AUTHORS**

*Julia A. Dilley is with the Multnomah County Health Department and Oregon Health Authority Public Health Division, Portland. Robert G. Hendrickson is with Oregon Health and Science University and Oregon Poison Center, Portland.*

**See also Myran et al., p. 1166.**

The effects on youths from legalizing adult-use (nonmedical) cannabis have been a primary concern in any discussions about cannabis policy, given the known harms of early initiation.[1,2] So far, the evidence is still inconclusive about how legalization may affect youth use and related harms.[3] Furthermore, following the COVID-19 pandemic, after disruptions in many established surveillance systems, youth cannabis and other substance use appears to have declined precipitously,[4] which—though welcome—makes it more difficult to determine the independent effects of legal cannabis marketplaces. One prevention approach that has been applied across all legalizing jurisdictions is an age threshold for legal cannabis possession and sales.

## CANNABIS HOSPITALIZATIONS IN DIFFERENT CONTEXTS

Legalization of nonmedical cannabis for adults is often treated as a binary condition, but, in fact, there are many different regulatory elements that could affect cannabis use and related outcomes. We offer a comparison of cannabis-related hospitalization trends by age group in Oregon to enrich understanding of findings from Canada.

Canada legalized cannabis for adult use in October 2018, with ages for legal cannabis purchases determined by individual provinces and territories, ranging from 18 to 21 years. Myran et al. (p. 1166) report 34% postlegalization decreases through mid-2022 in cannabis-related hospitalizations among people below the minimum legal age (MLA), relative to those of legal age to purchase, compared with expected rates based on prelegalization trends. Their findings were consistent across different MLAs applied by Canadian jurisdictions.

Voters in the state of Oregon legalized cannabis for adult use, with MLA defined as ages 21 and older, in November 2014. We used Oregon data to examine trends in semiannual cannabis-related hospitalizations using the same definitions and age groupings as the Canadian study (Figure 1). Based on visual inspection, Oregon's cannabis-related hospitalizations in 3 age groups (ages 18–20, 21–44, and 45–64 years) all appeared to increase over the early legalization implementation period and then declined after the full market opening in 2016. The group aged 15 to 17 years similarly increased during early implementation but to a lesser degree, and then also showed gradual declines after 2016. In contrast, the group aged 65 years or older increased with legalization implementation, and rates stayed about the same for the following years.

Oregon's data do not appear to show the same clear pattern as Canada of postlegalization reductions among minors (people aged younger than age 21 years) in comparison with older adults, based on expected trends from prelegalization. However, Oregon's longer-term trends—up to 7 years following the full market opening, versus Canada's data from fewer years after market opening—do suggest greater long-term reductions in rates among those aged 18 to 20 years in comparison with those aged 21 to 44 years, as well as relatively stable hospitalization trends among those aged 15 to 17 years in comparison with other age groups. This may be an indication of the effectiveness of minors' access laws, but to a lesser degree than observed in Canada.

Like Canada, Oregon applied a "staged" implementation of legalization: adult possession became legal in July 2015, sales of flower began through established medical dispensaries in October 2015, sales of low-dose edibles and concentrates were added in July 2016, and full retail sales of all product types through nonmedical licensees began in October 2016. However, Oregon differs in some other respects relevant to preventing use among young people. For example, Oregon may have twice as many retail cannabis sales outlets as Canada (e.g., 16.8 per 100 000 in Oregon in June 2022[5] vs 8.0 per 100 000 in Canada in September 2021[6]). Canada also

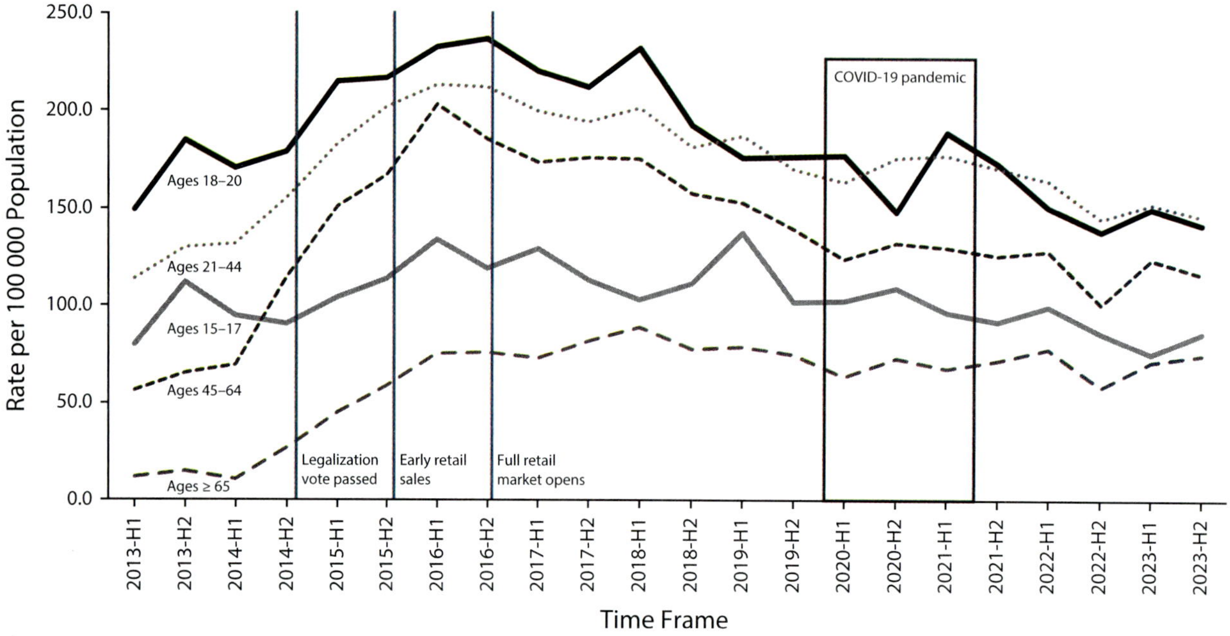


**FIGURE 1— Semiannual Cannabis-Related Hospitalizations by Age Group: Oregon, 2013–2023**

*Note.* H1 = first half of year (January–June); H2 = second half of year (July–December).
*Source.* Oregon Health Authority, hospital discharge data.

restricts advertising to a greater degree than US legal states,[7] and survey data indicate that population-level exposure to cannabis advertising is lower in Canada than in US legal states.[8]

The evolution of retail cannabis markets to offer increasingly higher-concentration tetrahydrocannabinol (THC) products is another policy-relevant factor, with evidence emerging that higher-concentration products may have more adverse health effects.[3] Relative to the United States, Canada has more restrictions on retail products with higher THC concentration. For example, Canada allows only 10 milligrams of THC per package for cannabis edibles sold in the retail marketplace, versus 100 milligrams of THC per package allowed in Oregon.[9] Although use of higher-THC products has grown in both the United States and Canada, the percentage of Canadians who use high-THC-concentration products is lower than in the United States.[10]

Furthermore, conditions like cannabis use disorder and CHS may result from longer-term cannabis use and higher-THC-concentration products. So, because of different restrictions on and use patterns of higher-THC products, there could be differential lags in observed cannabis-related health outcomes related to policy.

Finally, although the Canadian study did not report on people aged 65 years and older, in Oregon, this is one age group for which cannabis-related hospitalizations—although lower than for other age groups—have not declined in the long term. Thus, older adults are another important age group to be considered in the development of policies intended to protect public health.

## INTERPRETING CANNABIS HOSPITALIZATION TRENDS

We also note that the postimplementation period in Canada largely includes time periods that might have been affected by the global COVID-19 pandemic, which could have differentially limited access to cannabis among young people below the MLA who obtain products from social sources. Oregon's data provide a perspective on health effects observed among minors more separated from the independent effect of the pandemic and show a short-term decrease among people aged 18 to 20 years, specifically during the pandemic period. Thus, longer-term monitoring of data in Canada will be useful.

In terms of outcome measurement, it is difficult to know whether there are differences in how *International Classification of Diseases, 10th Edition, Clinical Modification* (*ICD-10-CM*) codes are used in different countries, especially when evidence about the contribution of cannabis to many health outcomes is still mixed and evolving.[4] Cannabis hyperemesis syndrome (CHS, or cyclic vomiting) is one example of a health outcome that is directly caused by cannabis use, but currently, there is no *ICD-10-CM* code for this specific condition. As a result of causal uncertainties, assignment of cannabis-related codes by providers may be inconsistent. Indeed, the actual contribution of cannabis to hospitalizations may be underestimated: a 2018–2019 study in Oregon asked providers to answer the question "Do you think that cannabis use was a significant factor leading to today's ED visit?" (answers: yes, no) as part of the patient electronic health record for about 48 000 individual emergency department visits, and found that more than four times as many cases were identified as at least partly cannabis-attributable based on provider reports than based on *ICD-10-CM* codes alone.[11] Furthermore, given that cannabis use is still illegal for young people, and that the United States does not have universal health care coverage as Canada does, motivation for young people to seek care and for providers to ask about or document cannabis use could be different for minors versus people of legal age, and potentially differentially underestimated in the United States relative to Canada.

## PUBLIC HEALTH IMPLICATIONS

In sum, Oregon's data suggest that MLA policy effectiveness could operate differently in the context of other factors. In the absence of more comprehensive prevention-supporting policies, such as restricting the number and location of cannabis retailers, associated advertising, and the composition of products sold in a legal marketplace, the effects of MLA policies might be diminished.

We suggest that the public health implications are that MLAs can reduce cannabis-related harms for young people in regions pursuing cannabis legalization as part of a comprehensive approach to mitigate effects, including regulations on cannabis access, products, and promotion. We also strongly encourage long-term monitoring of cannabis-related health effects for specific populations, including age groups. AJPH

### CORRESPONDENCE

Correspondence should be sent to Julia Dilley, Program Design and Evaluation Services (PDES), 800 NE Oregon St, Suite 260, Portland, OR 97232 (e-mail: julia.dilley@multco.us). Reprints can be ordered at https://ajph.org by clicking the "Reprints" link.

### PUBLICATION INFORMATION

Full Citation: Dilley JA, Hendrickson RG. Minimum legal age restrictions on cannabis sales: just one important tool for prevention. *Am J Public Health*. 2025;115(7):979–981.

Acceptance Date: April 13, 2025.

DOI: https://doi.org/10.2105/AJPH.2025.308157

ORCID iDs:

Julia A. Dilley https://orcid.org/0000-0002-1926-9750

Robert G. Hendrickson https://orcid.org/0000-0002-5998-3908

### CONTRIBUTORS

J. A. Dilley and R. G. Hendrickson jointly conceptualized the original work. J. A. Dilley provided the first draft. J. A. Dilley and R. G. Hendrickson jointly revised and finalized the paper.

### ACKNOWLEDGMENTS

The authors would like to thank Erik Everson for conducting the hospital data analysis. J. A. Dilley was supported by the National Institute on Drug Abuse of the National Institutes of Health (award 1R01DA039293, PI: Dilley).

**Note.** The opinions in this editorial are those of the authors entirely and do not necessarily represent those of the National Institute on Drug Abuse or other agencies.

### CONFLICTS OF INTEREST

The authors have no conflicts to disclose.

### HUMAN PARTICIPANT PROTECTION

The parent study (1R01DA039293) was reviewed and approved by the Washington State institutional review board and Oregon Public Health institutional review board.

### REFERENCES

1. National Academies of Sciences, Engineering, and Medicine. 2017. *The Health Effects of Cannabis and Cannabinoids: The Current State of Evidence and Recommendations for Research.* Washington, DC: The National Academies Press; 2017. https://doi.org/10.17226/24625.
2. Volkow ND, Baler RD, Compton WM, Weiss SRB. Adverse health effects of marijuana use. *N Engl J Med.* 2014;370(23):2219–2227. https://doi.org/10.1056/NEJMRA1402309
3. National Academies of Sciences, Engineering, and Medicine. *Cannabis Policy Impacts Public Health and Health Equity.* Washington, DC: The National Academies Press; 2024. https://doi.org/10.17226/27766.
4. Miech RA, Johnston LD, Patrick ME, O'Malley PM. Monitoring the Future national survey results on drug use, 1975–2024: overview and key findings for secondary school students. Monitoring the Future Monograph Series. Institute for Social Research, University of Michigan. 2024. Available at: https://monitoringthefuture.org/results/annual-reports. Accessed April 2, 2025.
5. Dilley JA, Johnson JK, Colby AM, et al. Cannabis retail market indicators in five legal states in the United States: a public health perspective. *Clin Ther.* 2023;45(8):778–786. https://doi.org/10.1016/j.clinthera.2023.06.015
6. Fataar F, Driezen P, Owusu-Bempah A, Hammond D. Distribution of legal retail cannabis stores in Canada by neighbourhood deprivation. *J Cannabis Res.* 2024;6(1):5. https://doi.org/10.1186/s42238-023-00211-x
7. Cannabis Act (S.C. 2018, c. 16). Government of Canada. Available at: https://laws-lois.justice.gc.ca/eng/acts/c-24.5/page-3.html#h-77141. Accessed April 1, 2025.
8. Rup J, Goodman S, Hammond D. Cannabis advertising, promotion and branding: differences in consumer exposure between "legal" and "illegal" markets in Canada and the US. *Prev Med.* 2020;133:106013. Available at: https://doi.org/10.1016/j.ypmed.2020.106013
9. Dilley JA, Hendrickson RG, Everson EM, Jeanne TL. Monitoring cannabis adverse events: lessons from edible packaging policies and child poisonings. *Am J Public Health.* 2024;114(suppl 8):S631–S634. https://doi.org/10.2105/AJPH.2024.307789
10. Hammond D, Goodman S, Wadsworth E, et al. Trends in the use of cannabis products in Canada and the USA, 2018–2020: findings from the International Cannabis Policy Study. *Int J Drug Policy.* 2022;105:103716. https://doi.org/10.1016/j.drugpo.2022.103716
11. Hendrickson RG, Dilley JA, Hedberg K, Jeanne TL, Love JS, Thompson JA, Choo EK. The burden of cannabis-attributed pediatric and adult emergency department visits. *Acad Emerg Med.* 2021;28(12):1444–1447. Available at: https://doi.org/10.1111/ACEM.14275

# Masking the Health Impacts of Anti-LGBTQ+ Policies by Political Suppression of Data and Informational Erasure

Joseph R. Cimpian, PhD, and Mollie T. McQuillan, PhD

**ABOUT THE AUTHORS**

*Joseph R. Cimpian is with the Department of Applied Statistics, Social Science, and Humanities, Steinhardt School of Culture, Education, and Human Development, New York University, New York, NY. Mollie T. McQuillan is with the Department of Educational Leadership & Policy Analysis, School of Education, University of Wisconsin-Madison.*

**See also Mittleman, p. 1137.**

AJPH July 2025, Vol. 115, No. 7

Youths who identify as lesbian, gay, bisexual, transgender, questioning, or other noncisgender or nonheterosexual (LGBTQ+) face greater health risks than their non-LGBTQ+ peers, as demonstrated by Mittleman's study in this issue of *AJPH* (p. 1137) using data from the National Youth Risk Behavior Survey (YRBS). This finding reinforces decades of health disparities research related to sexual orientation and gender identity.[1,2] What distinguishes this new work is its utilization of the first National YRBS data set to include a gender identity measure—filling a critical gap in our ability to examine transgender adolescents' health with this population-based youth sample. Including the gender identity measure provides empirical confirmation of what previous state- and district-level YRBS analyses suggested: transgender youths experience particularly elevated risks for adverse childhood experiences, even beyond the already heightened risks faced by cisgender LGBQ youths.

These new YRBS findings emerge at a troubling moment. LGBTQ+ youths—especially transgender youths—face intensifying state-level legislative restrictions and federal-level executive orders subverting evidence-based medical, educational, and research practices.[3] More specifically, these documents attempt to only recognize a binary sex while rejecting gender identity, regulate LGBTQ+-representative curricula, limit access to safe school adults and facilities, and ban school-based athletic participation aligned with gender identity rather than sex assigned at birth. We aim to highlight the legitimate concerns that these governmental actions will inflict additional harm on LGBTQ+ youths. Research using quasi-experimental designs has found that pro-LGBTQ+ policies lower suicide attempts for LGBTQ+ youths and improve overall youth well-being.[4,5] That is, the majority of youths fared better when state laws treated LGBTQ+ people more equitably. Thus, there is reason to suspect that the latest wave of government measures restricting LGBTQ+ rights will have the opposite effect, possibly worsening health outcomes for LGBTQ+, cisgender, and heterosexual youths alike.

As political rhetoric targeting transgender youths intensified, public support for transgender individuals declined between 2022 and 2025, according to Pew Research data.[6] Although readers may hold varying views on specific policy questions such as athletic inclusion, the scientific research presented here focuses on adolescent mental health and well-being descriptions. Empirical evidence consistently shows that transgender youths (and LGBTQ+ youths more broadly) experience elevated average health risks and face significantly greater rates of social stressors than their cisgender and heterosexual peers. These studies point to not only "culture war" topics but serious concerns about mental health, physical abuse, emotional abuse, and suicidality. While opinions on culture war issues may vary, the health evidence indicates political attacks targeting LGBTQ+ youths may exacerbate already elevated risks at precisely the time when increased—not decreased—support is needed.

Erasing gender identity data collection from some of the most rigorously designed, large, population-based studies as policymakers remove protections for transgender youths may reflect a coordinated strategy to erase transgender people. Even before the Trump administration's Executive Order 14168, which called for the ban of federally collected gender identity data, several states that passed bans on LGBTQ+-inclusive education and gender-affirming medical care had already withdrawn from the YRBS—one of the only surveys that produces reliable state comparisons of adolescent health outcomes.

Just as researchers began assessing transgender–cisgender disparities at the national level, continued collection and processing of these data were indefinitely suspended. This severely limits our ability to evaluate health risks and strengths among an extremely vulnerable population of American youths. Eliminating measurement capacity does not eliminate the underlying risks—rather, the data suppression further harms transgender youths by restricting researchers' ability to describe risks, who is disproportionally at risk, and how effective different interventions are. Informational erasure occurs when people within organizations lack awareness about gender diversity, and it underlies "the assumption that little information exists to guide gender diversity reforms of policies, procedures, or practices."[3(p649)] The availability of gender identity data, such as the 2023 YRBS, combats informational erasure by enabling nuanced descriptions of adolescents' experiences and needs rather than relying on assumptions and stereotypes. Without such data, governmental and public health organizations may struggle to assess needs, allocate resources effectively, and maintain operational efficiency.

Importantly, data suppression and informational erasure are fundamentally different from implementing data validity checks regarding potentially invalid, careless, and mischievous responses. Suppressing data enables misinformation and misconceptions about stigmatized populations, such as trans and nonbinary youths, whereas validity checks aim to capture the authentic experiences of stigmatized groups.[7,8] Mittleman implements a machine learning–based validity checking technique that Cimpian et al. developed,[8] and finds that the patterns of elevated adverse childhood experiences for LGBTQ+ youths are robust to this validity-checking procedure. What we have consistently found through research implementing rigorous validity checks is that LGBTQ+ youths require greater protections in schools and society.[7–9] The elevated discrimination, bullying, and harassment these youths experience remains robust to validity checks, and with these additional checks we can be more confident in the genuine policy and societal need to support LGBTQ+ youths. We have also discovered that some disparities that might give the public a distorted impression of LGBTQ+ youths—such as dramatically elevated illicit drug use, extreme alcohol use, and certain sexual risk behaviors—are often substantially reduced when potentially invalid data are accounted for.[7,8] This indicates that health risks most closely associated with stigma and social stressors represent the most reliable findings, further supporting the need to protect all LGBTQ+ youths.

Additionally, our recent analysis of repeated cross-sectional National YRBS data reveals that over one third of high school females now identify as LGBQ.[10] Importantly, we could not include transgender youths in the study because the gender identity item was not part of the national survey until 2023. This lack of previous gender identity data contributes to informational erasure in assessing national trends for transgender youths over time. Our findings indicate that LGBQ people constitute a substantial segment of today's high school population—not a marginal group—meaning that governmental actions restricting LGBQ rights, protections, data, and research-based reports on government Web sites affect a growing proportion of American youths. These restrictions could be especially consequential because LGBQ youths consistently report higher rates of suicidality across time periods.[10] Recent focus on increasing suicide risk among US high school females over the past decade—which has received extensive media attention—may overlook a key factor: the growing percentage of females identifying as LGBQ,[10] who likely experience stigmatization and stressors earlier in development than previous generations.[11] This insight highlights why continued measurement of sexual identity in the YRBS is essential—without it, we may miss crucial explanations for increased suicide risk among adolescent girls more generally. With over one third of high school females now identifying as LGBQ, informational erasure of LGBTQ+ populations is indefensible, especially given its connection to life-threatening outcomes. Eliminating the gender item in the YRBS makes a similar analysis by gender identity impossible.

Without comprehensive, systematic evidence, policymakers cannot make evidence-based policies. Collectively, the public health research evidence clearly demonstrates that LGBTQ+ youths consistently face elevated risks for adverse experiences, from child mistreatment to suicidality.[1,2,7–10] But these health outcomes are not inevitable. As more youths feel comfortable disclosing their LGBTQ+ identities and as data collection has expanded, researchers have gained better understanding of risks, benefits, and protective factors. For instance, laws concerning LGBTQ+ people likely causally affect LGBTQ+ health outcomes, including among youths.[4,5] Recent governmental actions rescinding LGBTQ+ protections and reversing gender identity data collection will likely negatively affect health—only now, we may lack the data needed to detect these effects and inform evidence-based policymaking and health practices. AJPH

## CORRESPONDENCE

Correspondence should be sent to Joseph R. Cimpian, PhD, New York University, Kimball Hall, 246 Greene Street, New York, NY 10003 (e-mail: joseph.cimpian@nyu.edu). Reprints can be ordered at http://www.ajph.org by clicking the "Reprints" link.

## PUBLICATION INFORMATION

Full Citation: Cimpian JR, McQuillan MT. Masking the health impacts of anti-LGBTQ+ policies by political suppression of data and informational erasure. *Am J Public Health.* 2025;115(7):982–984.

Acceptance Date: March 31, 2025

DOI: https://doi.org/10.2105/AJPH.2025.308141

ORCID iDs:

Joseph R. Cimpian https://orcid.org/0000-0001-6111-8895

Mollie T. McQuillan https://orcid.org/0000-0002-2522-3871

## CONTRIBUTORS

J. R. Cimpian and M. T. McQuillan wrote this editorial.

## CONFLICTS OF INTEREST

J. R. Cimpian reports no potential or actual conflicts of interests. M. T. McQuillan has been hired by the American Civil Liberties Union to provide expert testimony in court cases.

## REFERENCES

1. Austin A, Herrick H, Proescholdbell S. Adverse childhood experiences related to poor adult health among lesbian, gay, and bisexual individuals. *Am J Public Health.* 2016;106(2):314–320. https://doi.org/10.2105/AJPH.2015.302904
2. Hughes PM, Ostrout TL, Perez Jolles M, Thomas KC. Adverse childhood experiences across birth generation and LGBTQ identity, Behavioral Risk Factor Surveillance System, 2019. *Am J Public Health.* 2022;112(4):662–670. https://doi.org/10.2105/AJPH.2021.306642
3. McQuillan MT, Lebovitz BA, Harbin L. The disruptive power of policy erasure: how state legislators and school boards fail to take up trans-affirming policies while leaning into anti-LGBTQ+ policies. *Educational Policy.* 2024;38(3):642–699. https://doi.org/10.1177/08959048231218206
4. Raifman J, Moscoe E, Austin SB, McConnell M. Difference-in-differences analysis of the association between state same-sex marriage policies and adolescent suicide attempts. *JAMA Pediatr.* 2017;171(4):350–356. https://doi.org/10.1001/jamapediatrics.2016.4529
5. Lee WY, Hobbs JN, Hobaica S, DeChants JP, Price MN, Nath R. State-level anti-transgender laws increase past-year suicide attempts among transgender and non-binary young people in the USA. *Nat Hum Behav.* 2024;8(11):2096–2106. https://doi.org/10.1038/s41562-024-01979-5
6. Pew Research Center. Americans have grown more supportive of restrictions for trans people in recent years. February 26, 2025. Available at: https://www.pewresearch.org/short-reads/2025/02/26/americans-have-grown-more-supportive-of-restrictions-for-trans-people-in-recent-years. Accessed March 11, 2025.
7. Cimpian JR, Timmer JD, Birkett MA, Marro RL, Turner BC, Phillips GL. Bias from potentially mischievous responders on large-scale estimates of lesbian, gay, bisexual, or questioning (LGBQ)–heterosexual youth health disparities. *Am J Public Health.* 2018;108(S4):S258–S265. https://doi.org/10.2105/AJPH.2018.304407
8. Cimpian JR, Timmer JD, Kim TH. Mitigating invalid and mischievous survey responses: a registered report examining risk disparities between heterosexual and lesbian, gay, bisexual, or questioning youth. *Child Dev.* 2023;94(5):1136–1161. https://doi.org/10.1111/cdev.13957
9. McQuillan MT, Cimpian JR, Lebovitz BA, Gill EK. Transgender adolescent school climate, mental health, and adult social support. *JAMA Pediatr.* 2024;178(10):1082–1084. https://doi.org/10.1001/jamapediatrics.2024.3079
10. Cimpian JR, McQuillan MT. An overlooked explanation for increasing suicidality: LGBQ stressors felt by more students. *Educ Res.* 2025;54(1):56–60. https://doi.org/10.3102/0013189X241305329
11. Fish JN, Russell ST. The paradox of progress for sexual and gender diverse youth. *Curr Opin Psychol.* 2022;48:101498. https://doi.org/10.1016/j.copsyc.2022.101498

# On The Efficacy and Legality of Vaccine Mandates

James G. Hodge Jr., JD, LLM

**ABOUT THE AUTHOR**

*James G. Hodge Jr. is with the Center for Public Health Law and Policy, Sandra Day O'Connor College of Law, Arizona State University, Phoenix.*

**See also Dullea et al., p. 1146.**

The long-standing legal history of vaccines is intrinsically tied to the use of mandates: requirements that persons be inoculated for infectious diseases as a condition of eligibility or participation in employment, education, service, travel, or other activities. Time and again, federal, state, tribal, and local public health officials, legislators, and policymakers have turned to vaccine mandates to promote the public's health, safety, and security. With rare exceptions, such mandates are adjudged constitutionally—and otherwise legally—sound. When confronted directly with rights-based challenges to an early smallpox vaccine mandate in 1905, the US Supreme Court endorsed state and local governmental powers to require vaccination among able-bodied adults in Cambridge, Massachusetts.[1] It later affirmed the soundness of school vaccination requirements in 1922.[2]

Although the Supreme Court rejected the authority of the federal Occupational Safety and Health Administration (OSHA) to require large businesses to set employee mandates for COVID-19 vaccines under a Biden era regulation in 2022,[3] it did so largely on the grounds of observed limitations of federal commerce powers. The value of COVID-19 vaccine mandates was not questioned so much as the scope of governmental powers. Thus, the same day that the court rejected OSHA's authority, it allowed a similar federal vaccine mandate affecting health care workers authorized via constitutional spending—and not commerce—powers.[4]

## VACCINE MANDATES WORK

Consistent legislative and judicial recognitions of governmental powers to conditionally require vaccination are premised on a simple fact: vaccine mandates work. When authorized at the appropriate levels of government (e.g., states) for specific entities (e.g., hospitals) or persons (e.g., children attending day care or school), mandates raise vaccination rates. Infectious disease rates subsequently decrease, resulting in improved personal health outcomes and enhanced public health and safety. What Dullea et al. reveal in their article "COVID-19 Vaccine Mandate and Vaccination Rates in the US Military, 2020–2022" (p. 1146) in this issue of *AJPH* is how well-timed mandates for military members during the pandemic (1) vastly improved their rates of vaccination (especially compared with the general population), and (2) contributed to greater equities across subgroups among the US armed forces.

Notwithstanding administrative, religious, and medical vaccine exemptions available to all active military personnel, the authors demonstrate how President Biden's COVID-19 mandate increased rates of vaccination among this population by more than 35% in just over four months between August 21, 2021, and January 1, 2022. As a result, more than 95% of US military personnel were vaccinated by the beginning of 2022 compared with less than 75% of the US general population. Better yet, the military's mandate greatly helped reduce existing disparities in vaccinations among Blacks, Hispanics, and other races who all sought inoculations more extensively than White military members. Essentially, minorities in armed forces caught up to majority immunization rates after the mandate was implemented. Conversely, military women's vaccination rates lagged slightly behind men's, owing in part to pregnancy statuses that may have led women to seek medical exemptions. Still, the authors' research based on data from the COVID-19 pandemic sustains their key, long-term conclusion: "US military must retain the authority to mandate safe and effective vaccines as an important tool to promote health, readiness, and national security" (p. 1154).

## POLITICIZATION AND LEGAL CHALLENGES TO VACCINE MANDATES

Incredibly, many federal, state, and local law- and policymakers have, in fact, taken the opposite view. Imposition of vaccine mandates has approached a level of political and legal toxicity rarely seen in US history. The military's mandate, effectuated via executive order during the Biden administration, was legislatively rescinded by Congress in January 2023 as the pandemic largely wound down.[5] Just days into office, on January 27, 2025, President Trump signed an executive order reinstating service members discharged solely because of their nonexempted refusal to receive the COVID-19 vaccine.[6] He followed up this pronouncement with an order on February 14 forbidding federal funding of schools or universities requiring COVID-19 vaccines as a condition of attendance.[7] Repercussions of the president's order were minimal, as few schools still required such vaccines. Yet the clear policy objective of derailing mandates has been buttressed by progressive antivaccination sentiments among national, state, and local officials.

Department of Health and Human Services secretary, Robert F. Kennedy Jr., has seriously questioned the risks of COVID-19 vaccines overall as well as routine vaccine requirements specifically for children—even as one of the worst outbreaks of measles in decades has surfaced in Texas and other areas, killing two children to date. His administration has defrocked vaccine advisory committees, terminated prominent vaccine experts, and initiated studies into the repeatedly disproven link of childhood vaccines with increased rates of autism. Manifold state and local governments have adopted antivaccination stances to perpetuate immunization misinformation and inhibit mandates.[8] In 2023, Florida, Texas, and multiple other states forbade employer-based COVID-19 vaccine mandates.[9] In December 2024, Louisiana's surgeon general instructed state and local health officials to de-emphasize mass vaccinations entirely.[10] On March 29, 2025, Idaho governor Brad Little had to defy his own Republican party to veto Senate Bill 1023, which would have prohibited vaccine mandates in any setting, including schools, statewide.[11]

## RISKS OF BANNING VACCINE MANDATES

These and multiple other legal and policy maneuvers run counter to decades of existing vaccination practices designed to ensure the health of populations. Provided vaccines are safe, effective, and accessible—as is the case of most US Food and Drug Administration authorized or approved vaccines—their uptake carries substantial communal and personal health benefits. Conversely, their rejection leads to profound harms. In the case of the US military, Dullea et al. rightly observe the potential diminutions in readiness extending from insufficiently vaccinated troops. Vaccination among the military is historically and currently a national security priority, not a threat against personal liberty. For all Americans, ensuring sufficiently high rates of vaccinations for preventable diseases—such as measles, mumps, rubella, polio, and, prospectively, avian flu—is not just about protecting others: it is also vital to individual health.

Those willing to risk exposure to infectious conditions by forgoing vaccines face profound long-term chronic or other conditions (e.g., long COVID) for which diagnoses and treatments may be lacking. According to the World Health Organization (WHO), extended impacts from unvaccinated exposure to measles include brain damage, pneumonia, deafness, and blindness. And, of course, deaths attributable to vaccine-preventable diseases are inevitable absent immunization. Among the more than seven million COVID-19 deaths globally, nearly four million (57%) might have been prevented if vaccines were fully available and used at the commencement of the pandemic, according to a 2024 WHO European study.[12]

Whether in the US military or in the general population, politicizing vaccine mandates as a social evil and infringement on personal liberties or choice defies science, ethics, security, and communal health. Objections may be sustained if mandates actually physically compelled people to get vaccinated—but they do not. Rather, as noted, vaccine legal mandates convey options conditioned on receipt of specific privileges. What undergirds such mandates is our shared choice to live freely in societies unburdened by the constant threat of preventable infectious diseases as well as the concurrent risks to national security by a weakened military plagued by illness. Americans refuting the civic option to seek safe and effective vaccinations face the very real possibility that the next life succumbing to infectious conditions will be their own. AJPH

### CORRESPONDENCE

Correspondence should be sent to James G. Hodge Jr., JD, LLM, Sandra Day O'Connor College of Law, Arizona State University, 111 E. Taylor St, MC 9520, Phoenix, AZ 85004 (e-mail: james.hodge.1@asu.edu). Reprints can be ordered at https://www.ajph.org by clicking the "Reprints" link.

### PUBLICATION INFORMATION

Full Citation: Hodge Jr JG. On the efficacy and legality of vaccine mandates. *Am J Public Health*. 2025;115(7):985–987.

Acceptance Date: April 12, 2025.

DOI: https://doi.org/10.2105/AJPH.2025.308161

ORCID iD:

James G. Hodge Jr. https://orcid.org/0000-0001-6928-8645

### ACKNOWLEDGMENTS

The views expressed are those of the author and not of his institution.

## CONFLICTS OF INTEREST

The author has no financial, personal, academic, or other conflicts of interest to disclose.

## REFERENCES


1. *Jacobson v Massachusetts*, 197 US 11 (1905).
2. *Zucht v King*, 260 US 174 (1922).
3. *National Federation of Independent Business v Department of Labor, Occupational Safety and Health Administration*, 595 US 109 (2022).
4. *Biden v Missouri*, 595 US 87 (2022).
5. James M. Inhofe National Defense Authorization Act for Fiscal Year 2023. Pub L no. 117–263. Available at: https://www.congress.gov/bill/117th-congress/house-bill/7776. Accessed May 1, 2025.
6. Exec. Order No. 14,184, 90 *Fed. Reg.* 8761 (January 27, 2025).
7. White House. Fact sheet: President Donald J. Trump prohibits federal funding for COVID-19 vaccine mandates in schools. February 14, 2025. Available at: https://www.whitehouse.gov/fact-sheets/2025/02/fact-sheet-president-donald-j-trump-prohibits-federal-funding-for-covid-19-vaccine-mandates-in-schools. Accessed April 1, 2025.
8. National Academy for State Health Policy. State efforts to limit or enforce COVID-19 vaccine mandates. February 26, 2025. Available at: https://nashp.org/state-tracker/state-efforts-to-ban-or-enforce-covid-19-vaccine-mandates-and-passports. Accessed April 1, 2025.
9. Ravitsky G, Houston Pope J. Texas joins Florida in prohibiting private employers from imposing vaccine mandates. December 20, 2023. Available at: https://www.workforcebulletin.com/texas-joins-florida-in-prohibiting-private-employers-from-imposing-vaccine-mandates. Accessed April 1, 2025.
10. Hilburn G. Bill Cassidy condemns new Louisiana vaccine policy after confirming vaccine skeptic RFK Jr. *Shreveport Times*. February 18, 2025. Available at: https://www.shreveporttimes.com/story/news/2025/02/18/senator-bill-cassidy-condemns-new-louisiana-vaccine-policy-but-confirmed-vaccine-skeptic-rfk-jr/79063797007. Accessed April 1, 2025.
11. Komatsoulis C. Gov. Little boasts "medical freedom" in Idaho, vetoes bill to ban vaccine mandates. *East Idaho News*. March 29, 2025. Available at: https://www.eastidahonews.com/2025/03/gov-little-boasts-medical-freedom-in-idaho-vetoes-bill-to-ban-vaccine-mandates. Accessed April 1, 2025.
12. World Health Organization. COVID-19 vaccinations have saved more than 1.4 million lives in the WHO European region, a new study finds. January 16, 2024. Available at: https://www.who.int/europe/news/item/16-01-2024-covid-19-vaccinations-have-saved-more-than-1.4-million-lives-in-the-who-european-region–a-new-study-finds. Accessed April 1, 2025.

# An Effective HIV Response Means HIV Decriminalization

*Joanne Csete, PhD, MPH*

**ABOUT THE AUTHOR**

*Joanne Csete is with the Mailman School of Public Health, Columbia University, New York NY.*

**See also Listerud et al., p. 1157.**

Incarceration carries obvious threats to mental and physical health for both the person deprived of liberty and the families and communities involved. Excessive, arbitrary, or discriminatory application of carceral sanctions is a public health issue as much as a social justice issue.

Under most legal systems, for a person to be judged guilty of a criminal offense there must be proof of (1) intent to do wrong, (2) actually having acted on that intent, and (3) demonstrable harm caused by the act.[1] In too many jurisdictions worldwide, including many US states, people can face criminal punishment for the "willful" transmission of HIV and the nondisclosure of HIV status before engaging in an act that could transmit HIV.

The Joint United Nations Program on HIV/AIDS (UNAIDS) has long asserted that there is no need for HIV-specific laws on transmission, exposure, and nondisclosure. As UNAIDS puts it, criminal prosecution can be warranted only when a person knows he or she is living with HIV, that person acts with the intention of transmitting HIV, and transmission does in fact take place.[1] In such extremely rare cases, UNAIDS states that general criminal law can handle the matter without recourse to HIV-specific law. From an evidentiary perspective, intent to transmit HIV is likely to be difficult to prove beyond reasonable doubt. The fact of HIV being transmitted by any given sexual act is likely to be virtually impossible to prove.[2]

In this issue of *AJPH*, Listerud et al. (p. 1157) conclude that in numerous US states, HIV criminal law has been applied disproportionately against Blacks, especially against Black gay and transgender persons. Stigma and discrimination faced by people with HIV, LGBTQI (lesbian, gay, bisexual, transgender, queer or questioning, or intersex) persons, people who use drugs, and sex workers remain a central challenge for the HIV response in the United States and worldwide.[3] When those prejudices come together with racism and motivate the unjust application of criminal law, the carceral implications are catastrophic.

Although prosecutions under HIV-specific criminal laws in the United States are few compared with the millions affected by the criminal legal system, media coverage of these prosecutions has been shown in many cases to contribute on a wide scale to the several forms of discrimination noted.[4] Moreover, even a small number of cases in which transgender women—who now face the threat of being housed in men's prisons in the United States[5]—are incarcerated can result in sexual violence, a heinous outcome on any scale.

Most HIV criminalization statutes in the United States date from the time before advances in HIV treatment made the virus undetectable in the bloodstream and therefore untransmissible by anyone receiving effective therapy. The science behind "U=U" (undetectable = untransmissible) is incontrovertible and has been used in many countries to reform or repeal HIV criminal statutes.[6] As denial of the fundamental tenets of HIV science has crept back into serious public discourse in the United States,[7] the disregard for science reflected in the continued existence of these statutes is of deep concern.

In the United States and elsewhere, most successful efforts to repeal HIV criminal statutes have been led by networks of people with HIV, often allied with organizations of LGBTQI persons, sex workers, and others concerned with human rights related to HIV. Globally, the HIV Justice Network has led the charge; it has also compiled the most reliable international data on reform and repeal efforts.[8]

Although considerable attention has been paid to the cutting of the President's Emergency Plan for AIDS Relief funding as it affects HIV treatment and prevention, the withdrawal of US support of HIV-related policy and legislative advocacy is also of great concern.[8] Curtailing the efforts of the HIV Justice Network, the US-based Center for HIV Law and Policy, and other organizations seeking repeal of these ill-originated laws would have long-term detrimental effects. Allowing HIV criminalization to thrive would compromise HIV testing, treatment, and prevention efforts over time by making people afraid to know their HIV status.

Civil society groups in the United States praised the action of the US Department of Justice in a 2024 challenge to a Tennessee law that allowed harsher prosecution of sex workers in the state if they were living with HIV.[9] The law was challenged as a violation of the Americans With Disabilities Act. The current Trump administration ended similar cases the Department of Justice was about to bring. The promise of this unusual alliance between government and civil society to confront HIV-based legal discrimination was short-lived.

But governments have an obligation to join this fight. The unanimously adopted 2021 UN General Assembly Political Declaration on HIV and AIDS, which established goals for 2030, includes a commitment to review and reform "discriminatory laws and practices that create barriers or reinforce stigma and discrimination, such as . . . laws related to HIV non-disclosure, exposure and transmission."[10(p14/19)]

These laws do not deter HIV transmission or nondisclosure, and they may make people fear seeking HIV testing and care. Criminal punishment is an expression of social repugnance for a criminal act, but the repugnance that these laws express is misplaced and discriminatory.

In the United States and beyond, the cases of persons incarcerated for HIV transmission and nondisclosure, including those serving long sentences, should be reviewed. Prosecutions not conforming to the UNAIDS guidelines—that is, virtually all prosecutions—should cease. The organizations working to repeal HIV criminalization statutes should be adequately funded. An effective, rights-based response to HIV in the United States and globally requires HIV decriminalization. AJPH

## CORRESPONDENCE

Correspondence should be sent to Joanne Csete, Columbia University Mailman School of Public Health, Department of Population and Family Health, 60 Haven Ave, B2, New York, NY 10032 (e-mail: jc1188@cumc.columbia.edu). Reprints can be ordered at https://www.ajph.org by clicking the "Reprints" link.

## PUBLICATION INFORMATION

Full Citation: Csete J. An effective HIV response means HIV decriminalization. *Am J Public Health*. 2025;115(7):988–989.

Acceptance Date: April 12, 2025.

DOI: https://doi.org/10.2105/AJPH.2025.308162

## CONFLICTS OF INTEREST

The author has no conflicts of interest to report.

## REFERENCES

1. Joint United Nations Programme on HIV/AIDS. Ending overly broad criminalization of HIV non-disclosure, exposure and transmission: critical scientific, medical and legal considerations. May 2013. Available at: https://www.unaids.org/sites/default/files/media_asset/20130530_Guidance_Ending_Criminalisation_0.pdf. Accessed May 1, 2025.
2. Barré-Sinoussi F, Abdool Karim SS, Albert J, et al. Expert consensus statement on the science of HIV in the context of criminal law. *J Intl AIDS Soc.* 2018;21(7):e25161. https://doi.org/10.1002/jia2.25161
3. Joint United Nations Programme on HIV/AIDS. *The Path That Ends AIDS: 2023 UNAIDS Global AIDS Update.* 2023. Available at: https://www.unaids.org/sites/default/files/media_asset/2023-unaids-global-aids-update_en.pdf. Accessed May 1, 2025.
4. Campbell CK, Rojo F, Khanna N, Dworkin SL. Sex, lies and videotape: a content and textual analysis of media coverage of the HIV criminal prosecution of Michael Johnson. *Crime Media Cult.* 2022;18(1):52–69. https://doi.org/10.1177/1741659020971000
5. Del Ray M. Transgender women moved to men's prisons despite rulings against Trump order. *Independent.* March 8, 2025. Available at: https://www.the-independent.com/news/world/americas/crime/trans-women-federal-prisons-b2711335.html. Accessed May 1, 2025.
6. Symington A. Expert consensus statement on the science of HIV in the context of criminal law—five-year impact report: bringing science to justice. 2023. Available at: https://www.hivjustice.net/publication/ecs. Accessed May 1, 2025.
7. McNeil DG Jr. RFK Jr. mimics AIDS denier Thabo Mbeki. *Washington Post.* April 3, 2025. Available at: https://www.washingtonpost.com/opinions/2025/04/03/kennedy-mbeki-aids-measles-denial. Accessed May 2, 2025.
8. Bernard EJ. Zimbabwe's victory: a beacon of hope for HIV justice amid global challenges. March 28, 2025. Available at: https://www.hivjustice.net/news/zimbabwes-victory-a-beacon-of-hope-for-hiv-justice-amid-global-challenges. Accessed May 1, 2025.
9. Rhodes A. Activists fighting HIV criminalization laws say they've lost federal government as a partner. March 5, 2025. Available at: https://prismreports.org/2025/03/05/hiv-criminalization-laws-trump. Accessed May 1, 2025.
10. United Nations General Assembly. Political declaration on HIV and AIDS: ending inequalities and getting on track to end AIDS by 2030. Document no. A/RES/75/284. June 9, 2021. Available at: https://digitallibrary.un.org/record/3928975?v=pdf. Accessed May 1, 2025.

# The Need for Comprehensive and Timely City-Level Fatal and Nonfatal Firearm Injury Surveillance

Anthony A. Braga, PhD, MPA

**ABOUT THE AUTHOR**

*Anthony A. Braga, PhD, MPA, is the Jerry Lee Professor of Criminology and Director of the Crime and Justice Policy Lab at the University of Pennsylvania in Philadelphia.*

**See also Smart et al., p. 1106.**

In this issue of *AJPH* (p. 1106), Smart et al. make an important contribution to firearm injury prevention policy and practice by developing a publicly available data set on state-level estimates of nonfatal firearm injury hospitalizations between 2000 and 2021. States' firearm laws and gun violence reduction programming vary tremendously across the United States and provide the context for state-level variation in firearm availability and community gun violence. This new data source will be valuable to descriptive research on regional risk factors associated with shootings and rigorous evaluations of state legislation and policies intended to reduce gun violence. Nevertheless, interpersonal gun violence is highly concentrated at specific high-risk places and among high-risk people within cities.[1] As such, city-level databases on fatal and nonfatal shootings are also desperately needed to provide a more refined picture of community gun violence and evaluate interventions that seek to reduce the risk of gun violence in local settings.

## AVAILABLE SHOOTING INJURY DATA

Considerable overlap exists in the characteristics and underlying circumstances of fatal and nonfatal shooting injuries with mortality determined by the number and location of wounds and by the size and weight of the bullets, among other variables.[2] Reforms are needed to generate timely, accurate, and publicly accessible nonfatal shooting data from local police departments and hospitals. Such a data set would serve as an important complement to the firearm homicide and firearm suicide data available from the Centers for Disease Control and Prevention's (CDC's) National Violent Death Reporting System (NVDRS), Web-based Injury Statistics Query and Reporting System (WISQARS), and Wide-ranging Online Data for Epidemiologic Research (WONDER) online databases.

Nonfatal firearm injury inpatient hospitalizations data do not capture patients who suffer minor gunshot injuries and are treated and released. Nonfatal firearm injury inpatient hospitalizations data also miss cases involving gunshot wound survivors who do not seek treatment. Local police department databases include nonfatal gunshot victims regardless of treatment status but are limited to criminal assaults rather than cases involving self-inflicted and accidental circumstances. No current system adequately captures accurate national data on nonfatal shootings emanating from criminal circumstances, some of which involve injuries that are not treated at hospitals and elude existing injury surveillance systems.[3] The Federal Bureau of Investigation's efforts to launch its National Incident-Based Reporting System (NIBRS) that shifts crime reporting from simple counts to more detailed incident-level data have, unfortunately, resulted in a drop in law enforcement agency participation that prevents valid national nonfatal shooting estimates.[3] NIBRS aggravated gun assault data can include blunt trauma from pistol whippings and, as such, do not report whether victims suffered actual gunshot wounds.

The Gun Violence Archive (GVA) is an independent research and data collection organization that attempts to provide real-time data on assaultive gun violence by accessing public records. GVA provides within-city data on gun homicides, nonfatal shootings, mass murders and shootings, officer-involved shootings, unintentional shootings, and defensive gun uses. Studies support the use of GVA data as an information source for gun violence research in large US cities.[4] The availability of city police department shooting databases was credited as an important factor in improving the comprehensiveness of GVA data. Another inquiry found that a local police database was more accurate than the GVA, as it captured a higher percentage of emergency department–presenting patients with gunshot wounds.[5] However, relative to hospital injury data, the study suggested that gunshot victims were less likely to be included in police records when they self-presented to the emergency department or were injured outside of the city. Police shooting databases can serve as valuable sources of timely and comprehensive city-level data on fatal and nonfatal shootings emanating from criminal assaults when used with caution and routinely compared with hospital emergency department records for accuracy. Philadelphia, Pennsylvania, provides an important example.

The authors estimate that the Commonwealth of Pennsylvania had a 2021 rate of 1.71 nonfatal firearm injuries per 10 000 residents (most recent year available in their study). This suggests that roughly 2217 people suffered nonfatal gunshot wounds that year ([12 964 056 population/10 000] * 1.71). The CDC further documented an additional 874 gunshot injury deaths in Pennsylvania resulting from criminal assaults and legal interventions in 2021.[6] Nearly 57% (494 of 874) of these fatal gunshot injuries occurred in the City of Philadelphia, which represents only 12% of the Commonwealth's population (1 576 251 residents in 2021).

## CONCENTRATED RISKS OF SHOOTING INJURIES

As part of the city's Open Government Initiative, the Philadelphia Police Department (PPD) posts real-time data on fatal and nonfatal shooting victimizations that involve gunshot wound injuries from criminal assaults and officer-involved shootings.[7] Official police data have some well-known limitations, with incomplete citizen reporting of crime and officer decision-making bias as to whether an incident should be recorded as a crime among the most pressing concerns. However, because of the presence of a cadaver, police-generated homicide data are generally viewed as reliable and valid sources of information on fatal gun injuries. In 2021, the CDC and PPD reported very similar numbers of fatal gun assaults (494 and 508, respectively). PPD fatal and nonfatal shooting data have also been validated by comparisons to hospital emergency department records.[8]

Table 1 presents the annual counts of fatal and nonfatal gunshot injury victimizations in Philadelphia. Like other US cities, community gun violence peaked during the COVID-19 pandemic (2020–2022) and then decreased in subsequent years. The overall case fatality rate for gun assaults with injury was almost 21% (3401 of 16 315), with a low of little more than 18% in 2015 (233 of 1271) and a high of nearly 23% in 2023 (375 of 1659). There were 3.8 nonfatal shooting victims for every firearm homicide between 2015 and 2024. Nonfatal interpersonal gun assaults in Philadelphia accounted for about 82% (1826 of 2217) of all nonfatal gun injuries in Pennsylvania, estimated by the authors in 2021.

Gun violence is highly concentrated at specific locations within Philadelphia. Spatial analyses show that only 3% of city street blocks accounted for 50% of fatal and nonfatal shootings between 2019 and 2023, and the top decile of census block groups experienced 36% of the shooting increase during the COVID-19 pandemic.[9]

Philadelphia fatal and nonfatal shooting victims during the 2015–2024 period were described in the data set as approximately 90% male (14 723 of 16 315), 82% Black (13 362), and 12% Latino (2008), and having a mean age of 29 years. In 2021, Black males between the ages of 18 and 34 years represented only 5% of the city population (80 532 of 1 576 251) but accounted for half of the fatal (252) and nonfatal (887) shooting

**TABLE 1— Annual Counts of Fatal and Nonfatal Shooting Victims in Philadelphia, PA: 2015–2024**

| Year | Nonfatal Shootings, No. | Fatal Shootings, No. | Total, No. | Case Fatality Rate, % |
|---|---|---|---|---|
| 2015 | 1038 | 233 | 1271 | 18.3 |
| 2016 | 1057 | 262 | 1319 | 19.9 |
| 2017 | 990 | 262 | 1252 | 20.9 |
| 2018 | 1137 | 298 | 1435 | 20.8 |
| 2019 | 1152 | 312 | 1464 | 21.3 |
| 2020 | 1795 | 449 | 2244 | 20.0 |
| 2021 | 1826 | 508 | 2334 | 21.8 |
| 2022 | 1780 | 474 | 2254 | 21.0 |
| 2023 | 1284 | 375 | 1659 | 22.6 |
| 2024 | 855 | 228 | 1083 | 21.1 |
| Total | 12 914 | 3401 | 16 315 | 20.8 |

victims. Shootings in disadvantaged city neighborhoods tend to arise from interpersonal disputes in high-risk social networks that include gangs, drug-selling organizations, robbery crews, and other criminally active groups.[10] Further analyses can be applied to consider how population denominators at small spatial units influence the hyperconcentration and racial stratification of gun violence.

The Philadelphia data suggest that statewide fatal and nonfatal shooting trends are driven by assaultive gun violence in cities that are further concentrated among a small number of risky places and risky people. Comprehensive and timely city-level databases are clearly important to monitor trends, launch new epidemiological inquiries, and evaluate programs and policies. Gun violence imposes heavy economic and social costs in the United States. A recent study suggests US citizens are willing to pay nearly $100 billion for a 20% reduction in gun violence.[11] Government investment in a national fatal and nonfatal firearm injury surveillance system that draws upon existing national mortality data sources, local police data sets, and hospital information could go far in achieving such a reduction. AJPH

## CORRESPONDENCE

Correspondence should be sent to Anthony Braga, Department of Criminology, University of Pennsylvania, 558 McNeil Building, 3718 Locust Walk, Philadelphia, PA 19104-6286 (e-mail: abraga@upenn.edu). Reprints can be ordered at https://www.ajph.org by clicking the "Reprints" link.

## PUBLICATION INFORMATION

Full Citation: Braga AA. The need for comprehensive and timely city-level fatal and nonfatal firearm injury surveillance. *Am J Public Health*. 2025;115(7): 990–992.

Acceptance Date: April 16, 2025.

DOI: https://doi.org/10.2105/AJPH.2025.308167

ORCID iD:

Anthony A. Braga https://orcid.org/0000-0002-5815-3734

## CONFLICTS OF INTEREST

The author declares no conflicts of interest.

## REFERENCES

1. Braga AA, Cook PJ. *Policing Gun Violence*. New York, NY: Oxford University Press; 2023.
2. Braga AA, Cook PJ. The association of firearm caliber with likelihood of death from gunshot injury in criminal assaults. *JAMA Netw Open*. 2018;1(3):e180833. https://doi.org/10.1001/jamanetworkopen.2018.0833
3. Barber C, Cook PJ, Parker S. The emerging infrastructure of US firearms injury data. *Prev Med*. 2022;165 (pt A):107129. https://doi.org/10.1016/j.ypmed.2022.107129
4. Gobaud AN, Mehranbod CA, Kaufman E, et al. Assessing the gun violence archive as an epidemiologic data source for community firearm violence in 4 US Cities. *JAMA Netw Open*. 2023;6(6):e2316545. https://doi.org/10.1001/jamanetworkopen.2023.16545
5. Anchan MG, Harris J, Natale-Short S, Georges MR, Pino EC. Assessing the gun violence archive and public police data as comprehensive sources for gun violence. *JAMA Netw Open*. 2025;8(1): e2458054. https://doi.org/10.1001/jamanetworkopen.2024.58054
6. Centers for Disease Control and Prevention. Underlying cause of death by single race 2018–2023 (WONDER online database). Available at: http://wonder.cdc.gov/ucd-icd10-expanded.html. Accessed February 26, 2025.
7. Open Data Philly. Shooting victims. Available at: https://opendataphilly.org/datasets/shooting-victims. Accessed February 26, 2025.
8. Kaufman E, Holena DN, Yang WP, et al. Firearm assault in Philadelphia, 2005–2014: a comparison of police and trauma registry data. *Trauma Surg Acute Care Open*. 2019;4(1):e000316. https://doi.org/10.1136/tsaco-2019-000316
9. MacDonald JM, Mohler G, Brantingham PJ. Association between race, shooting hot spots, and the surge in gun violence during the COVID-19 pandemic in Philadelphia, New York and Los Angeles. *Prev Med*. 2022;165 (pt A):107241. https://doi.org/10.1016/j.ypmed.2022.107241.
10. Roman CG, Link NW, Hyatt JM, Bhati A, Forney M. Assessing the gang-level and community-level effects of the Philadelphia focused deterrence strategy. *J Exp Criminol*. 2019;15 (4):499–527. https://doi.org/10.1007/s11292-018-9333-7
11. Cook PJ, Jeuland M, Ludwig J. Valuing the benefits of reducing firearm violence in the US. *Proc Natl Acad Sci*. 2025;122(4):e2419864122. https://doi.org/10.1073/pnas.2419864122

# Equity as a Pragmatic Application of Ethics: Considerations for Scarce Resource Allocation During a Pandemic

Rachel Gur-Arie, PhD, MS

**ABOUT THE AUTHOR**

*Rachel Gur-Arie, PhD, MS, is with Edson College of Nursing and Health Innovation, Arizona State University, Phoenix, AZ.*

**See also Emanuel and Jung, p. 1085.**

Debates surrounding the prioritization of scarce resources like personal protective equipment and vaccines dominated most of the ethics discourse during the early phases of the COVID-19 pandemic (https://bit.ly/32rhHPb).[1,2] Today, COVID-19 vaccines are available globally, and severe acute respiratory syndrome coronavirus 2 (SARS-CoV-2) is endemic. Accordingly, in their *AJPH* Analytic Essay, Emanuel and Jung (p. 1085) ask the important and timely question: "Was the allocation of COVID-19 vaccines globally fair and equitable?"

## STANDARDS OF ETHICAL VACCINE ALLOCATION

Emanuel and Jung focus on comparing two standards for COVID-19 vaccine allocation: (1) the population-based standard (PBS), which guided the World Health Organization's COVAX initiative (https://bit.ly/32rhHPb), and (2) the health-burden standard (HBS), proposed in the Fair Priority Model (FPM).[2] Table 1 outlines some key characteristics of the equitable vaccine allocation standards.

Under the HBS and FPM paradigm, middle-income countries like Mexico were treated in the most unfair and inequitable fashion during COVID-19 vaccine allocation, given that they had the most excess deaths and did not receive sufficient vaccine supply. Emanuel and Jung also emphasize that low-income countries and sub-Saharan Africa had low excess deaths despite high infection rates and, therefore, did not need to be prioritized for vaccine allocation.

Accordingly, Emanual and Jung conclude that after witnessing the shortcomings of the PBS in COVAX, the global consensus is that the HBS is the superior ethical standard for assessing fair allocation of scarce resources and vaccines.

However, it is crucial to examine potential assumptions, tradeoffs, and limitations associated with HBS and FPM.

Arguably, one of the central ethical concerns that arises with embracing HBS is the notion that HBS relies on excess deaths data to guide scarce resource allocation. Inherently, this assumes that all countries have excess deaths data available, even during emergencies like pandemics. There are significant equity-related limitations associated with accepting that excess deaths are a "better" ethical standard than the direct number of deaths that PBS relies on.[3]

First, this inequitably favors countries that have health care systems with strong enough infrastructure to gather excess deaths data. Emanuel and Jung state how countries with weaker infrastructure probably are less well-positioned to distribute scarce resources, anyway—another assumption that is country- and context-dependent. Where data are lacking, modeling is suggested to appropriately fill the gaps. Research consistently shows that models are biased and disproportionately represent certain groups over others.[4] Relying too heavily on models when data are unavailable (like HBS does) for scarce resources allocation could exacerbate inequities[5] by perpetuating assumptions built into models.

Second, the authors positively recognize how HBS places the onus on countries to improve their health infrastructure when excess deaths as a metric is centralized during scarce resource allocation. Though optimistic, this premise may or may not be realistic. It is unclear if and how countries with weaker health infrastructures could and should improve their health infrastructures. After all, it is reasonable to assume that these improvements would come at a potential cost to other important national needs. Before celebrating how centralizing HBS and the FPM in scarce resource allocation would automatically improve weaker health systems and infrastructure around the world, it is important to understand how, to be aware and ready for unintended consequences.[6] Accordingly, it is necessary to better understand the logic underlying Emanuel and Jung's assumption that

**TABLE 1— Comparison of Population-Based Standard and Health-Burden Standard for Equitable Vaccine Allocation**

| | Population-Based Standard | Health-Burden Standard |
|---|---|---|
| Origin | COVAX (World Health Organization) | Fair Priority Model[2] |
| Equity metric of fair distribution | Number of COVID-19 cases | Where the most lives or standard expected life-years will be saved (excess deaths) |
| How should vaccine supply be allocated? | Vaccines per person until initially 3% and then up to 20% of a given country's population is vaccinated | Proportional to how many deaths or life years lost in a country each additional vaccine can prevent |
| Which countries should be prioritized for COVID-19 vaccine allocation? | Low- and middle-income countries | Middle-income countries |

health care system and infrastructure improvements will automatically happen when adopting HBS. While possible, critical empirical, ethical, and policy examination should justify such a conclusion—otherwise, it is likely to perpetuate assumptions and health inequities.

## INTERTWINED AND CONTEXT-DEPENDENT ETHICS AND EQUITY

HBS is an impressive and important ethical standard that is a significant contribution to scarce resource allocation during a pandemic. However, in Emanuel and Jung's essay, both PBS and HBS are presented as relatively inflexible metrics. Pandemics require adaptation.[7] HBS and FPM can be adapted to the next pandemic, just like PBS might be adapted. Instead of framing PBS and HBS as competition in scarce resource allocation, it is worth considering them as tools in the ethical standard "toolbox" for scarce resource allocation decision-making, among other standards.[8,9]

At the theoretical level, there are strong ethics and equity strengths associated with prioritizing HBS and FPM during scarce resource allocation. In the context of COVID-19, in hindsight, Emanuel and Jung's conclusion that HBS and FPM's equity justifications are stronger than those associated with PBS and COVAX is reasonable. However, FPM and HBS are not, by definition, ethical or equitable.[10] The application of FPM and HBS is what will be judged to be ethical or equitable when the next pandemic or emergency comes. In considering the use of ethical standards and frameworks for scarce resource allocation, the different ways in which infectious diseases are transmitted and the different impacts of these diseases (e.g., different severity of morbidity vs mortality) impact the ethical considerations and frameworks used (or not). HBS might be a better fit for a future pandemic, but maybe not.

Ethics, when "done right," usually does not offer absolute answers—but rather outlines a spectrum of potential choices with associated tradeoffs to be made.[11] There were tradeoffs to relying on PBS in the way the COVAX program did. This does not mean that pivoting to fully rely on HBS is the answer. There are inevitably limitations to excess death data, despite it having equity-related strengths over population-based data.

Emanuel and Jung state that equity is a matter of ethics and not pragmatics, and that pragmatism does not target inequity. What if the future application and implementation of FPM and HBS during scarce resource allocation embraced the notion that equity can be the pragmatic application of ethics?

To have effective, ethical, and equitable emergency and pandemic management is to execute evidence-based decision-making that meets the moment. This means meeting people (and countries) where they are at, not forcing them to fit into standards and models (https://bit.ly/42N3nkz). Pragmatism may not be the full determinant of equity, but it certainly is an important part.

While HBS may be a compelling ethical standard to take into consideration in scarce resource allocation, it is ethically problematic to frame it as the superior one. Like all ethical standards and equity metrics, it has its strengths and weaknesses (https://bit.ly/4dijZzt). Adopting it in the future allocation of scarce health resources should be considered in the context of what it can offer, while also remaining cognizant of what it cannot. AJPH

### CORRESPONDENCE

Correspondence should be sent to Rachel Gur-Arie, PhD, MS, Edson College of Nursing and Health Innovation, 500 N 3rd St, Phoenix, AZ 85004 (e-mail: rgurarie@asu.edu). Reprints can be ordered at https://www.ajph.org by clicking the "Reprints" link.

### PUBLICATION INFORMATION

Full Citation: Gur-Arie R. Equity as a pragmatic application of ethics: considerations for scarce resource allocation during a pandemic. *Am J Public Health*. 2025;115(7):993–995.

Acceptance Date: April 16, 2025.

DOI: https://doi.org/10.2105/AJPH.2025.308172

ORCID iD:
Rachel Gur-Arie https://orcid.org/0000-0002-0868-7682

## CONFLICTS OF INTEREST

The author reports no conflicts of interest.

## REFERENCES


1. Emanuel EJ, Persad G. The shared ethical framework to allocate scarce medical resources: a lesson from COVID-19. *Lancet.* 2023;401(10391):1892–1902. https://doi.org/10.1016/s0140-6736(23)00812-7
2. Emanuel EJ, Persad G, Kern A, et al. An ethical framework for global vaccine allocation. *Science.* 2020;369(6509):1309–1312. https://doi.org/10.1126/science.abe2803
3. Krieger N. Health equity and the fallacy of treating causes of population health as if they sum to 100%. *Am J Public Health.* 2017;107(4):541–549. https://doi.org/10.2105/ajph.2017.303655
4. Delgado JL. Beyond diversity—time for new models of health. *N Engl J Med.* 2022;386(6):503–505. https://doi.org/10.1056/NEJMp2115149
5. Giang A, Edwards MR, Fletcher SM, et al. Equity and modeling in sustainability science: examples and opportunities throughout the process. *Proc Natl Acad Sci U S A.* 2024;121(13):e2215688121. https://doi.org/10.1073/pnas.2215688121
6. Woolf SH. Potential health and economic consequences of misplaced priorities. *JAMA.* 2007;297(5):523–526. https://doi.org/10.1001/jama.297.5.523
7. Corpuz JCG. Adapting to the culture of 'new normal': an emerging response to COVID-19. *J Public Health (Oxf).* 2021;43(2):e344–e345. https://doi.org/10.1093/pubmed/fdab057
8. Xiao M, Molina KC, Aggarwal NR, et al. A machine learning method for allocating scarce COVID-19 monoclonal antibodies. *JAMA Health Forum.* 2024;5(9):e242884. https:/doi.org/10.1001/jamahealthforum.2024.2884
9. Romney D, Fox H, Carlson S, Bachmann D, O'Mathuna D, Kman N. Allocation of scarce resources in a pandemic: a systematic review of US state crisis standards of care documents. *Disaster Med Public Health Prep.* 2020;14(5):677–683. https://doi.org/10.1017/dmp.2020.101
10. Pauly B, Revai T, Marcellus L, Martin W, Easton K, MacDonald M. "The health equity curse": ethical tensions in promoting health equity. *BMC Public Health.* 2021;21(1):1567–1511. https://doi.org/10.1186/s12889-021-11594-y
11. Gur-Arie R, Jamrozik E, Kingori P. No jab, no job? Ethical issues in mandatory COVID-19 vaccination of healthcare personnel. *BMJ Glob Health.* 2021;6(2):e004877. https://doi.org/10.1136/bmjgh-2020-004877

# Health Inequalities, Disparities, Equity: What's in a Name?

*Paula Braveman, MD, MPH*

**ABOUT THE AUTHOR**

*Paula Braveman is with the Department of Family and Community Medicine at the University of California, San Francisco.*

"Health inequalities," "health disparities," and "health equity" are hardly everyday household words, but they have become increasingly familiar in the realms of public health and medicine globally. Figure A (available as a supplement to the online version of this article at https://ajph.org) shows the dramatic increase in their appearance in peer-reviewed health and medical literature from 2000 to 2023. While these terms are often not defined explicitly, the implicit—or explicit if stated—definitions vary markedly; Box 1 displays selected examples reflecting a range of approaches. As discussed previously in this journal[19] and elsewhere,[3] some definitions are clear, some are eloquent, some are both, and some fail to capture crucial concepts adequately or at all. Although some federal agencies have markedly improved their definitions over time, some definitions of health inequalities or disparities lack relevance to health equity,[1,3,4,5,8,20] and some definitions of health equity are so general that they do not guide measurement or reflect principles central to the concept of equity.[19]

These are not matters of stylistic preference or academic hair-splitting. Whether wielded consciously or not, concepts shape and justify actions. Concepts guide measurement and, hence, accountability for policies' effects. Lack of clarity about the concepts of health inequalities, disparities, and equity can—intentionally or not—promote and sustain inequitable policies and practices by obscuring or drawing attention and resources away from the pervasive and often profound differences hidden beneath the surface of population averages. Box 2 gives a few examples of how resource allocation might vary based on the prevailing understanding of health inequalities/disparities and equity. Clarity regarding these concepts may be especially important at present, given ongoing White House strongarm efforts to force public and private institutions to cease using these and related terms and to cease addressing the concepts they represent.[21,22]

This article aims to clarify the concepts of health inequalities, disparities, equity, and inequity; to stimulate discussion among scholars and advocates; and, ultimately, to contribute to greater consensus regarding their meaning. After defining the terms, four consequential and sometimes contentious issues regarding their meaning are discussed.

## DEFINING HEALTH INEQUALITIES/ DISPARITIES AND EQUITY

Health inequalities and disparities are differences in health that are associated with social (including economic) advantage; they adversely affect excluded, marginalized, or disenfranchised groups of people.

"Health inequalities" is used globally except in the United States, where "health disparities" is far more common. "Health inequalities" originally referred specifically to socioeconomic differences in health but has come to encompass health inequalities by social advantage or disadvantage considered more broadly, including, for example, differences by racialized or ethnic group, gender, migrant status or national origin, sexual orientation, gender identity, religion, disability status, and other characteristics historically associated with discrimination, exclusion, marginalization, or disenfranchisement.[23–26] "Health disparities" originally referred specifically to health differences across different racialized/ethnic groups. Like "health inequalities," however, over time, it evolved to refer more broadly to health differences across diverse dimensions of social advantage.

Given the evolution of both concepts, health disparities and health inequalities now are synonyms. Both refer to health differences associated with social advantage, adversely affecting socially disadvantaged (marginalized, excluded, disenfranchised) groups. Although some individuals may attach different meanings to the two terms, multiple dictionary definitions of inequality and disparity offer one as a synonym for the other,[27–34] which is consistent with their usage in the literature.

AJPH July 2025, Vol. 115, No. 7

## BOX 1— Examples of Definitions of Health Inequality, Disparity, Equity, and Inequity

**Health inequality**

Some authors have proposed defining health inequalities as any avoidable differences in health among any individuals, who should not be grouped a priori according to social characteristics (except possibly geographic location) because doing so could prejudge causation.[1]

Health inequalities are "systematic differences in the health of groups and communities occupying unequal positions in society."[2(p101)]

A health inequality/disparity "is a particular type of difference in health or in the most important influences on health that could potentially be shaped by policies; it is a difference in which disadvantaged social groups (such as the poor, racial/ethnic minorities, women, or other groups that have persistently experienced social disadvantage or discrimination) systematically experience worse health or greater health risks than more advantaged groups."[3(p180)]

**Health disparity**

Health disparities include "differences . . . by gender, race or ethnicity, education or income, disability, geographic location, or sexual orientation."[4(p11)]

Health disparities are "differences in the incidence, prevalence, mortality, and burden of disease and other adverse health conditions that exist among specific population groups in the United States."[5]

See definitions of health inequality/disparity above.[3]

Healthy People 2020 defines a health disparity as "a particular type of health difference that is closely linked with social, economic, and/or environmental disadvantage. Health disparities adversely affect groups of people who have systematically experienced greater obstacles to health based on their racial or ethnic group; religion; socioeconomic status; gender; age; mental health; cognitive, sensory, or physical disability; sexual orientation or gender identity; geographic location; or other characteristics historically linked to discrimination or exclusion."[6]

"Health disparities definitions vary, but they all address differences in health status between one population group in comparison to a more advantaged group and most address issues of social justice and equity."[7]

"Health disparities are preventable differences in health status and outcomes that adversely affect certain populations." "Disparity populations" are "defined as racial/ethnic minority, low socio-economic status, rural, and sexual and gender minority populations in the United States."[8]

"Health disparities are preventable differences in the burden of disease, injury, violence, or opportunities to achieve optimal health that are experienced by socially disadvantaged populations . . . Health disparities are inequitable and are directly related to the historical and current unequal distribution of social, political, economic, and environmental resources."[9]

"A health disparity is a health difference that adversely affects disadvantaged populations."[10]

**Health equity**

Equity in health means that all persons have fair opportunities to attain their full health potential, to the extent possible.[11]

Pursuing equity in health means trying to reduce avoidable gaps in health status and health services between groups with different levels of social privilege.[12]

Equity in health is operationally defined as minimizing avoidable disparities in health and its determinants—including but not limited to health care—between groups of people who have different levels of underlying social advantage.[13]

Equity in health is "the absence of systematic and potentially remediable differences in one or more aspects of health across populations or population subgroups defined socially, economically, demographically, or geographically."[14(p546)]

"For the purposes of measurement and operationalisation, equity in health is the absence of systematic disparities in health (or in the major social determinants of health) between groups with different levels of underlying social advantage/disadvantage—that is, wealth, power, or prestige . . . Assessing health equity requires comparing health and its social determinants between more and less advantaged social groups."[15(p254)]

"Health equity means that everyone has a fair and just opportunity to be as healthy as possible. This requires removing obstacles to health such as poverty, discrimination, powerlessness, and their consequences, including lack of access to good jobs with fair pay; quality education, health care, and housing; and safe environments. For the purposes of measurement, health equity means reducing and ultimately eliminating disparities in health and its determinants that adversely affect excluded or marginalized groups."[16]

"Health equity is the attainment of the highest level of health for all people . . . Achieving health equity requires valuing everyone equally with focused and ongoing societal efforts to address avoidable inequalities, historical and contemporary injustices, and social determinants of health—and to eliminate disparities in health and health care."[17(p2)]

"Equity is the absence of unfair, avoidable or remediable differences among groups of people, whether those groups are defined socially, economically, demographically, or geographically or by other dimensions of inequality (e.g. sex, gender, ethnicity, disability, or sexual orientation) . . . Health equity is achieved when everyone can attain their full potential for health and well-being."[18]

**Health inequity**

"The term 'inequity' has a moral and ethical dimension. It refers to differences which are unnecessary and avoidable, but in addition are considered unfair and unjust. So, in order to describe a certain situation as inequitable the cause has to be examined and judged to be unfair in the context of what is going on in the rest of society."[11(p431)]

One way to define health equity (Box 1 notes others) is as follows: equity means justice. Health equity means that everyone has a fair and just opportunity to be as healthy as possible. This requires removing obstacles to health, such as poverty, discrimination, powerlessness, and their consequences, including lack of access to good jobs with fair pay, safe environments, and quality education, housing, and health care. Pursuing health equity

**BOX 2— Resources May Be Allocated Differently Based on How Health Inequalities/Disparities Are Defined**

| |
|---|
| If health inequalities/disparities are not defined as health differences associated with social advantage: |
| If well-off residents of a certain area have less convenient geographic access to dental care than their counterparts in another area, they may advocate for that to be addressed as a health inequalities/disparity issue. |
| Resources designated for reducing inequalities/disparities in maternal mortality could be used to address slightly higher maternal mortality among White women in one state than among White women in another. This could divert resources from addressing dramatically higher rates of maternal mortality among African American women compared with White women, which are observed virtually everywhere. |
| Resources to reduce reproductive health inequalities/disparities could be used to address higher rates of fertility problems among affluent than poor couples in one geographic area. |
| If health inequalities/disparities were defined simply as health differences without normative content, all of the health differences listed here would qualify as "health inequalities/disparities," and resources would be directed to better-off groups. In each case, policymakers might allocate resources differently based on their understanding of health equity and inequalities/disparities. In each of these fictitious examples, the problems noted should receive attention—however, according to the criteria presented here, not as health equity/inequalities issues and not using resources intended to address health inequalities/disparities. |

means reducing and ultimately eliminating inequalities or disparities in health and its determinants that adversely affect excluded, marginalized, or disenfranchised groups of people (adapted from Braveman et al.[16]).

Although longer than ideal, this definition's strengths are that it is relatively explicit, unambiguous, and concrete; it explicitly guides measurement; and it highlights structural and upstream factors as well as medical care. The definition's second sentence is an adaptation of Whitehead's eloquent and oft-cited definition.[11] The third sentence reduces ambiguity by providing concrete examples of what it would mean in general policy terms to pursue fair and just opportunities for everyone to be as healthy as possible. The final sentence further guides action and measurement, specifying inequalities/disparities in health and its (major) determinants as crucial metrics for assessing health equity. The aim of the specificity is to minimize confusion about or cooptation of the concept—for example, to prevent its interpretation in ways that could justify actions that do not prioritize the health of disadvantaged groups or that limit the scope of action to medical care alone without addressing social, including structural, influences on health.

## FOUR CONTENTIOUS ISSUES

The following text examines four important issues regarding the concepts noted previously, on which consensus has been elusive.

### A Fundamentally Normative Concept

"Health inequalities/disparities," often used interchangeably with "social inequalities in health," is a fundamentally normative concept. It implicitly but unequivocally refers to health differences associated with social advantage, adversely affecting marginalized, excluded, or disenfranchised groups.

At times, proposals have surfaced to treat health inequalities or disparities as purely mathematical or technical concepts without a normative (i.e., ethical, moral, or legal) dimension.[1,4,5,35] From the inception of European initiatives calling for the elimination of health inequalities, however, the concept's moral and ethical dimension has been clearly expressed.[11,36] Similarly, the profound concern of the health disparities movement in the United States with racial injustice has been clear from the beginning. Since both movements were launched in the early 1990s, "health inequalities" and "health disparities" have been understood, albeit often implicitly, to mean health differences among social groups with different levels of social advantage, with socially disadvantaged groups experiencing worse health; the term "social inequalities in health" is often used interchangeably. Underscoring the fundamentally normative nature of health inequalities/disparities, furthermore, some dictionary definitions of "inequality" and "disparity" refer to fairness explicitly[27,28,37,38]; others are less explicit in the definition itself but feature social inequality in the illustrative examples.[29–31,39–44]

If health inequalities/disparities were construed simply as health differences, or even as health differences by demographic or geographic characteristics without normative criteria, virtually all health differences—the realm of the science of epidemiology—would be called health inequalities/disparities. They would include, for example, higher rates of fractures among people who ski than nonskiers and infectious disease outbreaks afflicting luxury cruise passengers but not people who cannot afford to take a cruise. Viewing health inequalities/disparities without normative criteria could be used in the United States to justify directing resources earmarked for health equity toward the higher incidence of breast cancer in White women, despite higher breast cancer mortality among African American women. In each case, resources would likely be directed to more advantaged groups. These health differences deserve attention but not as health disparities or inequalities (i.e., not using resources intended for health equity; see Box 2 for more examples).

## Ethical Concepts Grounded in Human Rights

Health equity and, by extension, health inequalities/disparities are ethical concepts, grounded in human rights principles and laws. Ethical and human rights principles are at the core of the concepts of health inequality, disparity, and equity.[3,15,19] The ethical principle of distributive justice calls for the resources and conditions (such as education, health care, shelter, nutritious food, clean water, and sanitation) that are essential for human welfare to be distributed fairly. The human rights principle of nondiscrimination prohibits not only intentional interpersonal discrimination (e.g., deliberate race-based name-calling or physical violence) but also unintended or structural biases (e.g., in laws, policies, and entrenched practices) that systematically put certain groups of people at a disadvantage regardless of current or conscious intent. Also of importance is the human rights principle of indivisibility—that is, that all rights are intrinsically interconnected and that no single right, such as the right to health, can be realized without the realization of all other rights, such as the rights to education, food, housing, clean water, and civil rights.[15,45] The indivisibility of all rights obligates governments and societies to strive not only for equitable health care but also for equity in all conditions that significantly influence health.

The conceptual basis of health equity and inequalities/disparities in ethics and international human rights laws and agreements reflects universal values. Virtually every country in the world has signed on to (although not necessarily ratified) international human rights laws and agreements articulating relevant principles; this reflects global consensus on the values, which is a powerful conceptual basis for the definitions proposed here.

## "Inequities" vs "Inequalities/Disparities"

Health inequalities/disparities raise concerns about equity (fairness, justice) because of their social patterning—that is, they are systematically (repeatedly, not randomly) and closely linked with social advantage; it also must be plausible, according to the best available scientific knowledge, but not necessarily proven, that the differences under consideration are at least in theory modifiable. A causal role for social advantage in an observed health inequality/disparity need not be established; observing systematically worse health in a socially disadvantaged (compared with a more advantaged) group is sufficient to call that health difference a health inequality/disparity. By contrast, a health inequity is a health difference whose causes are judged to be unfair and unjust. All health inequities are health inequalities/disparities, but not all health inequalities/disparities are necessarily inequities.

Some discussions of health disparities/inequalities avoid using those terms, instead using "inequities" to refer to all observed health differences associated with social advantage, regardless of whether the etiology of the difference is known. Proving that a health difference is an inequity (i.e., determining the causes and demonstrating that they are unjust) can be difficult, given the stringent standards for causal inference in medical science. Consider, for example, the United States' large and persistent Black:White inequalities/disparities in preterm birth, a strong predictor of infant mortality, childhood disability, and adult chronic disease. There are many hypotheses about the causes of the inequalities/disparities, including scientifically plausible hypotheses implicating racism in various forms as a likely upstream factor activating multiple downstream causes[46]; however, there is no scientific consensus about the causes (except that they are complex). Given lack of consensus on the causes, it seems inappropriate to call this inequality/disparity an inequity; yet, referring to it simply as a difference fails to acknowledge the marked and consistent social patterning and plausible role for racism. "Inequalities/disparities" seems a good fit here and with many other health outcomes for which neither "inequity" nor simply "differences" seems appropriate.

One might argue, however, that even without knowing the etiology of a disparity/inequality, the presence of systematically worse health in a socially disadvantaged group is intrinsically an inequity because it puts a group that is already at a social disadvantage (e.g., because of poverty) at further disadvantage with respect to its health; this seems particularly unfair, given that good health is often needed to escape social disadvantage. Thus, one could claim that a separate "health inequality/disparity" category is unnecessary, because "inequity" could include both suspected and proven injustices. Eliminating the separate category for inequalities/disparities and calling all inequalities/disparities associated with social disadvantage "inequities" would, however, be ill-advised, because the theoretical arguments justifying it are likely to be challenged by other researchers and unlikely to be very comprehensible or compelling for policymakers and the public. "Health inequalities/disparities" should be kept in the lexicon with a meaning distinct from the meanings of both "health differences or variations" and "health inequities."

### "Health Equity," "Health Justice," or Both

The term "health justice" has been used by some scholars instead of or in addition to "health equity."[47,48] "Justice" is a synonym for "equity."[49,50] For many people, "justice" may be more familiar and clear and less abstract than "equity," particularly given other unrelated uses (e.g., "home equity," "private equity"). One might therefore argue for substituting "health justice" for "health equity." Considerable hard-won momentum has been built globally for "health equity" across more than three decades, however, and widespread recognition for "health equity" has been achieved within health and medicine. It seems unwise to jeopardize that momentum by abandoning the term. Both terms are valuable.

## FINAL REMARKS

It is hoped that this article will stimulate discussion, which, in turn, will produce greater clarity and, ideally, greater consensus in using the terms "health inequalities, disparities, and equity." In particular, it is hoped that the article and subsequent discussion will put to rest the recurrent and mistaken notion that "health inequalities" and "health disparities" are purely technical terms devoid of normative content. Dictionary definitions support the ways in which these terms have been understood in health and medicine for more than three decades—namely, as referring not to all possible health differences but to a specific subset of health differences associated with social advantage, warranting concern because of ethical and human rights considerations. They are suspected—but not necessarily proven—of being unfair or unjust based on their social patterning. They are essential metrics for assessing health equity. Health inequalities/disparities and equity are not the only important health considerations; populations' average health levels also warrant concern, as do some health differences between groups that may not differ on social advantage—but not as health equity, inequality, or disparity issues. While not the only legitimate considerations, health inequalities/disparities and equity are crucial considerations in any society that cares about justice.

If there is no clarity about the nature of health inequalities/disparities and equity, they will not be measured or understood, and there will be no accountability for policies' differential effects on the health of more and less socially advantaged groups. It is far more challenging to measure social inequalities/disparities in health than average levels of health; measuring inequalities/disparities requires data on health disaggregated by relevant social characteristics. Without clarity, the path of least resistance for those who assess populations' health will not include measuring social inequalities/disparities in health, and we will lack data vitally needed to assess the extent of health equity and how it changes over time in relation to policies. Lack of data and confusion or lack of understanding of data on health inequalities/disparities serve the interests of those who control the wealth and power and, hence, to a large extent, the health of societies.

Researchers should always ask themselves and their colleagues these questions: To assess population health, have we compared health and the key factors that influence it across more and less socially advantaged groups? If we lack the requisite data now, what needs to be done to obtain it? Policymakers should insist on routinely having that comparative information; like researchers, they should always use an equity lens (i.e., assess differential effects of policies on more and less advantaged groups).

Lack of clarity and consensus can make well-intentioned efforts vulnerable to being detoured away from health equity. Lack of clarity and consensus about definitions is not the most important barrier to health equity; in all societies, political will and power are its preeminent determinants. Clarity and consensus among scholars and advocates about the nature and measurement of health equity, inequalities, and disparities can, however, influence political will by influencing public and policymaker opinion and discourse. Let us be clear. AJPH

## CORRESPONDENCE

Correspondence should be sent to Paula Braveman, 25 Hill St, San Francisco, CA 94110 (e-mail: paula.braveman@ucsf.edu). Reprints can be ordered at https://www.ajph.org by clicking the "Reprints" link.

## PUBLICATION INFORMATION

Full Citation: Braveman P. Health inequalities, disparities, equity: what's in a name? *Am J Public Health*. 2025;115(7):996–1002.

Acceptance Date: February 3, 2025.

DOI: https://doi.org/10.2105/AJPH.2025.308062

## ACKNOWLEDGMENTS

Nicole Holm made major contributions to the research.

## CONFLICTS OF INTEREST

There are no conflicts of interest.

## REFERENCES

1. Murray CJ, Gakidou EE, Frenk J. Health inequalities and social group differences: what should we measure? *Bull World Health Organ*. 1999;77(7):537–543.
2. Graham H. Social determinants and their unequal distribution: clarifying policy understandings. *Milbank Q*. 2004;82(1):101–124. https://doi.org/10.1111/j.0887-378X.2004.00303.x
3. Braveman P. Health disparities and health equity: concepts and measurement. *Annu Rev Public Health*. 2006;27(1):167–194. https://doi.org/10.1146/annurev.publhealth.27.021405.102103
4. *Healthy People 2010: Understanding and Improving Health*. Washington, DC: US Department of Health and Human Services; 2000: 8–16.
5. National Institutes of Health. Addressing disparities: the NIH program of action. What are health disparities? Available at: http://healthdisparities.nih.gov/whatare.html. Accessed August 14, 2024.
6. US Department of Health and Human Services. Healthy People 2020: About disparities. Available at: https://www.healthypeople.gov/2020/about/disparitiesAbout.aspx. Accessed August 14, 2024.
7. American Psychological Association. Fact Sheet: Health disparities. Available at: https://www.apa.org/topics/racism-bias-discrimination/health-disparities-defined. Accessed August 21, 2024.
8. National Institutes of Health. Minority health and health disparities research. August 25, 2022. Available at: https://www.nih.gov/ending-structural-racism/minority-health-health-disparities-research. Accessed August 14, 2024.
9. Centers for Disease Control and Prevention. Health disparities. May 26, 2023. Available at: https://www.cdc.gov/healthyyouth/disparities/index.htm#1. Accessed August 14, 2024.
10. National Institute on Minority Health and Health Disparities. Minority health and health disparities: definitions and parameters. January 12, 2024. Available at: https://www.nimhd.nih.gov/about/strategic-plan/nih-strategic-plan-definitions-and-parameters.html. Accessed August 14, 2024.
11. Whitehead M. The concepts and principles of equity and health. *Int J Health Serv*. 1992;22(3):429–445. https://doi.org/10.2190/986L-LHQ6-2VTE-YRRN
12. Braveman PA, Tarimo E. *Equity in Health and Health Care: a WHO/SIDA Initiative*. Geneva, Switzerland: World Health Organization; 1996.
13. Braveman P. *Monitoring Equity in Health: A Policy-Oriented Approach in Low- and Middle-Income Countries*. Geneva, Switzerland: World Health Organization; 1998.
14. Starfield B. Improving equity in health: a research agenda. *Int J Health Serv*. 2001;31(3):545–566. https://doi.org/10.2190/DGJ8-4MQW-UP9J-LQC1
15. Braveman P, Gruskin S. Defining equity in health. *J Epidemiol Community Health*. 2003;57(4):254–258. https://doi.org/10.1136/jech.57.4.254
16. Braveman P, Arkin E, Orleans T, Proctor D, Plough A. What is health equity? And what differences does a definition make? Robert Wood Johnson Foundation. 2017. Available at: https://www.rwjf.org/en/insights/our-research/2017/05/what-is-health-equity-.html
17. US Department of Health and Human Services. Health equity in Healthy People 2030. Available at: https://health.gov/healthypeople/priority-areas/health-equity-healthy-people-2030. Accessed August 14, 2024.
18. World Health Organization. Health equity. Available at: https://www.who.int/health-topics/health-equity#tab=tab_1. Accessed August 14, 2024.
19. Braveman PA, Kumanyika S, Fielding J, et al. Health disparities and health equity: the issue is justice. *Am J Public Health*. 2011;101(suppl 1):S149–S155. https://doi.org/10.2105/AJPH.2010.300062
20. National Cancer Institute. Cancer health disparities definitions and examples. February 17, 2015. Available at: https://www.cancer.gov/about-nci/organization/cche/about-health-disparities/definitions. Accessed August 14, 2024.
21. Researchers at academic institutions nationwide say that US science is being dismantled. *New York Times*. March 31, 2025. Available at: https://www.nytimes.com/interactive/2025/03/31/health/scientists-letter.html. Accessed April 10, 2025.
22. Lantz PM. Death by a thousand federal cuts: Trump administration actions will not make America healthy again. *Millbank Quarterly Opinion*. April 8, 2025. Available at: https://www.milbank.org/quarterly/opinions/death-by-a-thousand-federal-cuts-trump-administration-actions-will-not-make-america-healthy-again. Accessed April 10, 2025.
23. Bleich SN, Jarlenski MP, Bell CN, LaVeist TA. Health inequalities: trends, progress, and policy. *Annu Rev Public Health*. 2012;33(1):7–40. https://doi.org/10.1146/annurev-publhealth-031811-124658
24. Read JG, Gorman BK. Gender and health inequality. *Annu Rev Sociol*. 2010;36(1):371–386. https://doi.org/10.1146/annurev.soc.012809.102535
25. Brown TH. Racial stratification, immigration, and health inequality: a life course-intersectional approach. *Soc Forces*. 2018;96(4):1507–1540. https://doi.org/10.1093/sf/soy013
26. McDermott E, Nelson R, Weeks H. The politics of LGBT+ health inequality: conclusions from a UK scoping review. *Int J Environ Res Public Health*. 2021;18(2):826. https://doi.org/10.3390/ijerph18020826
27. Cambridge Dictionary. Disparity. 2024. Available at: https://dictionary.cambridge.org/us/dictionary/english/disparity. Accessed July 30, 2024.
28. Cambridge Dictionary. Inequality. 2024. Available at: https://dictionary.cambridge.org/us/dictionary/english/inequality. Accessed July 30, 2024.
29. Dictionary.com. Disparity. 2024. Available at: https://www.dictionary.com/browse/disparity. Accessed August 14, 2024.
30. Dictionary.com. Inequality. 2024. Available at: https://www.dictionary.com/browse/inequality. Accessed August 14, 2024.
31. Merriam-Webster. Disparity. 2024. Available at: https://www.merriam-webster.com/dictionary/disparity. Accessed August 14, 2024.
32. Merriam-Webster. Inequality. 2024. Available at: https://www.merriam-webster.com/dictionary/inequality. Accessed August 14, 2024.
33. Thesaurus.com. Disparity. 2024. Available at: https://www.thesaurus.com/browse/disparity. Accessed July 31, 2024.
34. Thesaurus.com. Inequality. 2024. Available at: https://www.thesaurus.com/browse/inequality. Accessed July 31, 2024.
35. *The World Health Report 2000: Health Systems: Improving Performance*. Geneva, Switzerland: World Health Organization; 2000:215.
36. Dahlgren G, Whitehead M. Policies and strategies to promote social. Institute for Futures Studies. 1991. Available at: http://s2.medicina.uady.mx/observatorio/docs/eq/li/Eq_2007_Li_Dahlgren.pdf. Accessed April 9, 2025.
37. The Britannica Dictionary. Disparity. 2024. Available at: https://www.britannica.com/dictionary/disparity. Accessed August 5, 2024.
38. The Britannica Dictionary. Inequality. 2024. Available at: https://www.britannica.com/dictionary/inequality. Accessed August 5, 2024.
39. *Oxford English Dictionary*. Disparity. 2024. Available at: https://www.oed.com/dictionary/disparity_n. Accessed August 14, 2024.
40. *Oxford English Dictionary*. Inequality. 2024. Available at: https://www.oed.com/dictionary/inequality_n. Accessed August 14, 2024.

41. Vocabulary.com. Disparity. 2024. Available at: https://www.vocabulary.com/dictionary/disparity. Accessed August 14, 2024.
42. Vocabulary.com. Inequality. 2024. Available at: https://www.vocabulary.com/dictionary/inequality. Accessed August 14, 2024.
43. Collins Dictionary. Disparity. 2024. Available at: https://www.collinsdictionary.com/us/dictionary/english/disparity. Accessed August 5, 2024.
44. Collins Dictionary. Inequality. 2024. Available at: https://www.collinsdictionary.com/us/dictionary/english/inequality. Accessed August 5, 2024.
45. Gruskin S, Braveman P. Addressing social injustice in a human rights context. In: Levy BS, Sidel VW, eds. *Social Injustice and Public Health*. 4th ed. New York, NY: Oxford University Press; 2024.
46. Braveman P, Dominguez TP, Burke W, et al. Explaining the Black–White disparity in preterm birth: a consensus statement from a multidisciplinary scientific work group convened by the March of Dimes. *Front Reprod Health*. 2021;3:684207. https://doi.org/10.3389/frph.2021.684207
47. Borras AM. Toward an intersectional approach to health justice. *Int J Health Serv*. 2021;51(2):206–225. https://doi.org/10.1177/0020731420981857
48. Ward MC. Health justice as a tool to fight existing and future pandemics. Atlanta, GA: Centers for Disease Control and Prevention; 2023.
49. Merriam-Webster Thesaurus. Equity. 2024. Available at: https://www.merriam-webster.com/thesaurus/equity. Accessed August 3, 2024.
50. Thesaurus.com. Equity. 2024. Available at: https://www.thesaurus.com/browse/equity. Accessed August 14, 2024.

# Integrating Reproductive Justice in Public Health Practice, Research, and Advocacy: An Imperative to Advance Health Equity

Marissa Velarde, PhD, MPH, and Asha Hassan, PhD, MPH

**ABOUT THE AUTHORS**

*Marissa Velarde is with the Department of Maternal and Child Health, UNC Gillings School of Global Public Health, Chapel Hill, NC. Asha Hassan is with the Department of Obstetrics, Gynecology, and Women's Health at the University of Minnesota Medical School, Minneapolis.*

The year 2024 marked the 30th anniversary of 12 Black women convening in Chicago, Illinois, to develop "Reproductive Justice," an organizing framework created to address issues that Black women and women of color faced that extended beyond the narrow focus of the reproductive rights movement. Reproductive justice holds that all people have the human right to (1) own their bodies and control their future, (2) have children, (3) not have children, and (4) parent their children in safe and sustainable communities.[1]

Over the past few decades, the reproductive justice framework has been adopted by numerous activists, organizations, and disciplines, including health care, law, psychology, social work, social policy, sociology, and public health. For example, as of the writing of this article, 109 *AJPH* articles have referred to reproductive justice. Undeniably, there has been increased discussion about reproductive justice in the field of public health in recent years, particularly after the Supreme Court decision in *Dobbs v Jackson Women's Health Organization*, which overturned the federal right to abortion care. However, the majority of public health discussion on reproductive justice deals with topics related to sexual and reproductive health, mainly abortion and contraception. When employing a reproductive justice lens, public health has rarely addressed the right to parent children in secure communities, a key component of the framework and an element that most clearly distinguishes it from reproductive rights. Thus, the field of public health has not applied the full potential of the reproductive justice framework, which offers a compelling lens for examining health inequities. Advancing health equity in the United States is a longstanding priority for the National Institutes of Health (NIH) as well as a core value of the American Public Health Association (APHA) and a commitment for the Centers for Disease Control and Prevention (CDC). This is particularly important considering that many health inequities have persisted in the past few decades, and some have widened in this country, most notably maternal mortality.[2]

In this article, we trace the roots of reproductive justice and reflect on its intersections with public health as well as their shared goals. Next, we apply the reproductive justice lens to two public health issues that address structural determinants of health that influence people's ability to parent children in safe and healthy environments. Finally, we issue a call to action for the public health community to recognize all pillars of reproductive justice when incorporating it in their work to advance health equity and offer recommendations for doing so.

## THE FOUNDING OF REPRODUCTIVE JUSTICE

In June 1994, a group of Black women gathered at a national prochoice conference in Chicago to discuss the unique needs of marginalized women, including women of color and those living on low incomes, that were not being addressed by the women's and reproductive rights movements, which were led by middle-class and wealthy White women.[3] They dubbed themselves "Women of African Descent for Reproductive Justice" (WADRJ), a name chosen to underscore the injustices of the health system faced by Black women, combining the concepts of reproductive rights and social justice. This name also sought to be inclusive. Reproductive justice articulates that restricting abortion is only one of many institutionalized barriers that women, people with the capacity for pregnancy, and their families faced in being healthy. The convening drafted a letter to members of Congress calling for a health care reform system that provided universal coverage and equal access to health services, including the full range of reproductive health services.[4] This letter was signed by 836 Black women and appeared as full-page ads in the *Washington Post* and the Congressional newsletter *Roll Call* in August 1994.[5]

Later that year, some members of WADRJ attended the United Nations International Conference on Population and Development in Cairo, Egypt. There, they learned from women in the Global South to use a human rights framework to strengthen their claims for women's full human rights.[5] Thus, reproductive justice came to integrate the concepts of reproductive rights, social justice, and human rights, acknowledging that health and wellness are not solely individual choices but, rather, are shaped by structural forces, including poverty, racism, and the built environment.[6] While the term reproductive justice was coined during this time, the concept was not a new one; rather, it was a product of a rich legacy of feminist activism within communities of color, including Black Feminist theory.[7]

In addition, reproductive justice is intersectional in its approach; that is, it considers how multiple social identities overlap and interact, resulting in unique combinations of oppression and privilege.[8] Reproductive justice has evolved in the decades since its inception but has always centered the experiences of the most marginalized people and applied an intersectional analysis to achieve human rights.[5]

## SHARED GOALS OF REPRODUCTIVE JUSTICE AND PUBLIC HEALTH

In recent decades, the field of public health has moved away from a focus on individual-level drivers of health and increasingly recognized the role of the broader forces and systems that shape people's lives and influence their health, known as the social determinants of health (SDOH). These are the conditions in which people are born, grow, work, live, and age,[9] and include factors like socioeconomic status, housing quality, community context, and the health care system.[10] Addressing SDOH is critical to improving overall health as well as diminishing health inequities, which are often rooted in social and economic inequities. As such, there has also been a growing effort to focus on people's social needs within health care and incorporate health outcomes into non-health sectors.[10]

Similar to SDOH, reproductive justice examines the larger context of health and well-being and understands that different forces affect people's lives in diverse ways, requiring multipronged approaches to achieve equity and justice. By creating the reproductive justice framework, the founders sought to highlight "the institutionalized barriers that constrict individual choices"[11(p19)]; this concept has been established by research confirming that social and environmental factors influence individual health behavior. Reproductive justice further focuses on upstream factors that influence health through its fourth pillar—raising children in safe environments. The field of public health acknowledges the importance of this strategy through its emphasis on addressing the conditions in which people are born and live. Public health has also sought to reduce health inequities by incorporating a life course perspective, which considers how health is shaped within and across generations.[12] Reproductive justice stems from the distinct historical realities of women of color who have been subjected to racism, sexism, classism, homophobia, xenophobia, ableism, and other forms of discrimination and oppression.[11]

Although further inspection is needed to fully align the field of public health with reproductive justice, reflecting on the injustices perpetuated by our field and working to address missteps is a crucial first step. This includes protecting and preserving transgender and queer health, pursuing innovative contraceptive methods that work for people assigned male at birth, and championing family supportive social policies like universal paid family leave. Public health practitioners should seek to advance health equity in a way that guarantees individual agency while still supporting community drivers of public health. Integrating the goals of reproductive justice and public health means to consider the multitude of factors, including historical ones, that shape people's lives.

## REPRODUCTIVE JUSTICE BEYOND REPRODUCTIVE HEALTH

To make progress on achieving health equity, it is imperative that public health professionals address all pillars of reproductive justice, including promoting safe environments for raising children. There are numerous examples of public health issues pertaining to raising families that merit a reproductive justice lens, such as housing insecurity, the child welfare system, and the mass incarceration of Black and Brown families living on low incomes, to name a few. Here, we apply a reproductive framework to two examples that are often left out of this topic: addressing food security and keeping immigrant families together.

## Food Security

In 2022, 17% of households with children experienced food insecurity, meaning they did not have reliable access to a sufficient amount of nutritious food at some time during the year.[13] Families of color were disproportionately impacted by food insecurity, with 22% of Black and 21% of Latinx households experiencing hunger, more than double the proportion of White families (9%). In addition, households headed by single moms had the highest occurrence of food insecurity, with a prevalence of 33%. Child hunger is associated with a range of adverse health outcomes, such as developmental delays, poor academic performance, and increased risk for certain health conditions.[14]

Considering the critical impact of food insecurity on the health of children in the short and long term, addressing it is a public health concern. Offering free breakfast to all school-age children, similar to the Black Panther Party's program, would be beneficial for many families, especially those subject to discrimination and living on low incomes. Yet, food insecurity must also be addressed through structural and holistic solutions that recognize its root causes, including unaffordable housing, childcare, and health care, as well as nonlivable wages.[15]

## Keeping Immigrant Families Together

The US government has a long history of mistreating migrants and immigrants, which has been exacerbated by harsher immigration enforcement policies in the past few decades.[16] These policies have led to increased rates of raids, detention, and deportation by Immigration and Customs Enforcement, including separating families both at the border and within the interior of the country. Studies have shown that deportation is associated with trauma, economic instability, and housing insecurity among households with children,[17,18] and some children may even be placed in the foster care system.[19] Though migrant workers are not "forcibly" removed from their families, many experience long periods of physical separation, which affects the health and well-being of both the migrant and their children.[17,18] There is evidence that children separated from a parent who is a migrant worker in the United States experience an increased risk of psychological stress.[17]

A reproductive justice approach to the treatment of immigrant children and families directs us to the need for family-friendly immigration policies.[20,21] Thus, all efforts should be made to keep families together at the border and within the interior of the country, regardless of documentation status, and should take into consideration migrant workers. In addition, human rights norms dictate that immigrants benefit from a presumption of liberty and should not be detained.[22] Immigrant detentions are expensive to administer and subject to harmful and abusive conditions. Studies have proven that community-based alternatives are safer, less expensive, and more effective at ensuring compliance with government requirements.[22] These programs allow asylum seekers and migrants to reside and move freely in the community while waiting for resolution on their migration status. Most importantly, community-based programs allow migrants to preserve family unity and offer compassion and dignity during the immigration process.

## CALL TO ACTION

In the wake of the *Dobbs* decision, there has been an appeal within public health to reaffirm our commitment to reproductive justice by advocating for abortion rights.[23] While abortion rights are necessary to advancing reproductive justice, it is only one piece of a grander picture. We call on public health professionals to use reproductive justice as a framework to guide health education, policy, practice, and research while recognizing all four of its tenets.

To integrate reproductive justice into public health endeavors, we should consider the following four aspects to ensure we are realizing the full potential of this framework, based on the nonprofit SisterSong's recommendations[24]:

1. Analyze power systems to understand the context that leads to health inequities. This includes both understanding the historical injustices as well as examining our own role in maintaining current systems of oppression.
2. Apply an intersectional analysis to recognize and conceptualize the multiple intersections of social–structural factors that are responsible for people's oppression and inequality as well as to facilitate health policies and practices that are equitable.[8]
3. Center the knowledge, experience, and perspectives of the most marginalized communities through participatory research methods and generating practice-based evidence. By addressing the needs of the most disadvantaged people, we can shift the power dynamics that marginalize certain people and better serve all people.

AJPH July 2025, Vol. 115, No. 7

4. Develop health research, programs, and policies that are comprehensive and collaborative. All people need and deserve access to affordable health care services, including diagnostic, preventive, treatment, and long-term care. We must also address structural factors that have an impact on health outside public health, including racism, poverty, and nonlivable wages. It will take many different sectors working together to make this a reality.

## CONCLUSION

Reproductive justice is well suited to examine and address health inequities both domestically and globally because of its emphasis on the historical systems of oppression and human rights. As outlined in this article, public health has used a reproductive justice framework predominantly to discuss matters related to abortion, family planning, and other reproductive health topics while overlooking the right to parent children in safe and sustainable communities, concerns that touch nearly every aspect of public health. Furthermore, its application in public health fails to address the numerous ways in which reproductive justice may be a useful lens to understand other health issues. Through this narrow focus, the full potential of reproductive justice in public health is not realized. Moreover, it is a disservice to its founders who created this theory and praxis in response to how the prochoice movement was not adequately addressing the needs of women of color. They understood that their ability to determine their own reproductive destiny was directly linked to the living conditions of their families and communities.[11]

As the 31st year of reproductive justice approaches, let us collectively reimagine how, when, and where public health employs this critical framework. Furthermore, let us expand our understanding of public health's capacity to incorporate a reproductive justice framework into intersecting topics such as criminal justice, immigration justice, climate justice, and more. This will require us to center bodily autonomy as the primary and foundational tenet of reproductive justice, which will allow us to build solidarity between justice-oriented topics. In doing so, public health can work to advance health equity and social justice for our communities in sustainable ways. AJPH

### CORRESPONDENCE

Correspondence should be sent to Marissa Velarde, 135 Dauer Dr, 401 Rosenau Hall, CB #7445, Chapel Hill, NC 27599-7445 (e-mail: marissa.velarde@gmail.com). Reprints can be ordered at https://www.ajph.org by clicking the "Reprints" link.

### PUBLICATION INFORMATION

Full Citation: Velarde M, Hassan A. Integrating reproductive justice in public health practice, research, and advocacy: an imperative to advance health equity. *Am J Public Health*. 2025;115(7): 1003–1007.

Acceptance Date: February 4, 2025.

DOI: https://doi.org/10.2105/AJPH.2025.308060

ORCID iD:

Marissa Velarde https://orcid.org/0000-0002-0736-9244

### CONTRIBUTORS

M. Velarde originated this work and drafted an initial version. A. Hassan provided critical revision for important intellectual content. Both authors approved of the final version to be published.

### ACKNOWLEDGMENTS

The primary author would like to thank Ariana Vigil for the opportunity to first conceptualize this work in her class.

### CONFLICTS OF INTEREST

The authors have no conflicts of interest to disclose.

### REFERENCES

1. Sister Song. Visioning New Futures for Reproductive Justice. Available at: https://www.sistersong.net/visioningnewfuturesforrj. Accessed December 15, 2024.
2. Chinn JJ, Eisenberg E, Artis Dickerson S, et al. Maternal mortality in the United States: research gaps, opportunities, and priorities. *Am J Obstet Gynecol*. 2020;223(4):486–492.e6. https://doi.org/10.1016/j.ajog.2020.07.021
3. Williams V. Why Black women issued a public demand for 'reproductive justice' 25 years ago. *Washington Post*. August 16, 2019. Available at: https://www.washingtonpost.com/nation/2019/08/16/reproductive-justice-how-women-color-asserted-their-voice-abortion-rights-movement. Accessed April 25, 2024.
4. Ross LJ. Reproductive justice as intersectional feminist activism. *Souls*. 2017;19(3):286–314. https://doi.org/10.1080/10999949.2017.1389634
5. Bond Leonard TM. Laying the foundations for a reproductive justice movement. In: Ross LJ, Roberts L, Derkas E, Peoples W, Bridgewater Toure P, eds. *Radical Reproductive Justice*. New York, NY: Feminist Press at CUNY; 2017:39–49.
6. Ross L, Gutiérrez E, Gerber M, Silliman J. *Undivided Rights: Women of Color Organizing for Reproductive Justice*. Chicago, IL: Haymarket Books; 2016.
7. Price K. What is reproductive justice?: How women of color activists are redefining the pro-choice paradigm. *Meridians*. 2020;19(suppl 1):340–362. https://doi.org/10.1215/15366936-8566034
8. Bowleg L. Evolving intersectionality within public health: from analysis to action. *Am J Public Health*. 2021;111(1):88–90. https://doi.org/10.2105/AJPH.2020.306031
9. World Health Organization. Social determinants of health. Available at: https://www.who.int/health-topics/social-determinants-of-health. Accessed May 1, 2024.
10. Artiga S, Hinton E. Beyond health care: the role of social determinants in promoting health and health equity. KFF. May 19, 2018. Available at: https://www.kff.org/racial-equity-and-health-policy/issue-brief/beyond-health-care-the-role-of-social-determinants-in-promoting-health-and-health-equity. Accessed May 1, 2024.
11. Ross LJ, Roberts L, Derkas E, Peoples W, Bridgewater Toure P, eds. Introduction. In: *Radical Reproductive Justice*. New York, NY: Feminist Press at CUNY; 2017:11–31.
12. Jones NL, Gilman SE, Cheng TL, Drury SS, Hill CV, Geronimus AT. Life course approaches to the causes of health disparities. *Am J Public Health*. 2019;109(suppl 1):S48–S55. https://doi.org/10.2105/AJPH.2018.304738
13. Rabbitt MP, Hales LJ, Burke MP, Coleman-Jensen A. Household food security in the United States in 2022. *Economic Research Report*. US Department of Agriculture. 2023. Available at: https://www.ers.usda.gov/publications/pub-details?pubid=107702&v=7814.4. Accessed May 1, 2024.
14. Hanson KL, Connor LM. Food insecurity and dietary quality in US adults and children: a systematic review. *Am J Clin Nutr*. 2014;100(2):684–692. https://doi.org/10.3945/ajcn.114.084525
15. Gaines-Turner T, Simmons JC, Chilton M. Recommendations from SNAP participants to improve wages and end stigma. *Am J Public Health*. 2019;109(12):1664–1667. https://doi.org/10.2105/AJPH.2019.305362

16. Hacker K, Chu J, Leung C, et al. The impact of immigration and customs enforcement on immigrant health: perceptions of immigrants in Everett, Massachusetts, USA. *Soc Sci Med*. 2011;73(4):586–594. https://doi.org/10.1016/j.socscimed.2011.06.007
17. Castañeda H, Holmes SM, Madrigal DS, Young MED, Beyeler N, Quesada J. Immigration as a social determinant of health. *Annu Rev Public Health*. 2015;36:375–392. https://doi.org/10.1146/annurev-publhealth-032013-182419
18. Dreby J. US immigration policy and family separation: the consequences for children's well-being. *Soc Sci Med*. 2015;132:245–251. https://doi.org/10.1016/j.socscimed.2014.08.041
19. Smith S, Martie G, Jasmine B, et al. Family separation in the Sunshine State: preparing for the traumatic impact and economic costs of immigrant parent deportation on Florida's Child Welfare System. *J Hum Rights Soc Work*. 2020;5(2):78–93. https://doi.org/10.1007/s41134-019-00105-0
20. Messing AJ, Fabi RE, Rosen JD. Reproductive injustice at the US border. *Am J Public Health*. 2020;110(3):339–344. https://doi.org/10.2105/AJPH.2019.305466
21. Fleming PJ, Lopez WD, Ledon C, et al. 'I'm going to look for you and take your kids': reproductive justice in the context of immigration enforcement. *PLoS One*. 2019;14(6):e0217898. https://doi.org/10.1371/journal.pone.0217898
22. Sampson R, Mitchell G. Global trends in immigration detention and alternatives to detention: practical, political and symbolic rationales. *J Migr Hum Secur*. 2013;1(3):97–121. https://doi.org/10.1177/233150241300100302
23. Kapadia F. Reproductive justice matters: a public health of consequence, August 2022. *Am J Public Health*. 2022;112(8):1107–1109. https://doi.org/10.2105/AJPH.2022.306959
24. Sister Song. Reproductive Justice. Available at: https://www.sistersong.net/reproductive-justice. Accessed May 6, 2024.

# Law and Policy Efforts to Dismantle Diversity, Equity, and Inclusion

Daniel G. Aaron, MD, JD, Fatima C. Stanford, MD, MPH, MPA, MBA, and Avery E. Emery, JD

**ABOUT THE AUTHORS**

*Daniel G. Aaron is with the University of Utah S.J. Quinney College of Law, Salt Lake City. Fatima C. Stanford is with the Harvard Medical School and Massachusetts General Hospital, Boston. Avery Emery is a recent graduate of the University of Utah S.J. Quinney College of Law, Salt Lake City.*

The impact of the ongoing attacks on public health has been undeniable, from reproductive health and gender-affirming care to vaccines.[1,2] Recently, the target has turned to diversity, equity, and inclusion (DEI) efforts in schools, businesses, and other institutions. Although a new spate of legal and policy efforts threatens the health system's ability to maintain a diverse workforce of physicians and public health practitioners, DEI opponents' success remains modest. To protect DEI—and the public health benefits of a diverse health workforce—proponents of DEI programs must understand the movement that seeks to challenge them and the tactics it employs. The second Trump administration's executive orders attempting to eliminate DEI in federal programs—and adjacent efforts targeting civil rights protections dating to the 1960s—heighten the importance of private institutions, communities, and state and local governments mounting cooperative efforts to defend DEI.

DEI programs aim to recognize humans' varying characteristics, highlight the uneven distribution of resources based on these characteristics, and foster an environment in which everyone is welcome and given the tools to succeed.[3] These programs represent a modest, if incomplete, effort to address unconscious bias, admissions, salary equity, workplace discrimination, and cultural competence, and they serve a desegregation role by fostering interidentity cooperation and community. Existing in some form for decades, DEI programs have increasingly been adopted by health system actors[4] including medical schools, hospitals, public health organizations, and professional organizations. Many recent programs are still collecting data on impact; however, a systematic review of studies of DEI training showed that 80% of the studies reported statistically significant improvements on at least one outcome measure.[5]

Data on admissions programs in medical education have revealed that terminating affirmative action programs is associated with drops in student body diversity.[6] White medical students in more diverse schools express feeling better prepared to treat minority populations, and they believe more strongly than White students in less diverse schools that access to care should be equitable.[7] Racial concordance between physician and patient is associated with better outcomes for patients of color, highlighting the need for physicians from underrepresented groups.[2] According to 2021 data the American Public Health Association (APHA) collected about its DEI programs, 80% of responding members agreed or strongly agreed that APHA fosters diversity and 67% agreed or strongly agreed that experiences at APHA increased their understanding of differences among their peers. Only 5% disagreed or strongly disagreed that members of differing backgrounds engage well together within APHA.[8]

Despite the significant benefits of DEI programs, the past five years have seen the rise of an anti-DEI movement. Between 2023 and April 2025, legislators introduced 132 bills in 29 states and Congress targeting common DEI initiatives such as DEI offices on college campuses, DEI training, and diversity statements.[9] In the same time frame, 16 states passed at least one anti-DEI law.[9] Many bills have not passed: only one of four anti-DEI bills introduced in North Carolina is now law, along with one of seven in Iowa, two of three in Texas, and one of four in Kentucky.[9]

The EDUCATE Act, a bill introduced in the House of Representatives in March 2024 by Representative Greg Murphy (R-NC), threatens to withhold federal funding from any medical school that does not eliminate its DEI initiatives. Senator John Kennedy (R-LA), who introduced the same bill in the Senate, declared that "[w]oke universities are forcing America's future doctors to care more about race and gender than saving lives."[10] Numerous health organizations, including the Association of American Medical Colleges, denounced the EDUCATE Act, noting that DEI initiatives are necessary to provide the highest standard of care to all patients, particularly those who are marginalized by society and continue to experience health inequities. Simultaneously, lawmakers are pressing other regressive tactics, including banning books by diverse authors or about diverse groups and prohibiting education at state-funded schools about "divisive concepts," including racism and sexism.[11]

Some of these efforts, in addition to combating DEI, go even further by targeting long-standing civil rights protections or aiming to embarrass or intimidate people of color. In February 2025, an organization called the American Accountability Foundation published a "DEI watchlist" consisting of full names and photographs primarily of Black people in federal service, most in the Department of Health and Human Services, who have worked on DEI-related issues or included pronouns in their bios.[12] Dr. Georges Benjamin, head of APHA, called the watchlist a "scare tactic" and "clear racism."[12]

Most recently, the Trump administration issued several executive orders purporting to curtail DEI, including by (1) terminating "DEIA" programs (which include accessibility programs) within the federal government, (2) ordering all federal agencies to enforce civil rights laws against institutions with DEI programs, and (3) revoking pro-DEI executive orders, including Executive Order 11246, a historic order from 1965 that prohibited discrimination in federal employment and federal contracting. In parallel, the administration's new orders instantiate plans to identify the "most egregious and discriminatory DEI practitioners" and require each federal agency to identify up to nine large corporations, organizations, and universities that could be targeted for enforcement.

In addition, the administration ordered the attorney general and the secretary of education to issue guidance to federally funded schools about compliance with federal civil rights law. Finally, the administration has attempted to freeze federal funding generally as well as specific outlays to institutions with DEI policies. For example, according to a letter to Harvard University, "[t]he University must immediately shutter all diversity, equity, and inclusion (DEI) programs." When Harvard refused this and other demands, the administration froze $2.2 billion in grant funding. Litigation over many of the administration's actions is ongoing.

The measures just described partially capture the evolving anti-DEI approaches of the new administration. Some of the administration's actions, which appear to be in violation of clearly established law, are likely aimed not to have legal effect but to generate fear. Indeed, federal law requires schools to maintain antidiscrimination programs, bars the president from impounding federal funds appropriated by Congress, and frequently imposes procedural guardrails on terminating funding. Yet, the climate generated by the administration's actions may matter more than their legality.

Before President Trump's inauguration, most of the country still favored DEI programs,[13] and many institutions refused efforts to roll back initiatives critical to building a more equal society. Therefore, anti-DEI organizations turned to two tactics: (1) pursuing aggressive public relations campaigns orchestrated by a small but vocal group of critics and (2) filing lawsuits (Table 1). By targeting name-brand institutions such as Harvard University, public relations campaigns and lawsuits have had some success. For example, in Students for *Fair Admission, Inc. v Harvard* (2023), the Supreme Court struck down Harvard's race-conscious admissions policies. Lawsuits carry the risks of incurring financial costs, diverting the attention of an institution's attorneys, and imparting reputational damage. Most important, lawsuits cause anxiety.

Since the inauguration, the administration has added the prospect of federal enforcement, largely targeting big-name institutions—per the terms of one executive order, nine top institutions per sector. Because it deviates from the law, the administration does not depend on lawsuits, which would subject its actions to judicial scrutiny. Rather, it has leveraged threats to withhold funding from—or otherwise punish—universities to secure "voluntary" concessions. For example, with $400 million at risk, Columbia University issued a four-page letter "reflect[ing] a stunning level of deference to the Trump administration from a top private research university," according to the *New York Times*.

Public health and medical experts must understand the arguments that anti-DEI activists have used to justify aggressive actions against DEI. Generally, anti-DEI activists have sought to frame DEI initiatives not as equality promoting but as inhibitors of equality, leveraging two arguments.

The first argument is that DEI programs do not promote equity but grant minorities "special privileges," thereby eliminating meritocracy. This argument is rooted in opposition to the Civil Rights Movement[14] and is exemplified by the lawsuit *Alliance for Equal Rights v Fearless Fund* (2023). The Alliance for Equal Rights lawsuit challenges as

**TABLE 1— Prominent Lawsuits Challenging DEI Initiatives**

| Case | DEI Program Being Challenged | Date Filed and Court |
|---|---|---|
| *John Doe v New York University* | New York University Law Review's consideration of race and sex for membership and editor positions | October 19, 2023, US District Court for the Southern District of New York |
| *National Center for Public Policy Research v Schultz et al.* | Starbucks's initiative to increase diversity in leadership and procurement from diverse suppliers | August 30, 2022, Washington State Court, Spokane County |
| *Correll v Amazon.com, Inc.* | Amazon's policies promoting minority sellers | October 28, 2021, US District Court for the Southern District of California |
| *American Alliance for Equal Rights v Fearless Fund Management et al.* | Fearless Fund's program giving grants to companies owned by Black women | August 2, 2023, US District Court for the Northern District of Georgia |
| *Daniel Suhr v Dean R. Dietrich et al.* | Wisconsin State Bar's Diversity Clerkship Program, which offers paid internships to minority law students | December 19, 2023, US District Court for the Eastern District of Wisconsin |
| *Do No Harm v Pfizer, Inc.* | Pfizer's fellowship program designed to increase diversity at all levels of the company | September 15, 2022, US District Court for the Southern District of New York |
| *Moses v Comcast Cable Communications Management* | Comcast's RISE program offering support to businesses owned by women or racial minorities | April 4, 2022, US District Court for the Southern District of Indiana |
| *Bolduc v Amazon.com, Inc.* | Amazon's practice of awarding a $10 000 bonus to delivery service partners of color | July 20, 2022, US District Court for the Eastern District of Texas |
| *Nuziard v Minority Business Development Agency (MBDA)* | MBDA's presumption that minority-owned businesses are disadvantaged and can therefore receive MBDA services | March 30, 2023, US District Court for the Northern District of Texas |
| *American Alliance for Equal Rights v Jorge Zamanillo et al.* | National Museum of the American Latino's internship program for Latinx individuals | February 22, 2024, US District Court for the District of Columbia |
| *American Alliance for Equal Rights v Winston & Strawn LLP* | Law firm Winston & Strawn's fellowship for law students who are part of historically underrepresented groups in law | October 30, 2023, US District Court for the Southern District of Texas |
| *American Alliance for Equal Rights v Morrison & Foerster LLP* | Law firm Morrison & Foerster's fellowship for law students who are people of color or members of the LGBTQ+ community | August 22, 2023, US District Court for the Southern District of Florida |
| *American Alliance for Equal Rights v Perkins Coie LLP* | Law firm Perkins Coie's fellowship for law students who are people of color, who are members of the LGBTQ+ community, or who have a disability | August 22, 2023, US District Court for the Northern District of Texas |
| *Californians for Equal Rights Foundation v City and County of San Francisco* | San Francisco's guaranteed income programs for certain Black, transgender, and undocumented individuals | May 31, 2023, California State Court, County of San Francisco |

*Note.* DEI = diversity, equity, and inclusion; LGBTQ+ = lesbian, gay, bisexual, transgender, and queer. Lawsuits regarding affirmative action in education are not included.

discriminatory a venture capital fund that awards funding to businesses owned by Black women. It relies on the Civil Rights Act of 1866, a law passed one year after the end of the Civil War that was intended to guarantee previously enslaved people the same economic rights as Whites. The Alliance for Equal Rights has flipped the law on its head, morphing the promise of nondiscrimination into a cudgel against programs designed to alleviate structural inequity. The idea that DEI provides special privileges ignores the baseline of systemic racism,[15] in which less than 1% of venture capital funding is awarded to businesses owned by Black women.

The second way that DEI is framed as undermining equality is by arguing that DEI initiatives hurt certain minority groups. For example, in 2024, a dermatologist and 92 coauthors put forward a resolution to sunset the American Academy of Dermatology's DEI programs, arguing that they hinder rather than help diversity. According to the resolution, the "DEI movement" has been perceived as antisemitic and has justified "extreme hate speech and violence" against Jews. But the resolution did not provide concrete examples of DEI being used to support antisemitism, instead citing a perception that it does so, and it failed after the advisory board heard testimony from a diverse group of dermatologists committed to DEI.[16] Jewish dermatologist Heidi Waldorf, who co-led the efforts to save the AAD's DEI initiatives, rebuked the resolution as misusing antisemitism to hide a "political agenda."[16]

A similar strategy was the basis for the Supreme Court cases curtailing race-based affirmative action, with those challenging the programs pointing to Harvard's alleged discrimination against Asian Americans.[2] Many Asian groups and individuals criticized these arguments as disingenuous attempts to discredit inclusionary policies by stoking division between racial groups.[17]

Anti-DEI activists have also suggested that DEI damages free speech by shutting down contrary views. However, DEI can increase free speech among those excluded from historical and contemporary conversations in public health and medicine. DEI can alleviate the self-censorship of those who have experienced marginalization and lead those with privilege to grant space to others.[18] Moreover, DEI is not intended to restrict speech, nor does it function to limit it. Perhaps the concern with free speech is that the ascendancy of a strong equality narrative has narrowed the space for previously tolerated views; yet, the First Amendment does not guarantee the right to state an opinion free of criticism.

There is also a deep irony in claiming that DEI infringes on speech: anti-DEI bills, sometimes purporting to guard free speech, have banned using terms such as diversity and equity or diversity training altogether, thereby curtailing speech. Part of Florida's Stop WOKE Act was held unconstitutional for this reason. A Trump-appointed judge wrote that Florida had penalized particular viewpoints, committing "the greatest First Amendment sin."[19] Often the same legislatures that advance anti-DEI bills have banned books or teaching on "divisive concepts," suggesting that the "free speech" argument may be in bad faith.

As noted, the most successful challenges to DEI have come via pressure campaigns built from lawsuits and public relations efforts. DEI's opponents have been less successful when forced to confront the majority of Americans in support of DEI programs[13] and public health and medical systems largely united in their defense of these programs. Indeed, Americans tend to underestimate the public level of support for DEI.[13] The seemingly successful backlash against DEI despite public support may be due, in part, to the dark money targeting DEI[20,21] and influencing the US Supreme Court,[22,23] which has empowered the wishes of six justices over the views of the many in cases ranging from environmental protection and voting rights to discrimination against lesbian, gay, bisexual, transgender, and queer (LGBTQ+) individuals and reproductive freedom.[24] In addition, voters in 2024, who were predominantly interested in improving the economy and mitigating inflation, likely did not intend to undo fundamental legal protections stemming from the Civil Rights Movement.

Despite legal and political efforts to drive a culture of fear and to pressure institutions to voluntarily retract their DEI commitments, institutions must not forget their legal obligations. Universities and employers are required to mitigate discriminatory bias, a critical role that DEI programs carry. If institutions resolve lawsuits or respond to federal pressure through fear, they paradoxically risk violating the law by fostering discrimination as well as experiencing significant reputational damage and lost morale, particularly among employees and students from marginalized backgrounds. Unnecessary compliance can actually exacerbate an institution's situation by encouraging more lawsuits and pressure.

Indeed, Harvard University continues to be pressured even as it resolves cases. In 2024, a conservative legal organization filed a lawsuit against the university for antisemitism that Harvard settled one day after the inauguration. Another conservative organization created a "watch list" on which it placed Harvard researchers examining the link between racism and ill health, and activist news outlets targeted Black women at Harvard—including its president, its chief DEI officer, and others—by publishing alleged episodes of plagiarism. Some Harvard faculty members and students perceived the university as responding to the pressure by taking a harsher approach to free speech, particularly regarding Gaza[25]; in 2024, the Foundation for Individual Rights and Expression rated Harvard as the worst institute of higher education with regard to free expression.

Meanwhile, perhaps in part because of the Supreme Court's constraints on DEI in university admissions, Harvard's undergraduate Black student enrollment dropped 4 percentage points in fall 2024, and Harvard Law School's Black student enrollment fell to a nadir not seen since the 1960s. Now in 2025 Harvard is again being targeted, this time by the administration.

There are several actions institutions can take to insulate themselves and their DEI programs. Given that DEI programs generally do not violate civil rights law, institutions should avoid offering ill-conceived settlements or unnecessary compliance to misunderstandings of the law. Lawsuits should be expected and managed in due course. Institutions should do what lawsuit defenders have done for years: file motions to transfer to a more friendly jurisdiction; raise additional issues; be open to the complexifying and prolongation of a legal proceeding; view litigation as a cost of doing business, as many institutions and corporations already do; and perhaps go on the offensive by filing defamation lawsuits against sources of misinformation where feasible.

Institutions might design cost-sharing agreements that spread litigation risk to defray efforts to target institutions with unmeritorious lawsuits. Institutions might also share information about legal proceedings and mutually provide advice on navigating this administration. Universities whose funding could be at risk should seek alternative funding sources; many have begun to issue debt. Clearly communicating the risks to alumni could galvanize donations. In four years, the skies may be clearer.

As they defend DEI programs internally and in court, institutions will be tempted to shrink from public discourse. Although understandable, this approach risks ceding public conversation to powerful groups that have seen some recent successes and appear to be determined to spread fear and misinformation about DEI. Institutions can serve as a corrective in public conversations about the ongoing impacts of racism and other forms of discrimination on health. Should misinformation go uncorrected and public opinion be turned against DEI, opponents could be empowered to usher in legislative changes that compromise DEI efforts—and the last 60 years of civil rights law with it.

In addition to supporting institutional DEI programs, individuals within the public health community can protect DEI by openly voicing their views and challenging bad-faith arguments invoking antiracism and free speech. Those whose identity groups are invoked in a bad-faith manner to paint DEI as racist should vocally oppose such disingenuous efforts. Those who have not been marginalized by society have a responsibility to join those under fire to nourish the seedling of equity in the United States.[26] We might also advocate for fairer voting structures that fulfill our nation's promise of democratic equality. A failure of the majority to vocalize its support for DEI could prompt institutions to bow in the face of pressure. DEI, if preserved, can open the halls of public health and medicine to those historically and currently excluded. AJPH

## CORRESPONDENCE

Correspondence should be sent to Daniel G. Aaron, MD, JD, University of Utah S.J. Quinney College of Law, 383 S University St, Salt Lake City, UT 84112 (e-mail: daniel.aaron@law.utah.edu). Reprints can be ordered at https://www.ajph.org by clicking the "Reprints" link.

## PUBLICATION INFORMATION

Full Citation: Aaron DG, Stanford FC, Emery AE. Law and policy efforts to dismantle diversity, equity, and inclusion. *Am J Public Health*. 2025; 115(7):1008–1013.

Acceptance Date: February 16, 2025.

DOI: https://doi.org/10.2105/AJPH.2025.308081

ORCID iDs:

Daniel G. Aaron https://orcid.org/0000-0003-4490-7504

Fatima C. Stanford https://orcid.org/0000-0003-4616-533X

Avery E. Emery https://orcid.org/0009-0003-6586-5128

## CONTRIBUTORS

All of the authors made substantial contributions to the conception and design of the article and worked on drafting the article and revising it critically for important intellectual content.

## CONFLICTS OF INTEREST

The authors report no conflicts of interest.

## REFERENCES

1. Ulrich MR. Practicing medicine in the culture wars—gender-affirming care and the battles over clinician autonomy. *N Engl J Med.* 2024;390(9): 779–781. https://doi.org/10.1056/NEJMp2313283
2. Aaron DG, Bajaj SS, Stanford FC. Supreme Court cases on affirmative action threaten diversity in medicine. *Proc Natl Acad Sci U S A.* 2023;120(17): e2220919120. https://doi.org/10.1073/pnas.2220919120
3. Association of American Medical Colleges. Importance of diversity in health care. Available at: https://www.aamc.org/about-us/mission-areas/medical-education/my-story-matters. Accessed January 2, 2025.
4. Dandar V, Fair M, Steinecke A, Sweeney N, Mallery T. *The Power of Collective Action: Assessing and Advancing Diversity, Equity, and Inclusion Efforts at AAMC Medical Schools.* Association of American Medical Colleges; 2022.
5. Wang ML, Gomes A, Rosa M, Copeland P, Santana VJ. A systematic review of diversity, equity, and inclusion and antiracism training studies: findings and future directions. *Transl Behav Med.* 2024;14(3):156–171. https://doi.org/10.1093/tbm/ibad061
6. Ly DP, Essien UR, Olenski AR, Jena AB. Affirmative action bans and enrollment of students from underrepresented racial and ethnic groups in U.S. public medical schools. *Ann Intern Med.* 2022; 175(6):873–878. https://doi.org/10.7326/M21-4312
7. Saha S. Student body racial and ethnic composition and diversity-related outcomes in US medical schools. *JAMA.* 2008;300(10):1135. https://doi.org/10.1001/jama.300.10.1135
8. American Public Health Association Committee on Health Equity. Equity, Diversity & Inclusion Survey. Available at: https://www.apha.org/-/media/Files/PDF/about/Committees/CHEQ_Diversity_and_Inclusion_Report.pdf. Accessed January 2, 2025.
9. Chronicle of Higher Education. DEI Legislation Tracker. Available at: https://www.chronicle.com/article/here-are-the-states-where-lawmakers-are-seeking-to-ban-colleges-dei-efforts. Accessed April 24, 2025.
10. Congressman Greg Murphy. Murphy's legislation to ban DEI in medicine introduced in Senate. Available at: http://murphy.house.gov/media/press-releases/murphys-legislation-ban-dei-medicine-introduced-senate. Accessed April 23, 2025.
11. Feingold J, Weishart JE. Discriminatory censorship laws. Available at: https://scholarship.law.bu.edu/cgi/viewcontent.cgi?article=4881&context=faculty_scholarship. Accessed January 2, 2025.
12. NBC News. Federal health workers terrified after "DEI" website publishes list of "targets." Available at: https://www.nbcnews.com/health/health-news/federal-health-workers-terrified-dei-website-publishes-list-targets-rcna190711. Accessed February 5, 2025.

13. Isenberg N, Brauer M. Diversity and inclusion have greater support than most Americans think. *Sci Rep.* 2024;14(1):28616. https://doi.org/10.1038/s41598-024-76761-8
14. Aaron DG, Francis LP. Health law and bigotry distractions. *J Law Med Ethics.* 2024;52(2):350–363. https://doi.org/10.1017/jme.2024.92
15. Aaron DG, Stanford FC. Medicine, structural racism, and systems. *Soc Sci Med.* 2022;298:114856. https://doi.org/10.1016/j.socscimed.2022.114856
16. NBC News. American Academy of Dermatology votes to keep its diversity policies after anti-DEI proposal. Available at: https://www.nbcnews.com/news/us-news/anti-dei-proposal-rejected-american-academy-dermatology-rcna142494. Accessed January 2, 2025.
17. Lee P. Rejecting honorary whiteness: Asian Americans and the attack on race-conscious admissions. *Emory Law J.* 2021;70(7):1475–1506.
18. Razzante R. Breanta Boss. DEI in the legal profession: identifying foundational factors for meaningful change. *Utah Law Rev.* 2022;2022(4):785–799. https://doi.org/10.26054/0D-Q1AP-Y9PD
19. Atterbury A. Appeals court slams Florida's "stop-woke" law for committing "greatest First Amendment sin." Available at: https://www.politico.com/news/2024/03/04/desantis-woke-law-court-00144801. Accessed November 22, 2024.
20. Harvard Crimson. SFFA funded by large conservative trusts, public filings show. Available at: https://www.thecrimson.com/article/2022/10/28/donors-sffa-conservative-trusts. Accessed January 2, 2025.
21. Nicol DJ. Activism for profit: America's "anti-affirmative action" industry. Available at: https://www.aljazeera.com/opinions/2021/2/28/activism-for-profit-americas-anti-affirmative-action-industry. Accessed January 2, 2025.
22. Warner J. The king of dark money effectively controls the US Supreme Court now. Available at: https://www.theguardian.com/commentisfree/2023/jun/30/supreme-court-leonard-leo-dark-money. Accessed January 2, 2025.
23. Kroll A, Bernstein A, Marritz, I. We don't talk about Leonard: the man behind the right's Supreme Court supermajority. Available at: https://www.propublica.org/article/we-dont-talk-about-leonard-leo-supreme-court-supermajority. Accessed January 2, 2025.
24. Aaron DG, Emery AE. US Supreme Court limits on the power of US health agencies. *JAMA.* 2024;331(17):1441–1442. https://doi.org/10.1001/jama.2024.3723
25. Tran J. Harvard temporarily bans faculty involved in "study-in" protests from using library. Available at: https://www.nbcboston.com/news/local/harvard-professors-banned-from-library-after-study-in/3532892. Accessed February 3, 2025.
26. Yearby R. The return of Jim Crow: government discrimination against women, LGBTQIA+ individuals, and racial/ethnic minority individuals. *Am J Public Health.* 2024;114(12):1331–1334. https://doi.org/10.2105/AJPH.2024.307884

# The American Public's Disengagement With Highly Pathogenic Avian Influenza (HPAI): Considerations for Vaccination and Dietary Changes

Rachael Piltch-Loeb, PhD, MSPH, Katarzyna Wyka, PhD, Trenton M. White, PhD, MPH, Shawn G. Gibbs, PhD, MBA, CIH, Sara Gorman, PhD, Ashish Joshi, PhD, MBBS, MPH, Spencer Kimball, JD, Jeffrey V. Lazarus, PhD, MIH, MA, John J. Lowe, PhD, Kenneth Rabin, PhD, Scott C. Ratzan, MD, and Ayman El-Mohandes, MBBCh, MD, MPH

AJPH July 2025, Vol. 115, No. 7

**ABOUT THE AUTHORS**

*Rachael Piltch-Loeb, Katarzyna Wyka, Jeffrey V. Lazarus, Kenneth Rabin, Scott C. Ratzan, and Ayman El-Mohandes are with the CUNY Graduate School of Public Health and Health Policy, New York, NY. Trenton M. White is with Barcelona Institute for Global Health (ISGlobal), Barcelona, Spain. Shawn G. Gibbs is with the Texas A&M University Graduate School of Public Health, College Station, TX. Sara Gorman is with Critica Science, Bronx, NY. Ashish Joshi is with the University of Memphis School of Public Health, Memphis, TN. Spencer Kimball is with Emerson College, Boston, MA. John J. Lowe is with University of Nebraska Medical Center College of Public Health, Omaha, NE.*

Since spring 2024, highly pathogenic avian influenza (HPAI) has reemerged as a significant threat to public health in the United States. There were 66 confirmed human cases of HPAI reported in the United States during 2024, with the first identified in Texas. Infections have predominately occurred among individuals with occupational exposure to sick or infected animals.[1] Notably, on September 6, 2024, the first case of HPAI without a known occupational exposure to sick or infected animals was diagnosed in Missouri, suggesting a potentially unknown transmission pathway or gaps in epidemiological and exposure data regarding this individual.[2] Despite the growing risks posed by HPAI, a concerning disconnect exists between public health experts' warnings and the public's awareness and response. This gap threatens the nation's ability to effectively manage and prevent further spread of the virus.

Recognizing the potential threat of HPAI, we conducted a population representative survey of US residents (n = 10 000) on August 5–15, 2024, which used an in-depth sampling framework and intentional oversampling of rural populations (n = 5000). The survey highlighted the public's lack of awareness regarding the threat posed by avian influenza, its potential to infect humans, and the necessary steps to protect oneself and others. Descriptive statistics for all variables are reported using weighted frequencies and percentages; they showed that whereas 64.4% of respondents had heard of HPAI, only 26.1% understood that it could spread to humans, and just 18.8% were aware that the H5N1 virus had been detected in cattle.

The findings indicated that 27% of respondents would be unwilling to modify their diet to reduce the risk of exposure to the virus, and 28.7% expressed reluctance to take a potential vaccine for H5N1, even if advised by the US Centers for Disease Control and Prevention (CDC) to do so to mitigate the consequences of the virus. This potential resistance to action could pose a serious obstacle to containing the virus and preventing a larger-scale public health crisis. Results varied by political party and geography, emphasizing the need for a proactive public health approach to addressing the issue. Here, we elaborate on specific findings and their implications for public health response (Table 1). A full description of methods and results, including sampling, survey items, analytic plan, descriptive statistics, and model results, can be found in the Appendix (available as a supplement to the online version of this article at http://www.ajph.org).

## LACK OF KNOWLEDGE ON AVIAN INFLUENZA AND FOOD SAFETY

Despite the increasing threat of H5N1, many Americans remain unaware of the virus's potential dangers. Nearly two thirds of the respondents (64.4%) had recently heard of HPAI; however,

**TABLE 1— Willingness to Take CDC-Recommended HPAI Vaccine and Change Dietary Behavior: United States, August 2024**

| | | If a Vaccine Were Recommended by the CDC to Prevent or Reduce Your Risk of Bird Flu, Would You Take That Vaccine? | | | If the CDC Recommended It, Would You Be Willing to Make Changes to Your Dietary Consumption of Milk or Eggs? | | |
|---|---|---|---|---|---|---|---|
| Reason for Vaccine Resistance | Overall, No. (%) | Yes, No. (%) | No/Unsure, No. (%) | P | Yes, No. (%) | No/Unsure, No. (%) | P |
| Overall | 6265 (100) | 2418 (38.6) | 3847 (61.4) | | 2782 (44.4) | 3483 (55.6) | |
| Recently heard of H5N1, sometimes called bird flu or avian flu | | | | | | | |
| Yes | 4036 (64.4) | 1706 (42.3) | 2330 (57.7) | <.001 | 1985 (49.2) | 2051 (50.8) | <.001 |
| No | 1828 (29.2) | 595 (32.5) | 1233 (67.4) | | 659 (36.1) | 1169 (64.0) | |
| Unsure | 402 (6.4) | 116 (28.9) | 285 (71.0) | | 138 (34.4) | 263 (65.5) | |
| Belief of populations affected this year (2024) | | | | | | | |
| Poultry, particularly chickens | 3090 (49.3) | 1324 (42.8) | 1766 (57.1) | <.001 | 1533 (49.6) | 1558 (50.4) | <.001 |
| Cattle, particularly dairy cows | 1175 (18.8) | 557 (47.4) | 618 (52.6) | <.001 | 626 (53.3) | 549 (46.7) | <.001 |
| People | 1636 (26.1) | 768 (46.9) | 868 (53.1) | <.001 | 820 (50.1) | 816 (49.9) | <.001 |
| Domestic cats | 214 (3.4) | 117 (54.7) | 97 (45.4) | <.001 | 113 (52.6) | 102 (47.4) | .003 |
| Wild fowl | 881 (14.1) | 411 (46.6) | 470 (53.5) | <.001 | 460 (52.2) | 421 (47.9) | <.001 |
| Unsure | 2258 (36.0) | 687 (30.4) | 1571 (69.6) | <.001 | 844 (37.4) | 1414 (62.6) | <.001 |
| Bird flu is a health threat to humans | | | | | | | |
| Strongly/somewhat agree | 3904 (62.3) | 1877 (48.1) | 2027 (51.9) | <.001 | 2083 (53.4) | 1821 (46.6) | <.001 |
| Unsure/no opinion | 1758 (28.1) | 434 (24.7) | 1325 (75.3) | | 510 (29.0) | 1249 (71.0) | |
| Strongly/somewhat disagree | 603 (9.6) | 107 (17.7) | 496 (82.3) | | 189 (31.3) | 414 (68.6) | |
| I am at risk for catching bird flu | | | | | | | |
| Strongly/somewhat agree | 1717 (27.4) | 987 (57.5) | 730 (42.5) | <.001 | 951 (55.4) | 766 (44.6) | <.001 |
| Unsure/no opinion | 2565 (40.9) | 858 (33.4) | 1707 (66.6) | | 1008 (39.3) | 1557 (60.7) | |
| Strongly/somewhat disagree | 1983 (31.6) | 573 (28.9) | 1410 (71.1) | | 823 (41.5) | 1160 (58.5) | |
| As far as you know, how safe is it to drink raw milk compared with pasteurized milk? | | | | | | | |
| Pasteurized milk is safer to drink | 3361 (53.7) | 1578 (46.9) | 1783 (53.1) | <.001 | 1796 (53.4) | 1565 (46.5) | <.001 |
| Raw milk is safer to drink | 421 (6.7) | 136 (32.3) | 285 (67.7) | | 116 (27.5) | 306 (72.5) | |
| All milk is equally safe to drink | 615 (9.8) | 182 (29.6) | 433 (70.5) | | 197 (32.0) | 418 (67.9) | |
| Unsure | 1868 (29.8) | 521 (27.9) | 1346 (72.1) | | 673 (36.0) | 1194 (63.9) | |
| As far as you know, can drinking unpasteurized milk improve your immunity against bird flu? | | | | | | | |
| Yes | 395 (6.3) | 228 (57.7) | 167 (42.3) | <.001 | 147 (37.1) | 248 (62.9) | <.001 |
| No | 2409 (38.5) | 1086 (45.1) | 1323 (54.9) | | 1237 (51.3) | 1172 (48.6) | |
| Unsure | 3461 (55.2) | 1103 (31.9) | 2358 (68.1) | | 1398 (40.4) | 2063 (59.6) | |
| Have you consumed unpasteurized (raw) milk in the past 12 months? | | | | | | | |
| Yes | 431 (6.9) | 197 (45.7) | 234 (54.3) | <.001 | 153 (35.5) | 278 (64.5) | <.001 |
| No | 5236 (83.6) | 2086 (39.8) | 3150 (60.1) | | 2488 (47.5) | 2748 (52.5) | |
| Unsure | 598 (9.5) | 135 (22.5) | 463 (77.4) | | 140 (23.5) | 457 (76.5) | |
| Cooking fish, eggs, chicken, or beef at high temperatures can kill bacteria and viruses that these animals may carry | | | | | | | |
| Strongly/somewhat agree | 4466 (71.3) | 1908 (42.7) | 2558 (57.3) | <.001 | 2130 (47.7) | 2335 (52.3) | <.001 |
| Unsure/no opinion | 1313 (21.0) | 367 (28.0) | 946 (72.0) | | 404 (30.8) | 909 (69.3) | |
| Strongly/somewhat disagree | 486 (7.8) | 143 (29.4) | 343 (70.6) | | 247 (50.8) | 239 (49.2) | |
| Political affiliation | | | | | | | |
| Democrat | 1997 (31.9) | 1159 (58.0) | 838 (41.9) | <.001 | 1238 (62.0) | 760 (38.1) | <.001 |
| Republican | 1865 (29.8) | 522 (28.0) | 1343 (72.0) | | 630 (33.8) | 1235 (66.2) | |
| Independent | 1560 (24.9) | 542 (34.7) | 1019 (65.2) | | 640 (41.0) | 920 (59.0) | |

*Continued*

## TABLE 1— Continued

| | | If a Vaccine Were Recommended by the CDC to Prevent or Reduce Your Risk of Bird Flu, Would You Take That Vaccine? | | | If the CDC Recommended It, Would You Be Willing to Make Changes to Your Dietary Consumption of Milk or Eggs? | | |
|---|---|---|---|---|---|---|---|
| Reason for Vaccine Resistance | Overall, No. (%) | Yes, No. (%) | No/Unsure, No. (%) | P | Yes, No. (%) | No/Unsure, No. (%) | P |
| None | 577 (9.2) | 132 (22.9) | 445 (77.1) | | 176 (30.5) | 401 (69.5) | |
| Prefer not to say | 266 (4.2) | 63 (23.7) | 203 (76.3) | | 98 (37.0) | 167 (63.0) | |
| Trust in CDC | | | | | | | |
| A great deal | 1129 (18.0) | 827 (73.2) | 302 (26.8) | < .001 | 797 (70.6) | 332 (29.4) | < .001 |
| A fair amount | 1982 (31.6) | 1042 (52.6) | 940 (47.5) | | 1132 (57.1) | 850 (42.9) | |
| Only a little | 1406 (22.4) | 359 (25.6) | 1047 (74.4) | | 525 (37.3) | 880 (62.6) | |
| None or almost none | 1215 (19.4) | 112 (9.2) | 1103 (90.8) | | 200 (16.5) | 1015 (83.6) | |
| Don't know | 344 (5.5) | 50 (14.5) | 294 (85.4) | | 70 (20.3) | 274 (79.6) | |
| I am not familiar with this agency | 190 (3.0) | 28 (14.8) | 161 (85.1) | | 57 (30.0) | 132 (70.0) | |
| Trust in US Food and Drug Administration | | | | | | | |
| A great deal | 969 (15.5) | 682 (70.4) | 287 (29.6) | < .001 | 629 (64.9) | 340 (35.1) | < .001 |
| A fair amount | 2221 (35.4) | 1116 (50.2) | 1105 (49.8) | | 1217 (54.8) | 1003 (45.2) | |
| Only a little | 1583 (25.3) | 438 (27.7) | 1146 (72.3) | | 612 (38.6) | 972 (61.4) | |
| None or almost none | 1010 (16.1) | 114 (11.3) | 897 (88.7) | | 215 (21.3) | 796 (78.7) | |
| Don't know | 342 (5.5) | 44 (12.8) | 299 (87.2) | | 70 (20.4) | 273 (79.6) | |
| I am not familiar with this agency | 139 (2.2) | 25 (18.0) | 114 (82.0) | | 39 (28.1) | 100 (71.9) | |
| Trust in US Department of Agriculture | | | | | | | |
| A great deal | 1002 (16.0) | 674 (67.3) | 328 (32.7) | < .001 | 623 (62.2) | 378 (37.8) | < .001 |
| A fair amount | 2373 (37.9) | 1078 (45.4) | 1295 (54.6) | | 1270 (53.5) | 1103 (46.5) | |
| Only a little | 1492 (23.8) | 439 (29.4) | 1053 (70.6) | | 562 (37.7) | 930 (62.3) | |
| None or almost none | 765 (12.2) | 110 (14.4) | 654 (85.6) | | 155 (20.3) | 609 (79.7) | |
| Don't know | 444 (7.1) | 80 (18.0) | 364 (82.0) | | 108 (24.3) | 336 (75.7) | |
| I am not familiar with this agency | 190 (3.0) | 37 (19.4) | 154 (80.6) | | 64 (33.7) | 126 (66.3) | |
| Living area | | | | | | | |
| Urban | 5000 (79.8) | 1989 (39.8) | 3011 (60.2) | < .001 | 2289 (45.8) | 2711 (54.2) | < .001 |
| Rural | 1265 (20.2) | 429 (33.9) | 836 (66.1) | | 493 (38.9) | 772 (61.0) | |
| Pandemic fatigue | | | | | | | |
| Yes | 2378 (38.0) | 861 (36.2) | 1517 (63.8) | < .001 | 948 (39.8) | 1430 (60.2) | < .001 |
| Unsure/no opinion | 1267 (20.2) | 344 (27.1) | 923 (72.9) | | 321 (25.3) | 946 (74.7) | |
| No | 2620 (41.8) | 1213 (46.3) | 1407 (53.7) | | 1513 (57.7) | 1107 (42.2) | |

*Note.* CDC = Centers for Disease Control and Prevention; HPAI = highly pathogenic avian influenza. Weighted No. and row % are reported. Bivariate associations were assessed by using the $\chi^2$ test. Willingness to take CDC-recommended flu vaccine and change dietary behavior by additional sample characteristics can be found in Appendix Table A (available as a supplement to the online version of this article at http://www.ajph.org).

only one in five (18.8%) believed the virus affected cattle and only one in four (26.1%) believed it affected humans. The majority (62.3%) agreed that HPAI is a health threat to humans, although only one in four (27.4%) believed they were at risk for catching it. These findings provide a baseline as of time of survey.

The survey also revealed that a majority of respondents were unaware of simple food safety practices that could reduce the risk of infection. Over half (53.7%) did not know that pasteurized milk is safer than raw milk, and fewer than three quarters (71.3%) understood that cooking meat at high temperatures could eliminate harmful bacteria and viruses like H5N1. This was of particular concern given that evidence from

California suggests H5N1 can be found in raw milk. The state issued a recent recall of contaminated raw milk.[3]

## RESISTANCE TO DIETARY CHANGES AND VACCINATION

The study posed hypothetical public health mitigation strategies to respondents, asking (1) would you be willing to take HPAI vaccine if one was recommended by the CDC (analyzed as yes, no, or unsure), and (2) would you be willing to change dietary behavior based on CDC recommendations (analyzed as yes = very or somewhat willing, no = unsure, no opinion, or somewhat or not at all willing).

In response to the question on vaccination, 28.7% of respondents were resistant to taking a potential H5N1 vaccine, with another 32.7% uncertain about whether they would accept it. The hesitancy to embrace vaccines is a serious barrier to public health efforts. Similar patterns of vaccine resistance were evident during the COVID-19 pandemic, where significant portions of the population rejected vaccination through misinformation, distrust of health authorities, and political polarization.[4,5] The H5N1 virus is a real and present danger, and a vaccine could be one of the most effective tools for preventing further spread. However, without broad public support, vaccine uptake will likely remain insufficient to stem the tide of the virus. This may be related to a low level of perceived risk and the level of knowledge at time of study. Similarly, 27% of respondents expressed unwillingness to follow a change in dietary guidelines. This hesitation reflects broader societal trends in which people are often unwilling to alter their behaviors in response to health risks.[6,7]

## POLITICAL POLARIZATION AND TRUST IN PUBLIC HEALTH INSTITUTIONS

The study also examined the relationship between political affiliation and public health attitudes. Americans' willingness to adopt preventive measures, such as getting vaccinated or changing their dietary habits, varied dramatically along partisan lines when sociodemographics were controlled for (Appendix Table). The study found that participants reporting to be Republicans (adjusted odds ratio [AOR] = 3.51 for vaccination and 1.56 for dietary changes) and Independents (AOR = 2.69 for vaccination and 1.43 for dietary changes) were significantly less likely to support both vaccination and dietary changes than Democrats. This political divide reflects broader societal trends. Skepticism of government recommendations, including those related to vaccinations and dietary changes, is particularly strong among conservative voters, further complicating efforts to promote widespread public health measures.[8–10] This should be taken into account in future public health communications plans.

Similarly, there was limited trust in government agencies like the CDC, the Food and Drug Administration, and the US Department of Agriculture reported by nearly 40.0% of the study's respondents. In the absence of trust, people are more likely to dismiss expert guidance and resist recommended actions, even if they are designed to protect their health and prevent the spread of dangerous diseases like H5N1. This indicates that significant efforts to reestablish the public's trust and use of trusted information pathways should be prioritized in prevention and response efforts.

## RURAL AMERICA AND VACCINE HESITANCY

There were also differences between urban and rural communities in terms of their response to public health guidance. Rural Americans, many of whom are more likely to work or live in agricultural areas or near livestock industries, are less likely to accept public health measures, including vaccination and dietary changes, compared with their urban counterparts. Only 33.9% of rural residents indicated a willingness to accept a CDC-recommended vaccine, compared with 39.8% of urban residents. Similarly, just 38.9% of rural respondents said they would be willing to change their dietary habits, compared with 45.8% of urban dwellers. These findings are consistent with the literature. There is also intersectionality between political affiliation and geography. Rural Americans often view government interventions as intrusive or unnecessary, making it more difficult to implement effective public health measures in these areas.[11] For public health efforts to be successful in controlling this outbreak, outreach to rural communities must be tailored to their unique needs and values.

## PANDEMIC FATIGUE AND PUBLIC HEALTH ENGAGEMENT

Pandemic fatigue continues to be a significant obstacle in managing new health threats. After years of grappling with the COVID-19 pandemic, many Americans are exhausted and disengaged from ongoing public health campaigns. This study found that 38.0% of respondents felt mentally and emotionally drained by the constant cycle of health warnings and changes to daily life. This fatigue can lead to apathy and resistance to new health measures, even when they are essential to controlling the spread of diseases like H5N1.[12]

## MOVING FORWARD: IMPROVING PUBLIC HEALTH COMMUNICATION

The findings of this study paint a picture of the American public's preparedness to address the avian influenza crisis and, when extrapolated, should cause concern for addressing other future outbreaks. General resistance to dietary changes and political polarization all contribute to the public's disengagement from the issue. To prevent further outbreaks and potential widespread illness, public health officials must find ways to bridge these gaps, engage communities more effectively, determine the root cause of distrust, and then rebuild trust. Clear, targeted messaging that engages local leaders and academic partners that are already working in the community, such as agricultural extension personnel, and that focuses on messages that resonate with a variety of political groups will be critical in helping people understand the risks posed by H5N1 and the importance of preventive measures. Sampling and self-report bias may have influenced these findings.

Managing this avian influenza threat (there are currently a growing number of human cases) and preparing the nation for future infectious disease challenges require urgent action. To prevent a full-scale public health crisis, the United States must strengthen its health agencies and surveillance and educate and engage the public and trusted health communicators on the risks of unpasteurized milk consumption and the benefits of vaccination to help those at risk protect themselves and their communities from the H5N1 threat. AJPH

### CORRESPONDENCE

Correspondence should be sent to Rachael Piltch-Loeb, PhD, MSPH, Assistant Professor, CUNY Graduate School of Public Health and Health Policy, 55 W 125th St, New York, NY 10027 (e-mail: Rachael.piltch-loeb@sph.cuny.edu). Reprints can be ordered at https://www.ajph.org by clicking the "Reprints" link.

### PUBLICATION INFORMATION

Full Citation: Piltch-Loeb R, Wyka K, White TM, et al. The American public's disengagement with highly pathogenic avian influenza (HPAI): considerations for vaccination and dietary changes. *Am J Public Health*. 2025;115(7):1014–1018.

Acceptance Date: February 16, 2025

DOI: https://doi.org/10.2105/AJPH.2025.308080

ORCID iDs:

Rachael Piltch-Loeb https://orcid.org/0000-0002-6813-1934

Katarzyna Wyka https://orcid.org/0000-0002-5699-2497

Trenton M. White https://orcid.org/0000-0002-0633-4445

Shawn G. Gibbs https://orcid.org/0000-0002-6041-5166

Spencer Kimball https://orcid.org/0009-0005-3072-8742

Jeffrey V. Lazarus https://orcid.org/0000-0001-9618-2299

### CONTRIBUTORS

R. Piltch-Loeb led the editorial writing and research question. K. Wyka led the analysis. A. El-Mohandes led the parent study design and acquisition of funding to support the study. All authors contributed to the overall design and interpretation of the data, as well as drafting and revisions to the writing. All authors approved the final manuscript.

### ACKNOWLEDGMENTS

Funding for this study was provided by the CUNY Graduate School of Public Health and Health Policy, New York, NY.

### CONFLICTS OF INTEREST

The authors declare no conflicts of interest.

### HUMAN PARTICIPANT PROTECTION

This study was found to be exempt by the institutional review board of Emerson College.

### REFERENCES

1. Garg S, Reinhart K, Couture A, et al. Highly pathogenic avian influenza A (H5N1) virus infections in humans. *N Engl J Med*. 2025;392(9):843–854.
2. US Centers for Disease Control and Prevention. CDC confirms human H5 HPAI case in Missouri. Available at: https://www.cdc.gov/media/releases/2024/s0906-birdflu-case-missouri.html#:~:text=September%206%2C%202024%20%2D%2D%20CDC,usual%20protocols%20and%20confirmed%20yesterday. Accessed September 19, 2024.
3. California Dept of Food and Agriculture. California Department of Food and Agriculture press release on the bulk tank findings and subsequent recall. December 14, 2024. Available at: https://pressreleases.cdfa.ca.gov/Home/PressRelease/63398203. Accessed December 16, 2024.
4. SteelFisher GK, Findling MG, Caporello HL, et al. Trust in US federal, state, and local public health agencies during COVID-19: responses and policy implications. *Health Aff (Millwood)*. 2023;42(3):328–337. https://doi.org/10.1377/hlthaff.2022.01204
5. Kaiser Family Foundation. Few firm beliefs and low trust: Americans not sure what's true in the age of health misinformation. Available at: https://kffhealthnews.org/news/article/few-firm-beliefs-low-trust-health-misinformation-kff-poll. Accessed September 19, 2024.
6. Nowak GJ, Cacciatore MA. State of vaccine hesitancy in the United States. *Pediatr Clin North Am*. 2023;70(2):197–210. https://doi.org/10.1016/j.pcl.2022.11.001
7. Middleton KR, Anton SD, Perri MG. Long-term adherence to health behavior change. *Am J Lifestyle Med*. 2013;7(6):395–404. https://doi.org/10.1177/1559827613488867
8. Rabin C, Dutra S. Predicting engagement in behaviors to reduce the spread of COVID-19: the roles of the health belief model and political party affiliation. *Psychol Health Med*. 2022;27(2):379–388. https://doi.org/10.1080/13548506.2021.1921229
9. Painter M, Qiu T. Political beliefs affect compliance with government mandates. *J Econ Behav Organ*. 2021;185:688–701. https://doi.org/10.1016/j.jebo.2021.03.019
10. Kiviniemi MT, Orom H, Hay JL, Waters EA. Prevention is political: political party affiliation predicts perceived risk and prevention behaviors for COVID-19. *BMC Public Health*. 2022;22(1):298. https://doi.org/10.1186/s12889-022-12649-4
11. Callaghan T, Kassabian M, Johnson N, et al. Rural healthy people 2030: new decade, new challenges. *Prev Med Rep*. 2023;33:102176. https://doi.org/10.1016/j.pmedr.2023.102176
12. Ford JL, Douglas M, Barrett AK. The role of pandemic fatigue in seeking and avoiding information on COVID-19 among young adults. *Health Commun*. 2023;38(11):2336–2349. https://doi.org/10.1080/10410236.2022.2069211

# The Unsettled PREEMIE Reauthorization Act and the Recalcitrant Challenge of Preterm Births

*Eli Y. Adashi, MD, MS, Daniel P. O'Mahony, MSLS, and I. Glenn Cohen, JD*

**ABOUT THE AUTHORS**

*Eli Y. Adashi is Professor of Medical Science and former Dean of Medicine and Biological Sciences at Brown University, Providence, RI. Daniel P. O'Mahony is Director of Library Planning and Assessment at the Brown University Library, Providence. I. Glenn Cohen is Deputy Dean and James A. Attwood and Leslie Williams Professor of Law at Harvard Law School, and faculty director at the Petrie-Flom Center for Health Law Policy, Biotechnology, and Bioethics at Harvard University, Cambridge, MA.*

In November 2024, the March of Dimes released its annual Report Card on the state of maternal and infant health for American families.[1] Among its leading observations, the Report Card makes note of the fact that the 2023 US preterm birth (≤37 completed weeks of gestation) rate, the leading cause of infant morbidity and death, remains alarmingly high at 10.4% (unchanged from 2022).[1] In all, more than 370 000 infants were born preterm.[1] The Report Card goes on to note that the preterm birth rate among babies born to Black mothers was 1.4 times higher than the rate among all other babies.[1] Moreover, the infant mortality rate increased for the first time in two decades in 2022, and babies born to Black mothers had a rate 1.9 times the national rate.[1] It follows that every effort must be made to bring this persistent crisis under control. The approach Congress has taken to address this crisis is the Prematurity Research Expansion and Education for Mothers Who Deliver Infants Early (PREEMIE) Reauthorization Act, the very objective of which is to expand research, education, and services with an eye toward reducing the recalcitrant annual incidence of preterm birth.[2] The objective of this editorial is to review the history of the PREEMIE Act and to discuss the prospects of the future enactment thereof.

As detailed in the March of Dimes Report Card, the highest annual national preterm birth rates were documented in the southern region of the United States[1]: Mississippi (15%), Louisiana (13.4%), West Virginia (13.1%), and Alabama (12.9%). A comparable analysis of US cities revealed Detroit, MI; Cleveland, OH; Mobile, AL; and New Orleans, LA, had the highest annual preterm birth rates in national urban centers at 15.6%, 14.8%, 14.6%, and 14.1%, respectively.[1] Established frequencies (% of all births) of preterm birth risk factors included, but were not limited to, diabetes (1.2%), hypertension (3.2%), smoking (3.8%), and unhealthy weight (34.7%).[1]

Recognizing the import of preterm births to the health of the nation, Congress passed the PREEMIE Act all of two decades ago. The brainchild of former Senator Lamar Alexander Jr (R-TN), the original bill was signed into law by President George W. Bush on December 22, 2006. Subsequently, Congress reauthorized the PREEMIE Act on November 27, 2013 (113th Congress) and on December 18, 2018 (115th Congress). Always considered bipartisan legislation, the reauthorization bills were enacted by Presidents Obama and Trump, respectively, and have come to be relied upon as a crucial investment in the health of our nation's children. At its core, the PREEMIE Act facilitates federal research, education, and intervention activities aimed at reducing preterm birth and infant mortality.[2] Aside from the plain desire to reduce preterm births and their complications—the second leading cause of infant deaths—Congress is also interested in lowering the attending societal economic costs associated with preterm birth in the United States, estimated in 2016 to be $25.2 billion.[2] Individually, the average first-year medical costs for premature infants are about four times greater than for term infants.[2]

With the PREEMIE Act set to expire on September 30, 2023, Representative Anna G. Eshoo (D-CA-16) and Senator Michael F. Bennet (D-CO), along with a contingent of 48 bipartisan congressional cosponsors, introduced the reauthorization bills for the 118th Congress. After hearings by the House Energy and Commerce Committee's Subcommittee on Health in June 2023, the House Bill (HR 3226) was passed unanimously by both the subcommittee

AJPH July 2025, Vol. 115, No. 7

(26–0) and the full committee (48–0) before ultimately being passed by the House on December 11, 2023.[2] The Senate companion bill (S 1573) received favorable treatment by the Senate Committee on Health, Education, Labor, and Pensions. Unfortunately, the PREEMIE Reauthorization Act was swept up in the now all-too-common end-of-year budgetary brinksmanship that Congress plays out. On December 20, 2024, Congress agreed on a second Continuing Resolution (HR 10545; Public Law 118-158) to extend federal spending and avert a government shutdown through March 14, 2025, and the provisions of the PREEMIE Reauthorization Act were removed from the final Continuing Resolution at the eleventh hour.[3] Still further, the PREEMIE Act remained excluded from the Full-Year Continuing Appropriations and Extensions Act (HR 1968) signed into law by the president on March 15, 2025.

When the new (119th) Congress convened in early 2025, Representative Robin L. Kelly (D-IL-2) and five of her House colleagues took up the mantle and introduced the latest version of the PREEMIE Reauthorization Act (HR 1197).[4] As written, the bill extends "research relating to preterm labor and delivery and the care, treatment, and outcomes of preterm and low birthweight infants" for the next five years, from fiscal year 2025 through fiscal year 2029.[4] In addition, the bill calls on the Secretary of the Department of Health and Human Services (HHS) to maintain an interagency working group intent on coordinating federal activities and programs related to preterm birth, infant mortality, and other adverse birth outcomes.[4] Furthermore, the bill instructs the HHS Secretary to work with the National Academies of Sciences, Engineering, and Medicine to convene a committee of experts to conduct a "Study on Preterm Births" that will examine the financial costs of premature births to society, the factors that impact preterm birth rates, and opportunities for earlier detection of premature birth risk factors.[4]

The PREEMIE Reauthorization Act of 2025 (HR 1197) takes a path-of-least-resistance approach to reauthorization, leaving intact the essential existing provisions found in previous reauthorizations. The Congressional Budget Office (CBO) assessment of a nearly identical earlier version of the bill (from the 118th Congress) stated that "Assuming appropriation of the authorized amounts and using historical spending patterns for those activities, CBO estimates that implementing [the bill] would cost $10 million over the [five year] period. Of that amount, $9 million would be for research and education."[5] Reauthorization continues to enjoy wide bipartisan and bicameral support; as of this writing, five additional bipartisan cosponsors are now included on the House Bill, and provisions of the PREEMIE Act are included in a broader Senate Bill, the Bipartisan Health Care Act (S 891), introduced by Senator Ron Wyden (D-OR) in early March. With this level of support, passage of the PREEMIE Reauthorization Act during the 119th Congress might generally seem assured; however, the heightened focus by President Trump's administration on cost-cutting and reducing federal government expenditures, including areas of scientific research, leaves the outcome of the bill anything but certain.

A strong advocacy constituency intent on ensuring Congressional passage worked throughout the 118th Congress. On June 29, 2023, the March of Dimes, along with 84 concerned organizations, wrote to Senators Bennet and John N. Boozman (R-AR) to express strong support for the PREEMIE Reauthorization Act, calling it "vital legislation to reauthorize and expand research, education and intervention activities related to preterm birth."[6] In her testimony on June 14, 2023, before the Subcommittee on Health of the House Committee on Energy and Commerce, Elizabeth Cherot, senior vice president and chief medical and health officer of the March of Dimes, warned that "The U.S. is one of the most dangerous places to give birth in the developed world, and there are unacceptable disparities in birth outcomes between women and infants of color and their White peers."[7] Among the successes of the PREEMIE Act that Cherot pointed to in her testimony was the Centers for Disease Control and Prevention's Pregnancy Risk Assessment Monitoring System, which tracks data on maternal attitudes and pregnancy experiences in 50 jurisdictions. This unique data set is used by researchers and governments to "plan and review programs and policies aimed at reducing health problems among mothers and infants" and "highlights the vital nature of this program in improving the understanding of the risks facing moms and babies."[7] Similar sentiments were articulated by maternal health care advocates when they descended on Capitol Hill on September 28, 2023, for the annual Cindy Pellegrini Maternal and Child Health Advocacy Day.[8] Such efforts no doubt will gear up again with the introduction of the new bill in the 119th Congress. Whether the efforts of these and like-minded groups will be able to convince both houses of Congress to pass the PREEMIE Reauthorization Act this time, and President Trump to continue these vital programs by signing such legislation, remains to be seen. AJPH

## CORRESPONDENCE

Correspondence should be sent to Eli Y. Adashi, MD, MS, Brown University, 222 Richmond St, Providence, RI, 02903 (e-mail: eli_adashi@brown.edu). Reprints can be ordered at https://www.ajph.org by clicking the "Reprints" link.

## PUBLICATION INFORMATION

Full Citation: Adashi EY, O'Mahony DP, Cohen IG. The unsettled PREEMIE Reauthorization Act and the recalcitrant challenge of preterm births. *Am J Public Health*. 2025;115(7):1019–1021.

Acceptance Date: March 22, 2025.

DOI: https://doi.org/10.2105/AJPH.2025.308139

## CONTRIBUTORS

All authors contributed to the writing and final approval of the article. E. Y. Adashi provided the initial conceptualization and writing of the original draft. D. P. O'Mahony provided original research and compilation of resources, as well as revising and editing of the final article. I. G. Cohen contributed to the writing, review, and editing.

## CONFLICTS OF INTEREST

I. G. Cohen is a member of the ethics advisory board for Illumina and the Bayer Bioethics Council and an advisor for World Class Health. He was also compensated for speaking at events organized by Philips with the *Washington Post* and attending the Transformational Therapeutics Leadership Forum organized by Galen Atlantica, and was retained as an expert in health privacy and reproductive technology and gender-affirming care lawsuits.

## REFERENCES

1. March of Dimes. 2024 March of Dimes Report Card for United States. November 2024. Available at: https://www.marchofdimes.org/report-card. Accessed March 13, 2024.
2. House of Representatives, Committee on Energy and Commerce. PREEMIE Reauthorization Act of 2023. House Report 118-164. August 25, 2023. Available at: https://www.congress.gov/congressional-report/118th-congress/house-report/164/1. Accessed March 13, 2024.
3. HR 10545, American Relief Act, 2025. December 21, 2024. Available at: https://www.congress.gov/bill/118th-congress/house-bill/10545. Accessed March 13, 2024.
4. HR 1197, PREEMIE Reauthorization Act of 2025. February 11, 2025. Available at: https://www.congress.gov/bill/119th-congress/house-bill/1197. Accessed March 13, 2024.
5. Congressional Budget Office. Cost Estimate: S. 1573, PREEMIE Reauthorization Act of 2023. January 26, 2024. Available at: https://www.cbo.gov/system/files/2024-01/s1573.pdf. Accessed March 13, 2024.
6. Letter to Senators Michael F. Bennet [D-CO] and John N. Boozman [R-AR] in support of the PREEMIE Reauthorization Act of 2023. June 29, 2023. Available at: https://www.boozman.senate.gov/public/_cache/files/8/1/81559bb5-3559-433c-a7ca-40653be27ef5/992D87A5EA4EB90577359463C37E21ED.preemie-letter.pdf. Accessed March 13, 2024.
7. House of Representatives. Committee on Energy and Commerce, Subcommittee on Health. Examining Proposals That Provide Access to Care for Patients and Support Research for Rare Diseases. June 14, 2023. Available at: https://d1dth6e84htgma.cloudfront.net/Elizabeth_Cherot_Witness_Testimony_06_14_23_20a6ab2dca.pdf?updated_at=2023-06-13T20:46:20.420Z. Accessed March 13, 2024.
8. Nemours Children's Health. Leading organizations advocate for better care for mothers and babies during Cindy Pellegrini Maternal & Child Health Advocacy Day. October 9, 2023. Available at: https://blog.nemours.org/2023/10/leading-organizations-advocate-for-better-care-for-mothers-and-babies-during-cindy-pellegrini-maternal-child-health-advocacy-day. Accessed March 13, 2024.

# Fluoride, Teeth, and Developing Brains: Dental Health in Tension With Environmental Health, Millions Affected

Howard Hu, MD, MPH, ScD, and Linda Birnbaum, PhD

**ABOUT THE AUTHORS**

*Howard Hu is with the Department of Population and Public Health Sciences, Keck School of Medicine, the University of Southern California, Los Angeles, CA. Linda Birnbaum is with the US National Institute of Environmental Health Sciences, Research Triangle Park, NC.*

AJPH July 2025, Vol. 115, No. 7

The recent transition in US presidential administrations may precipitate changes to the nation's policies on the fluoridation of water. Touted as a great public health achievement that dramatically reduced dental caries, water fluoridation has become the subject of intensifying environmental health research and a target for action as a threat to health by Robert F. Kennedy Jr, who was recently confirmed as the new Secretary of the Department of Health and Human Services. Fluoride was also the focus of a lawsuit by consumer groups against the US Environmental Protection Agency (EPA) that led a US District Court to conclude in September of 2024 that

> *"Plaintiffs have proven, by a preponderance of the evidence, that water fluoridation at the level of 0.7 mg/L—the prescribed optimal level of fluoridation in the United States—presents an unreasonable risk of injury to health or the environment, without consideration of costs or other non-risk factors, including an unreasonable risk to a potentially exposed or susceptible subpopulation under the conditions of use." 15 USC §2620(b)(4)(B)(ii)*[1]

The ruling was based on five years of deliberations, testimony from dozens of scientists, and the release by the US National Toxicology Program (NTP) in August 2024 of a systematic review of the literature contained in a State of the Science report[2] on fluoride. By contrast, the American Dental Association (ADA) subsequently issued an announcement stating that the court ruling provides no scientific basis for the ADA to change its endorsement of community water fluoridation,[3] a position also taken by the American Academy of Pediatrics.[4]

Unsurprisingly, this leaves the public health, medical, and dental communities, as well as the general public, confused. Policies regarding fluoridation have enormous implications for the 209 million Americans whose drinking water undergoes community fluoridation, as well as the many people whose tap water is naturally fluoridated (11 million whose fluoride concentration exceeds the current public health service recommendation of 0.7 milligrams per liter [mg/L]).

So, what are the facts and implications for science and policy?

## FLUORIDE AS A BENEFIT TO TEETH

In the 1930s and 1940s, the prevalence of dental caries (i.e., tooth decay) in the United States increased markedly following a general increase in sugar consumption.[5] This led to prospective field studies in selected US cities in the 1940s that showed that community water fluoridation was associated with a 50% to 70% reduction in caries.[6] Fluoride has been shown to prevent decay by slowing demineralization, promoting remineralization of enamel by enhancing the precipitation of hydroxyfluorapatite, and inhibiting bacterial metabolism and acid production.[7] In 1950, the ADA and the American Medical Association endorsed the widespread fluoridation of community water to a target level of 0.7 to 1.2 parts per million (mg/L). By 1969, 43.7% of the US population lived in communities supplied by fluoridated water.[8]

At the same time, however, many fluoride-containing consumer products had become available and were being used. A systematic review and meta-analysis published in 2003 found that the use of toothpastes, gels, and mouth rinses was associated with a 26% reduction in the number of decayed, missing, and filled tooth surfaces.[9] A subsequent Cochrane Collaboration systematic review and meta-analysis of 21 studies initiated after 1975 concluded that community water fluoridation led to a reduction in cavities, but with a much smaller effect size (equivalent to the prevention of one quarter of a cavity per individual) than had been seen in pre-1975 studies.[10] Research has also shown that, mechanistically, fluoride's beneficial effect predominantly occurs after tooth eruption and is a topical phenomenon (i.e., from contact of tooth surfaces with oral solutions of fluoride or fluoride that has been ingested, absorbed, and excreted into saliva).[11,12] An exception may be the pits and fissures of permanent molars, which are difficult for topical fluorides to reach and may benefit from pre-eruptive fluoride exposure.[13] On the other hand, a Cochrane Collaboration systematic review showed that fluoride supplements taken by pregnant women do not benefit the dental health of their offspring.[14]

## FLUORIDE AS A NEURODEVELOPMENTAL TOXICANT

In 2006, an expert panel convened by the US National Academies concluded that there was growing evidence that fluoride at levels of 2 to 4 mg/L in drinking water may increase the risk of skeletal fluorosis, bone fractures, IQ deficits, and assorted endocrine and other effects, and that more research was needed.[15] Such research has since accelerated, particularly with respect to epidemiology and toxicology studies relevant to neurodevelopment. In its August 2024 report, based on a detailed systematic review, the NTP concluded that fluoride exposures associated with drinking water levels exceeding 1.5 mg/L of fluoride, the limit recommended by the World Health Organization, are consistently associated with lower IQ in children.[2] Although 1.5 mg/L of fluoride is higher than the US Public Health Service's optimal water fluoride level since 2015 of 0.7 mg/L, in a meta-analysis NTP subsequently conducted of pooled data from the 13 best studies relevant to drinking water fluoride levels of less than 1.5 mg/L,[16] an increase in maternal or child urinary fluoride (a validated biomarker of fluoride exposure) of 1 mg/L was associated with a significant decrease in child IQ of 1.63 points (95% confidence interval [CI] = −2.33, −0.93). When confined to the three best studies that were prospective, rated as high quality and having a low risk of bias, and that focused on prenatal fluoride exposure, the estimated decrease in offspring IQ points associated with an increase in maternal urinary fluoride during pregnancy (MUF) was 1.70 points.

In a separate dose–response analysis by Grandjean et al. that focused on the previously mentioned three studies, an increase in maternal pregnancy urinary fluoride of 1 mg/L was associated with a decrease in IQ of 2.06 points.[17] Although the studies of fluoride and IQ lack data on US women, a recent prospective study of prenatal fluoride exposure among 490 pregnant US women living in Los Angeles, California, examined offspring behavioral outcomes and found that MUF was associated with significantly increased measures of anxiety and other internalizing behaviors.[18] The median MUF level among these US women of 0.76 mg/L is very close to 0.87 mg/L, the mean MUF level seen in both of the high-quality and low-risk-of-bias prospective studies included in the NTP and Grandjean et al. publications that found a significant negative association between prenatal fluoride exposure and offspring IQ.

In terms of biological plausibility, recent toxicological research indicates that the mechanism of fluoride's neurotoxicity may be exerted through impacts on oxidative stress, synaptic and neurotransmission dysfunction, disruption of mitochondrial and energy metabolism, and calcium channel dysregulation.[19] Another mechanism that may be at play relates to observations made in epidemiological studies that fluoride exposure is associated with reductions in maternal thyroid hormone levels[20] as well as clinical hypothyroidism,[21] which, in turn, are well-known risk factors for adverse neurodevelopmental outcomes.

## CONCLUSION

Clearly, more research is needed. We need to increase the base of evidence on the impacts on intelligence and behavior of prenatal and postnatal fluoride exposure at the levels seen in most communities. Research is needed on potential susceptibility factors, because from a policy perspective regarding risk, EPA is required to consider setting standards that provide a margin of safety, currently dramatically exceeded by EPA's regulatory limit of 4 mg/L, to protect potentially susceptible individuals. This includes pregnant women and children and, arguably, individuals who may be genetically susceptible (such as those recently found to have variants related to dopamine metabolism that are associated with amplified fluoride neurotoxicity effects[22]). Research is also needed that, apart from water fluoridation, compares the benefits in terms of caries prevention and risk of systemic ingestion of fluoride via various modes of fluoride application (e.g., the use of toothpastes, gels, and mouth rinses). New methods of fluoride application could potentially be developed that further minimize the risk of ingesting fluoride, especially in young children, while maximizing the benefit of fluoride for caries prevention.

In the meantime, however, we believe that the time has come for dental, medical, public health, environmental health, health policy, epidemiology, and risk assessment professionals to come together, weigh the evidence, and arrive at a consensus on policy recommendations and steps. As a first step, given that neither prenatal nor infant exposures to fluoride contributes toward the reduction of cavities in permanent teeth, whereas the major anticaries benefits of fluoride are from topical contact with posterupted teeth, it may be prudent to consider recommendations that minimize prenatal and infant fluoride exposure. We owe our young ones and future generations nothing less. AJPH

## CORRESPONDENCE

Correspondence should be sent to Howard Hu, MD, 2926 Graceland Way, Glendale, CA 91206 (e-mail: howard.hu@med.usc.edu). Reprints can be ordered at https://ajph.org by clicking the "Reprints" link.

## PUBLICATION INFORMATION

Full Citation: Hu H, Birnbaum L. Fluoride, teeth, and developing brains: dental health in tension with environmental health, millions affected. *Am J Public Health*. 2025;115(7):1022–1024.

Acceptance Date: April 15, 2025.

DOI: https://doi.org/10.2105/AJPH.2025.308166

ORCID iD:

Howard Hu https://orcid.org/0000-0002-3676-2707

## CONTRIBUTORS

H. Hu and L. Birnbaum discussed and agreed upon the topic, the arguments to be made, and the sources. H. Hu drafted the article, L. Birnbaum contributed edits, H. Hu drafted the revision, and L. Birnbaum contributed edits to that as well.

## ACKNOWLEDGMENTS

This work was supported by US National Institutes of Health grant R01ES021446.

**Note.** The contents of this article are solely the responsibility of the authors and do not necessarily represent the official views of the National Institute of Environmental Health Sciences or National Institutes of Health.

## CONFLICTS OF INTEREST

The authors are not aware of any affiliations, memberships, funding, or financial holdings that might be perceived as affecting the objectivity of this commentary. H. Hu served as a nonretained scientific expert witness for the recent federal trial on water fluoridation (*Food & Water Watch et al. v US Environmental Protection Agency*, US District Court for the Northern District of California at San Francisco).

## REFERENCES

1. *Food & Water Watch Inc v United States EPA*, No. 17-cv-02162-EMC, 2024 US Dist, LEXIS 172635 (ND Cal; September 24, 2024).
2. National Toxicology Program. *NTP Monograph on the State of the Science Concerning Fluoride Exposure and Neurodevelopment and Cognition: A Systematic Review.* Research Triangle Park, NC: National Institute for Environmental Health Sciences, National Institutes of Health; August 2024.
3. American Dental Association. Community water fluoridation at optimal levels is safe and effective. September 25, 2024. Available at: https://www.ada.org/about/press-releases/community-water-fluoridation-at-optimal-levels-is-safe-and-effective. Accessed November 21, 2024.
4. American Academy of Pediatrics. AAP, ADA stand by fluoride recommendations following court ruling. *American Academy of Pediatrics News*. September 26, 2024. Available at: https://publications.aap.org/aapnews/news/30299/AAP-ADA-stand-by-fluoride-recommendations?autologincheck=redirected. Accessed February 28, 2025.
5. Kearns CE, Glantz SA, Schmidt LA. Sugar industry influence on the scientific agenda of the National Institute of Dental Research's 1971 National Caries Program: a historical analysis of internal documents. *PLoS Med*. 2015;12(3):e1001798. https://doi.org/10.1371/journal.pmed.1001798
6. Centers for Disease Control and Prevention. Achievement in public health, 1990–1999. Fluoridation of drinking water to prevent dental caries. *MMWR Morb Mortal Wkly Rep*. 1992;48(41):933–940.
7. Featherstone JD. Prevention and reversal of dental caries: role of low level fluoride. *Community Dent Oral Epidemiol*. 1999;27(1):31–40. https://doi.org/10.1111/j.1600-0528.1999.tb01989.x
8. Centers for Disease Control and Prevention. Timeline for community water fluoridation. Available at: https://www.cdc.gov/fluoridation/timeline-for-community-water-fluoridation/index.html. Accessed February 28, 2025.
9. Marinho VC, Higgins JP, Logan S, Sheiham A. Topical fluoride (toothpastes, mouthrinses, gels or varnishes) for preventing dental caries in children and adolescents. *Cochrane Database Syst Rev*. 2003;2003(4):CD002782. https://doi.org/10.1002/14651858.CD002782
10. Iheozor-Ejiofor Z, Walsh T, Lewis SR, et al. Water fluoridation for the prevention of dental caries. *Cochrane Database Syst Rev*. 2024;10(10):CD010856. https://doi.org/10.1002/14651858.CD010856.pub3
11. Featherstone JD. The science and practice of caries prevention. *J Am Dent Assoc*. 2000;131(7):887–899. https://doi.org/10.14219/jada.archive.2000.0307
12. European Union. What role does fluoride play in preventing tooth decay? Scientific Committee on Fluoridation. Available at: https://ec.europa.eu/health/scientific_committees/opinions_layman/fluoridation/fr/l-3/5.htm. Accessed March 1, 2025.
13. Singh KA, Spencer AJ. Relative effects of pre- and post-eruption water fluoride on caries experience by surface type of permanent first molars. *Community Dent Oral Epidemiol*. 2004;32(6):435–446. https://doi.org/10.1111/j.1600-0528.2004.00182.x
14. Takahashi R, Ota E, Hoshi K, et al. Fluoride supplementation (with tablets, drops, lozenges or chewing gum) in pregnant women for preventing dental caries in the primary teeth of their children. *Cochrane Database Syst Rev*. 2017;10(10):CD011850. https://doi.org/10.1002/14651858.CD011850.pub2
15. National Research Council. *Fluoride in Drinking Water: A Scientific Review of EPA's Standards*. Washington, DC: The National Academies Press; 2006. https://doi.org/10.17226/11571
16. Taylor KW, Eftim SE, Sibrizzi CA, et al. Fluoride exposure and children's IQ scores: a systematic review and meta-analysis. *JAMA Pediatr*. 2025;179(3):282–292. https://doi.org/10.1001/jamapediatrics.2024.5542
17. Grandjean P, Meddis A, Nielsen F, et al. Dose dependence of prenatal fluoride exposure associations with cognitive performance at school age in three prospective studies. *Eur J Public Health*. 2024;34(1):143–149. https://doi.org/10.1093/eurpub/ckad170
18. Malin AJ, Eckel SP, Hu H, et al. Maternal urinary fluoride and child neurobehavior at age 36 months [erratum in: *JAMA Netw Open*. 2024;7(6):e2424057]. *JAMA Netw Open*. 2024;7(5):e2411987. https://doi.org/10.1001/jamanetworkopen.2024.11987
19. Zhang Y, Gao Y, Liu X. Focus on cognitive impairment induced by excessive fluoride: An update review. *Neuroscience*. 2024;558:22–29. https://doi.org/10.1016/j.neuroscience.2024.08.011
20. Hall M, Hornung R, Chevrier J, Ayotte P, Lanphear B, Till C. Fluoride exposure and thyroid hormone levels in pregnancy: The MIREC cohort. *Environ Int*. 2024;184:108442. https://doi.org/10.1016/j.envint.2024.108442
21. Peckham S, Lowery D, Spencer S. Are fluoride levels in drinking water associated with hypothyroidism prevalence in England? A large observational study of GP practice data and fluoride levels in drinking water. *J Epidemiol Community Health*. 2015;69(7):619–624. https://doi.org/10.1136/jech-2014-204971
22. Zhao L, Yu C, Lv J, et al. Fluoride exposure, dopamine relative gene polymorphism and intelligence: a cross-sectional study in China. *Ecotoxicol Environ Saf*. 2021;209:111826. https://doi.org/10.1016/j.ecoenv.2020.111826

# Yellow Power: Building Asian Student Community Voices Against Gender-Based Violence Through Public Health Research and Art

Eunhee V. Park, MPH

**ABOUT THE AUTHOR**

*Eunhee V. Park is with the Department of Community Health Sciences in the Fielding School of Public Health at the University of California, Los Angeles (UCLA).*

The Atlanta, Georgia, spa shooting in March 2021, where six of the eight victims were Asian women, stands as a chilling reminder of how racism and misogyny intersect to justify harm to Asian women.[1] Often objectified as submissive and hypersexualized, Asian women are frequently reduced to harmful stereotypes that take away their humanity. Since the COVID-19 pandemic, this objectification has intensified with anti-Asian rhetoric scapegoating Asians for the virus, amplifying hostility and bias.[2]

## AMPLIFYING COMMUNITY VOICES THROUGH RESEARCH

As a South Korean immigrant and public health student, I faced anti-Asian discrimination firsthand and witnessed the trauma it caused within my community. Experiencing this ongoing adversity compelled me to act. Starting in 2018, I joined the UC Speaks Up project, which addressed sexual violence on college campuses.[3] Leveraging this work, I focused my research on the Double Jeopardy Study, exploring the intersection of violence experienced by Asian students.[4] I worked with Jianchao Lai and Jennifer Wagman to create a trauma-informed environment within a public health research framework, where victim-survivors of sexual violence could safely share their experiences.[4] We conducted more than 50 in-depth interviews and collected more than 20 transmedia-photovoice pieces for this mixed-method study. The resilience and strength of the study participants came through as they shared their hopes for solutions to prevent violence and spare others from similar harms. I realized that my role as a public health scholar extends beyond research. I was inspired to take initiatives that supported recovery and solidarity of victim-survivors by creating beautiful community spaces.

## EXPRESSING RESILIENCE AND PAIN THROUGH CREATIVE ART

My team developed transmedia–photovoice, incorporating creative writing, painting, film, and sound narratives. This approach provided participants with a broad range of expressive tools to convey their stories. Through the art, I saw pain from gendered and racialized discrimination, violence, fetishization, silence, isolation, depression, and anxiety—alongside expression of gratitude, hope, love, resilience, and strength. These layered emotions were powerfully captured in art, revealing what numbers and words alone cannot show. The complexities of violence, the subsequent harms, and the coping processes were closely tied to participants' growth and identity formation.

## RESEARCH AND ART AS A CATALYST FOR DIALOGUE AND HEALING

We displayed interview quotes on yellow silk panels—our interpretation of "Yellow Power,"[5] inspired by 1970s Asian student activism—inviting the campus community to engage with narratives usually confined to academic journals. The installation, featuring quotes from interviews and transmedia–photovoice pieces, created a beautiful space that illuminated these experiences. The weeklong exhibition, culminating in a panel discussion, reached students and community members from UCLA and other campuses across Los Angeles, California, highlighting the power of creatively expressed lived experiences. Through this exhibition, we revealed the

AJPH July 2025, Vol. 115, No. 7

pervasive and often covert forms of violence against Asian communities. The open dialogue on stigmatized topics like sexual violence and racism was made possible by the art exhibition, which fostered respectful and empathetic discussion. The exhibit grounded participants in shared experiences and understanding as the community connected through the art, offering insights that will shape our future work in violence prevention and intervention.

## CONCLUSION

Art can feel intimidating in public health where there is no clear right or wrong answer and no *P* value to indicate significance. When I voiced these concerns, Lauren, an artist and a professor at UCLA Design Media Arts, simply said, "Have fun with it. Experiment with it and see where it takes you." That encouragement helped me embrace uncertainty and explore creatively with an open mind. As I continue to uplift often-silenced voices through research and art, I have found my own community of support—a network of shared resilience and hope. Together, we are forging a path toward healing and understanding, showing that public health can be a space not only for prevention but also for connection, reconciliation, and growth. AJPH


### CORRESPONDENCE

Correspondence should be sent to Eunhee V. Park, 650 Charles E Young S, 46-071 CHS, Los Angeles, CA 90095 (e-mail: eepark@g.ucla.edu). Reprints can be ordered at https://www.ajph.org by clicking the "Reprints" link.



### PUBLICATION INFORMATION

Full Citation: Park EV. Yellow power: building Asian student community voices against gender-based violence through public health research and art. *Am J Public Health*. 2025;115(7):1025–1026.

Acceptance Date: November 20, 2024.

DOI: https://doi.org/10.2105/AJPH.2024.307956



ORCID iD:
Eunhee V. Park https://orcid.org/0000-0001-6442-8119



### ACKNOWLEDGMENTS

Funding for the Double Jeopardy Study and exhibitions was provided by Center of Institutional Courage, UCLA Asian American Studies Center, UCLA Racial and Social Justice Grant, and AAPI Data.

I am grateful to the Double Jeopardy Study participants for sharing their experiences. Special thanks to my collaborators, Jianchao Lai and Jennifer Wagman, for their leadership and dedication, and to our incredible student researchers—Jenny Lee, Rhea Gandhi, Allison Massey, Madison Logan, Grace Nguyen, Sabrina Dou, and Sean Sugai. Nox Yang, Lauren Cramer, Anmol Gupta, and Lauren McCarthy played pivotal roles in the transmedia–photovoice project and community exhibitions. Thank you to UC Speaks Up, Center for Gender and Health Justice at UC Global Health Institute, Bruin Consent Coalition, UC Survivors and Allies, UCLA CARE, and the Oxy Sexual Assault Coalition for their invaluable partnership. Connect with us via Instagram: https://www.instagram.com/api.ucspeaksup.

### CONFLICTS OF INTEREST

The author has no conflicts of interest to report.


### REFERENCES


1. Anderson B. Prosecutor to seek hate crime charges, death penalty for spa shooting suspect. *NPR*. May 11, 2021. Available at: https://www.npr.org/2021/05/11/995915454/prosecutor-plans-to-seek-death-penalty-in-spa-shootings. Accessed August 31, 2024.
2. Chou RS. *Asian American Sexual Politics: The Construction of Race, Gender, and Sexuality*. Lanham, MD: Rowman & Littlefield; 2012.
3. Wagman JA, Amabile C, Sumstine S, et al. Student, staff, and faculty perspectives on intimate partner and sexual violence on 3 public university campuses: protocol for the UC Speaks Up study and preliminary results. *JMIR Res Protoc*. 2022;11(4):e31189. https://doi.org/10.2196/31189
4. Park E, Lai J, Gandhi R, et al. Double Jeopardy Study protocol: mixed-methods study to understand ANHPI college students at the intersection of sexual violence and anti-Asian racism after COVID-19. Preprint. Posted online November 5, 2024. Research Square. https://doi.org/10.21203/rs.3.rs-5272796/v1
5. Watkins R. *Black Power, Yellow Power, and the Making of Revolutionary Identities*. Jackson, MS: University Press of Mississippi; 2012.

# Disability Dream Work for the Public's Health

Vishal Sivamani and Stacy V. Lu, MSPH

**ABOUT THE AUTHORS**

*Vishal Sivamani (they/them) is with the Public Health Studies Program, Krieger School of Arts and Sciences, Johns Hopkins University, Baltimore, MD. Stacy V. Lu (she/her) is with the Department of Population, Family and Reproductive Health, Johns Hopkins Bloomberg School of Public Health, Baltimore, MD.*

The authors are two queer disabled people of color trained in public health at a large private research institution in the United States. The first author is an undergraduate student and the second author is a doctoral candidate.

Disability justice aims to achieve collective access and liberation for all people—leaving no body or mind behind.[1] Public health shares similar goals to protect and promote the health of people and their communities. However, disabled people and the disability community, especially those who are multiply marginalized, have often been harmed and forgotten in public health efforts.

Any discussion of advancing public health must consider the locus of where empirical knowledge is produced and where the producers of that knowledge gain their bearing. Issues related to disability representation are rife in the scientific community, as disabled people are underrepresented in higher faculty positions and earn lower salaries than nondisabled people.[2] Opportunities for public health graduate training and course offerings focused on disability and health disparities experienced by the disability community are limited.[3] These issues likely shape and are shaped by the dominant perspective in public health that disability is a problem that needs to be solved. As disabled students and researchers, we are not mere observers of the public health topics we learn about and investigate. We are part of the population that experiences disability health disparities, and we are the people represented in the prevalence of disparities many public health efforts strive to reduce.

The exclusion of disabled students and the exploitation of "disabled labor"[4] in public health education are silenced in common dialogue yet highly prescient in the content and form of knowledge production that begets public health innovation. Productivity is often considered a necessary attribute and important marker of success in the academy. Being disabled means that we have a different experience of time and pace of production living in "crip time."[5] Crip time is nonlinear and unpredictable, and we lose track of days and the sense of our surroundings when hyperfocusing on an idea that strikes. Crip time is collective wisdom gained from feeling and responding to the familiar signals in our bodies and minds that can be learned only through living. Crip time is life strategy, as we cannot thrive unless we survive and we cannot survive unless we slow down and rest.

However, educational institutions are structured in ways that inherently block out such modes of disabled knowledge production and existence. University accommodations are often inaccessible despite their intended purpose to meet students' access needs. We have personally encountered several bureaucratic barriers and costs—of money, time, and "spoons"[6] or disabled units of energy—in our experiences seeking disability accommodations. The consequences of these educational structures reproduce standardized lacunae surrounding the advancement of health and disability research. They further entrench these inequities by hindering recruitment and development of the next generation of disabled scholars along with their untapped potential to creatively reimagine the future of public health. This presents great harm not just to disabled scholars and the disability community but to members of the larger population who would all benefit from disability-led public health approaches.

An equitable future does not exist without achieving disability justice. We dare you to do the "dream work"[7] with us, to imagine a future where all bodies and minds are truly and wholly included and cared for[1] and make it a reality. We call you to question the norms we take for granted in public health. We invite you to join us in affirming and preserving disabled ways of being and doing, in all of our brilliance and messiness, to secure a more equitable future for all. AJPH

## CORRESPONDENCE

Correspondence should be sent to Stacy V. Lu, MSPH, Johns Hopkins Bloomberg School of Public Health, 615 N Wolfe St, Baltimore, MD 21205 (e-mail: slu47@jh.edu). Reprints can be ordered at https://www.ajph.org by clicking the "Reprints" link.

## PUBLICATION INFORMATION

Full Citation: Sivamani V, Lu SV. Disability dream work for the public's health. *Am J Public Health.* 2025;115(7):1027–1028.

Acceptance Date: December 8, 2024.

DOI: https://doi.org/10.2105/AJPH.2024.307972

ORCID iDs:
Vishal Sivamani https://orcid.org/0009-0006-2058-1932

Stacy V. Lu https://orcid.org/0000-0001-5941-533X

## CONTRIBUTORS

Both authors contributed substantially to all aspects of this work. V. Sivamani led the conceptualization, analysis, and writing of the original draft. As the project supervisor, S. V. Lu provided overall mentorship and support throughout the process and led the review and editing of the article.

## ACKNOWLEDGMENTS

The perspectives offered in this publication are those of the authors.

## CONFLICTS OF INTEREST

Both authors declare that they have no conflicts of interest.

## REFERENCES

1. Articulating a movement. In: *Skin, Tooth, and Bone: The Basis of Movement Is Our People.* 2nd ed. Berkeley, CA: Sins Invalid; 2019:10–27.
2. Castro F, Stuart E, Deal J, Varadaraj V, Swenor BK. STEM doctorate recipients with disabilities experienced early in life earn lower salaries and are underrepresented among higher academic positions. *Nat Hum Behav.* 2024;8(1):72–81. https://doi.org/10.1038/s41562-023-01745-z
3. Akakpo CW, Lobianco A, Lollar D. Inclusion of disability content in graduate public health curricula. *Am J Public Health.* 2020;110(10):1509–1511. https://doi.org/10.2105/AJPH.2020.305882
4. Wong A. Labor, care work, and disabled queer femmes. Available at: https://disabilityvisibilityproject.com/2017/10/22/ep-6-labor-care-work-and-disabled-queer-femmes. Accessed December 8, 2024.
5. Gauthier-Mamaril É. MedHums 101: what is crip time? Available at: https://thepolyphony.org/2024/01/26/medhums-101-what-is-crip-time. Accessed December 1, 2024.
6. Miserandino C. The spoon theory. Available at: https://butyoudontlooksick.com/articles/written-by-christine/the-spoon-theory. Accessed December 1, 2024.
7. Lewis TA. The birth of resistance: courageous dreams, powerful nobodies & revolutionary madness. In: Wong A, ed. *Resistance and Hope: Essays by Disabled People.* San Francisco, CA: Disability Visibility Project; 2018:33–38.

# Stride by Stride: How Run Clubs Foster Public Health

Lilian N. Bui

**ABOUT THE AUTHOR**

*The author is with the Feinberg School of Medicine, Northwestern University, Chicago, IL.*

On Instagram, the West Town Brew Crew,[1] a run club based in Chicago, Illinois, posted a screenshot of Robert Putnam's *New York Times* interview and captioned it "HEY POLITICAL PEOPLE IN TOWN if you support democracy then you should run outside with friends." In his interview, Putnam,[2] author of *Bowling Alone*, stated "How does having fun in a running club, for example, translate to democracy? How does that small germ of social connection in a club then translate to 'I believe in this whole experiment?'" Like the democratic experiment, public health relies on community building, which run clubs do remarkably well.

For me, running and community go hand in hand. Running is often considered a solitary activity. But if it was only that, I would never have started running for fun. Before college, I ran only when I had to for gym class. I started running out of my own free will as a Back on My Feet (BoMF)[3] volunteer. This nonprofit aims to "empower people to achieve economic independence through fitness and community." I volunteered weekly at BoMF morning runs throughout my entire undergraduate career, as did many other students once they joined.

Our commitment was not because we loved running at 5:30 on Friday mornings. We were college students, after all. It was because we loved spending time with each other and the program participants. An organization such as BoMF redefines volunteering and community engagement. It blurs power dynamics through an activity in which everyone is doing the same thing. An observer would not know who is running as a beneficiary of the nonprofit versus who is running for community service hours.

Through running with BoMF, I connected with people I would not have encountered on my college campus. I would not have appreciated the differences between the city streets and suburban sidewalks. BoMF models what Putnam called "doing with," relying on direct interpersonal engagement, as opposed to "doing for," which is aiding from a distance.[4] Although many other organizations provide housing and employment resources in the spirit of doing for, few break the barrier between those who are serving and those who are served. Of course, power differences still exist, but in the morning runs everyone is a runner.

Likewise, Walk with a Doc[5] and Walk with a Future Doc exemplify doing with. These nonprofit organizations create a space for community members and health care providers to discuss health topics while walking. As a medical student in my local chapter, I met Chicago residents who told me about free physical activity events for seniors, which I then shared with patients in my continuity clinic. We had a mutual exchange of information. I shared lifestyle medicine tips, and participants shared their deep knowledge of community resources. This demonstrates the relationship between social capital and public health. Participants later organized their own walks in addition to the ones led by Walk with a Future Doc. Social connection thus facilitated sustainable behavior change.

Independently organized, freestanding run clubs also create spaces for diverse people to gather without fees and prerequisites. Chicago Run Collective emphasizes its social component, making the club palpable for novice runners. With 436 000 Instagram followers, this run club could be mistaken for a major race event. It puts the "club" in run club with signs reading "Saturdays are for clubbin'" and dance music blasting. I met Turkish medical students, Lollapalooza concertgoers, laborers, and financial consultants who were all eager to converse with new people. I watched Allport's intergroup contact theory play out. Allport[6] proposed the idea of prejudice reduction through positive contact under four conditions: equal status within the situation, common goals, intergroup cooperation, and support of authorities, law, or custom. The trend of informal, recreational social clubs such as run clubs enacts Allport's theory. Run clubs, particularly large ones such as Chicago Run Collective, often fulfill Allport's conditions and provide a starting point for improving intergroup relations.

After a run, people often continue socializing whether through planning other runs, walking dogs together, or participating in potlucks. These are all wonderful extensions of Chicago's Shut Up and Run Club, for example. Run clubs cement outdoor urban spaces as third spaces where people can gather without spending money. They expand

AJPH July 2025, Vol. 115, No. 7

social networks that people long for outside of their professional lives. As Rebecca Solnit[7] wrote in *A Paradise Built in Hell: The Extraordinary Communities That Arise in Disaster*,

> We have, most of us, a deep desire for this democratic public life, for a voice, for membership, for purpose and meaning that cannot be only personal. We want larger selves and a larger world.

Run clubs connect people with each other and physical spaces, thus reminding individuals why they have a stake in public health interests.

Obviously, run clubs provide the health benefit of physical activity. What differentiates a run club from running alone, though, are the perks of social interaction: accountability for the physical activity and amplified mental health benefits. A review of recent longitudinal research[8] demonstrated that social connectedness, via strong support and expansive networks, protects adults from depression and anxiety disorders. From learning about a run club on social media, where many clubs post meeting times and locations, to getting outside to directly connect with others, run clubs combat social isolation in this digital age. Outdoor exercise, also known as green exercise, may have additive benefits for mood and enjoyment of the activity.[9] In alignment with the World Health Organization's definition of health, freestanding run clubs promote physical, mental, and social well-being.[10]

Across the country, run clubs have brought people of varying running abilities and backgrounds together. According to one runner from Stamford, Connecticut:

> [Runners Collective/Social Athletic Run Club] has such a diverse group of people. I never knew people from so many different career paths were even in my area. There's that saying about the company you keep, the circle you maintain—these people each inspire me to be and do more and better things in different ways—and I'd like to think I do the same. Whether it's physical or mental health, religion/spirituality, relationship advice, hobbies, following your passions—you name it—we've talked about it!

A runner in Chicago gave a shout out to Read and Run Chicago:

> it's an incredible run club that highlights local authors and books about Chicago in their runs, they broaden my perspective about the community and history of Chicago.

A Lakeview Run Club participant reported: "Run club is probably the only community event I attend. . . it's social suffering!" And to the West Coast, an avid runner in Eugene, Oregon, stated "Often I go to a run club to try new shoes or try running gear like hydration/electrolytes or learn new running routes."

Increased use of public spaces for running may, in turn, raise awareness of public space needs and encourage policymakers to develop safe, attractive running environments. Novice and experienced runners alike prefer lively, green, and comfortable running surfaces.[11] A plethora of cycling advocacy organizations such as Slow Roll Chicago[12] already exist to encourage the creation of safe bike lanes and cycling as a form of transportation and exercise. With a shared mission for mobility justice, run clubs and cycling groups could unite their political organizing power to advocate for urban planning aligned with public health interests.

Are run clubs the new bowling club? Perhaps, according to Putnam—but they are so much more. By inviting strangers to run in public spaces without cost, on a regular basis, run clubs foster new relationships, build social capital, and nurture our compassion, care, and interests in broader, inclusive communities. The accessibility of run clubs across communities is the crux of their power. Public health is invested not in individuals but, rather, in a collective people. Although run clubs do benefit the individual, their aggregate influence as a social phenomenon undeniably promotes and serves public interests. AJPH


## CORRESPONDENCE

Correspondence should be sent to Lilian Bui, 420 E Superior St, Chicago, IL 60611 (e-mail: lilian.bui@northwestern.edu). Reprints can be ordered at https://www.ajph.org by clicking the "Reprints" link.



## PUBLICATION INFORMATION

Full Citation: Bui LN. Stride by stride: how run clubs foster public health. *Am J Public Health*. 2025;115(7): 1029–1031.

Acceptance Date: December 8, 2024.

DOI: https://doi.org/10.2105/AJPH.2024.307973



ORCID iD:

Lilian N. Bui https://orcid.org/0000-0002-2664-4862



## ACKNOWLEDGMENTS

I thank Joseph Feinglass and Mita Goel for their mentorship, the runners who shared their insights, and run clubs for existing.


## CONFLICTS OF INTEREST

The author has been a student leader of Back on My Feet and Walk with a Future Doc and a participant in several run clubs, and she currently works a part-time job at Heartbreak Hill Running Company, which may be considered constituting a real, potential, or apparent conflict of interest.

## REFERENCES


1. westtownbrewcrew Instagram page. #HEY POLITICAL PEOPLE IN TOWN if you support democracy then you should run outside with friends Available at: https://www.instagram.com/p/C-3giAfvesa/?igsh=X2tXczdMYVM5&img_index=1. Accessed August 27, 2024.

2. Garcia-Navarro L. Robert Putnam knows why you're lonely. Available at: https://www.nytimes.com/2024/07/13/magazine/robert-putnam-interview.html. Accessed August 26, 2024.
3. Back on My Feet. About us. Available at: https://backonmyfeet.org/about-us. Accessed August 26, 2024.
4. Hudson A. Bowling alone at twenty. Available at: https://www.nationalaffairs.com/publications/detail/bowling-alone-at-twenty. Accessed August 27, 2024.
5. Walk with a Doc. Our mission. Available at: https://walkwithadoc.org/who-we-are/our-mission. Accessed August 27, 2024.
6. Allport G. *The Nature of Prejudice*. White Plains, NY: Addison-Wesley; 1954.
7. Solnit R. *A Paradise Built in Hell: The Extraordinary Communities That Arise in Disaster*. New York: Viking Adult; 2009.
8. Wickramaratne PJ, Yangchen T, Lepow L, et al. Social connectedness as a determinant of mental health: a scoping review. *PLoS One*. 2022;17(10):e0275004. https://doi.org/10.1371/journal.pone.0275004
9. Lahart I, Darcy P, Gidlow C, Calogiuri G. The effects of green exercise on physical and mental wellbeing: a systematic review. *Int J Environ Res Public Health*. 2019;16(8):1352. https://doi.org/10.3390/ijerph16081352
10. World Health Organization. Basic documents. Available at: https://apps.who.int/gb/bd. Accessed December 20, 2024.
11. Deelen I, Janssen M, Vos S, Kamphuis CBM, Ettema D. Attractive running environments for all? A cross-sectional study on physical environmental characteristics and runners' motives and attitudes, in relation to the experience of the running environment. *BMC Public Health*. 2019;19(1):366. https://doi.org/10.1186/s12889-019-6676-6
12. Shefsky J, Cornejo T. Slow Roll Chicago. Available at: https://news.wttw.com/2014/11/12/slow-roll-chicago. Accessed December 20, 2024.

# *AJPH* Project Examines the *Journal*'s Past Representation of Historically Marginalized Populations

*Theodore M. Brown, PhD, Marian Moser Jones, PhD, and Cassia Roth, PhD*

**ABOUT THE AUTHORS**

*Theodore M. Brown is professor emeritus of history and public health sciences, University of Rochester, Rochester, NY. Marian Moser Jones is with the College of Public Health, The Ohio State University, Columbus. Cassia Roth is with the Department of Society, Environment, and Health Equity, University of California, Riverside. All three authors are* AJPH *associate editors.*

AJPH July 2025, Vol. 115, No. 7

In conjunction with this year's celebration of *AJPH*'s 115th anniversary, we have undertaken a retrospective examination of how well *AJPH* has done with regard to publication on health issues in different groups that other scientific literature has identified as historically underrepresented or represented in a disrespectful or distorted manner. Initially, we examined the *Journal*'s past treatment of the health issues of Black, Hispanic/Latino/as, LGBTQ+ (lesbian, gay, bisexual, transgender, queer or questioning, and all subsects), and South Asian individuals. This initial examination is not intended to be exhaustive: the *Journal*'s past representation of health issues in connection with other historically marginalized US and non-US populations—American Indians and Alaska Natives, Native Hawaiian and other Pacific Islanders, East Asians and East Asian Americans, Arab Americans, veterans, and people with disabilities to name a few—also warrants retrospective study. However, we must start somewhere, and the health of the four population groups (or historically designated groups that approximate these contemporary categories) mentioned have been perennial topics for the journal.

We have worked on the preliminaries of this project for several months and have recruited students from The Ohio State University and the University of Rochester to work with us. Together we have begun to delve into *AJPH*'s publications in these areas over the 115-year span of its history. Theodore M. Brown continues to provide leadership for the project and will work with the students as we move into the next phase, which is to form close working partnerships with outstanding historical scholars who have known expertise and to pursue a series of collaborative studies of the *Journal*'s publication history in each of the four areas we have identified.

Brown has already noticed some dramatic historical trends. In the 1910s, several *AJPH* articles referred to "Negroes" as a major health problem for Whites because "Negro" populations were said to be particularly disease ridden owing to allegedly inferior inheritance, poor habits, and substandard levels of hygiene. Only certain *AJPH* authors focused on "Negro poverty" and other social challenges and their health consequences. In the 1920s the number of studies reflecting a more balanced and sympathetic perspective by White authors increased, and in the 1930s these authors were joined by self-identified "Negro" authors who also advanced that analytical perspective. By the 1940s and 1950s, issues of segregation, racial bias, and institutional discrimination became central concerns as both "Negro" and White authors contributed significant studies. In the 1960s many articles in the *Journal* reflected the concerns of the Civil Rights Movement. In 1968 the American Public Health Association elected its first Black president, and by the end of the 1960s there were intense debates in the pages of *AJPH* over the challenges of poverty and the hopes of Black families as well as the promise and threat embodied in calls for "Black Power."

These preliminary observations need to be explored and tested in collaboration with an established Black historical scholar, and the same needs to be done for *AJPH* publications on the health of Hispanic/Latino/as, LGBTQ+, and South Asian individuals. When we form our academic collaborations, we will work in teams to delve into the details and nuances of *AJPH*'s pattern and content of publication with regard to the health of these populations over the course of its history. This approach will make our project much like the project undertaken by the *New England Journal of Medicine*, which has launched an exploration of its own publication history with a series of articles on the theme "Recognizing Historical Injustices in Medicine and the Journal." Led by a group of Harvard historians of medicine and public health, the series was launched with the December 6, 2023, article "Slavery and the Journal—Reckoning With History and Complicity."[1] This was followed by other articles published at intervals in 2024.

*AJPH*'s self-reflective project will proceed via collaboration with specialty area historical scholars. Together we will look at our own publication history, both at moments that cause retrospective embarrassment and at moments that make us proud. We will publish the results of these studies when research and analysis for each is completed over the course of the next year. AJPH

## CORRESPONDENCE

Correspondence should be sent to Theodore M. Brown, Department of History, University of Rochester, 362B Rush Rhees Library, P.O. Box 270070, Rochester, NY 14627 (e-mail: theodore_brown@urmc.rochester.edu). Reprints can be ordered at https://www.ajph.org by clicking the "Reprints" link.

## PUBLICATION INFORMATION

Full Citation: Brown TM, Jones MM, Roth C. *AJPH* project examines the *Journal*'s past representation of historically marginalized populations. *Am J Public Health*. 2025;115(7):1032–1033.

Acceptance Date: February 19, 2025.

DOI: https://doi.org/10.2105/AJPH.2025.308093

## CONTRIBUTORS

T. M. Brown wrote the first draft of the editorial. M. Moser Jones wrote a second draft. C. Roth contributed several specific textual edits.

## CONFLICTS OF INTEREST

The authors have no conflicts of interest to disclose.

## REFERENCE

1. Jones DS, Podolsky SH, Bannon Kerr M, Hammonds E. Slavery and the journal—reckoning with history and complicity. *N Engl J Med*. 2023;389(23):2117–2123. https://doi.org/10.1056/NEJMp2307309

# Point of View: Portraits of Maternal Mental Health

Jennifer Glance, DO, and Jeffrey A. Nielson, MD, MS

The resilience of the human spirit is not easily summarized in words. The depiction of this complex, abstract concept can be communicated nonverbally through visual art. The ability to perceive and respond to others' emotions is an essential human trait. A painting from the series Point of View: Portrait With Still Life, oil on canvas, was exhibited at the 2024 American Public Health Association's (APHA's) Student Think Tank art exhibition. Viewers were encouraged to share their lived experiences through verbal or written storytelling during the exhibition.

My aim in exhibiting this artwork was to engage the viewer in exploring their own point of view regarding maternal mental health. By encouraging viewers to explore their own experiences with maternal mental health, I hoped to increase empathy to cultivate sustainable change. Health care workers who viewed the art were able to demonstrate cognitive empathy by seeing mental health through the subject's point of view. Viewers expressed empathy through shared storytelling of lived experiences with maternal mental health.

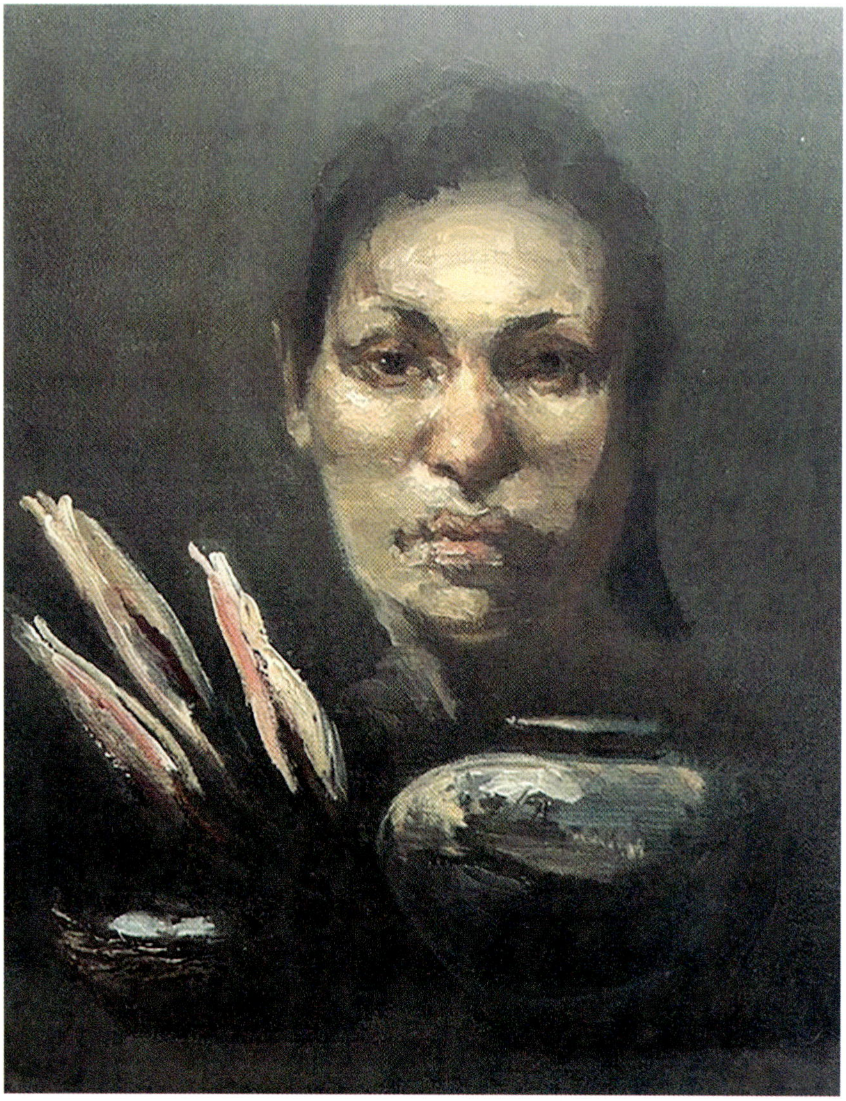

**FIGURE 1— Image From the Painting Series POV: Portrait With Still Life, Oil on Canvas, by Jennifer Glance, 2025**

## BACKGROUND

Resilient Beginnings is a Health Resources and Services Administration Rural Maternal Health Resident Education grant–sponsored activity that aims to increase resident training in maternal mental health.[1–7] The residency program offers obstetrical training, maternal mental health didactics, and an annual empathy training course. Owing to the anecdotal finding of health care workers' increased cognitive empathy at the APHA Student Think Tank art exhibition, it was felt that sharing art from the series might have measurable educational value for local family medicine residents. Secondarily, we sought to determine whether the activity had an impact on emotional and cognitive empathy.

## METHODS

A painting from the series POV: Portrait With Still Life along with a verbal description of the artwork were presented to Soin Family Medicine residents and Resilient Beginnings health care workers. The narrative was provided as the participants viewed the painting (Figure 1). The painting was described as a representation of a recently delivered mother who encountered a health crisis. A voluntary online survey was provided. Respondents were given a Likert scale to select how the painting made them feel. Options ranged from extreme negative emotions (e.g., anger, anxiety, and depression) to extreme positive feelings of happiness. Participants were asked whether they interpreted the painting from one of three perspectives: their own point of view (emotional empathy), the subject's point of view (cognitive empathy), or as the subject (also cognitive empathy). Respondents had the opportunity to provide a free text response.

## RESULTS

Twenty-nine family medicine residents and two additional health care workers viewed the painting. Fourteen responses (48.6%) were completed. Twelve responses were from residents and two were from the other health care workers; 78.6% of survey respondents demonstrated emotional empathy: the ability to share an emotion with the subject. On a Likert scale, 0% reported feelings of anger, contentedness, or happiness. Overall, 78.6% (n = 7) of respondents reported feeling some degree of sadness: 28.6% (n = 4) reported "I feel sad," 50% (n = 7) reported feeling "mildly sad," and the remaining 21.4% (n = 3) selected "I feel neutral." Free text responses included a "sense of desperation and loss." Another respondent stated, "I can't place why the painting makes me feel sad. I appreciate that it evoked an emotional response." Other comments included that the subject looked solemn and possibly depressed because of physical abuse or trauma; however, they did not see the connection with maternal mental health in the painting without the artist's narrative. Regarding the type of empathy invoked, 93% (n = 13) of respondents saw the painting from their own point of view, and 7% (n = 1) saw the painting from the subject's point of view.

Shared storytelling was elicited during the presentation of the painting. One participant revealed that she did not consider the postpartum client's point of view when discussing tobacco abuse. "I see now that was her only way to cope. I did not consider everything she had to deal with being a new mom. Smoking was her only way to deal with her stress." One health care worker had both affective and cognitive empathy. "She has a look of despair. Now I understand her point of view. She is saying, 'The health care policies that are supposed to protect me are barriers to my care. The system is against me.'" Cognitive empathy was increased during direct conversation with the artist during the viewing. The artist's narrative alongside the artwork increased viewer reflection, cognitive empathy, and increased awareness of previous medical bias in past patient or client encounters.

## DISCUSSION

Providing medical students with empathy training is an official goal of the American Medical Colleges. However, empathy training skills decline at the time of graduation.[8,9] Patient-centered care is one of the six aims for health care improvement of the National Academy of Medicine (formerly the Institute of Medicine).[10] Empathy is important in patient-centered care, but tools to measure and teach empathy vary in their impact.[9,11] Interaction with imagery followed by an artist's narrative is a unique method of demonstrating emotional and cognitive empathy in viewers.[9,11] This method may help providers debrief and gain insight into the patient's point of view. Our study showed that supplementary empathy training had positive results.

Another interesting concept is Health Equity Rounds: a case-based conference series that has been shown to mitigate medical bias among residents.[12] However, maternal mental health is not a topic that is generally covered. This might be an interesting future direction.

## CONCLUSIONS

This study shows that empathy training using a case study format is successful for resident and health care worker empathy training on maternal mental health[8]: 78.6% of survey respondents expressed affective empathy when viewing the painting with a verbal description, whereas 7% expressed cognitive empathy. This suggests that experiencing portraiture art accompanied by a case narrative is a unique and effective way to supplement empathy training in health care providers.[11] Incorporation of this form of empathy training may help health care providers sustain their ability to effectively read nonverbal cues and appreciate the patient's perspective.

The ability to perceive and respond to emotions is an essential human trait. Emotions can be difficult to communicate. Art, like emotions, can be abstract and difficult to describe. Art as a form of communication can facilitate discussions of emotions and promote empathy. Understanding the patient's point of view is an important aspect of patient-centered care. Cognitive empathy and seeing another person's perspective leads to successful patient–provider relationships. Physicians who can read and respond to nonverbal cues can address patient anxiety[8] and provide patient-centered care. In this way, health care providers will help to carry the human spirit and promote resilience. AJPH

## ABOUT THE AUTHORS

Jennifer Glance is a clinical informatics fellow and project director of the Health Resources and Services Administration Rural Maternal Health Resident Education grant, Kettering Health, Miamisburg, OH, and a clinical professor with the Department of Obstetrics and Gynecology, Wright State University, Dayton, OH. Jeffrey A. Nielson is the clinical informatics program director at Kettering Health, Miamisburg, OH.

## CORRESPONDENCE

Correspondence should be sent to Jennifer Glance, DO, Department of Medical Education, Soin Medical Center, 3535 Pentagon Blvd, Beavercreek, OH 45431 (e-mail: jennifer.glance@ketteringhealth.org). Reprints can be ordered at https://www.ajph.org by clicking the "Reprints" link.

## PUBLICATION INFORMATION

Full Citation: Glance J, Nielson JA. Point of view: portraits of maternal mental health. *Am J Public Health*. 2025;115(7):1034–1036.

Acceptance Date: February 4, 2025.

DOI: https://doi.org/10.2105/AJPH.2025.308064

ORCID iD:

Jennifer Glance https://orcid.org/0009-0006-6064-6091

## CONTRIBUTORS

J. Glance designed and conceptualized the study. J. A. Nielson contributed to draft revisions and provided final approval of the version to be published.

## ACKNOWLEDGMENTS

Funding for this work was provided by the Health Resources and Services Administration, Rural Maternal Health Resident Education (grant T34 HP 42126).

The subjects appearing in the paintings are fictional representations. Any resemblance to actual persons, living or dead, is coincidental.

## CONFLICTS OF INTEREST

The authors have no conflicts of interest to disclose.

## HUMAN PARTICIPANT PROTECTION

The Kettering Health institutional review board has determined this study to be exempt from institutional review board (IRB) oversight (IRB reference KHN-2025-3).

## REFERENCES

1. Curry SJ, Krist AH, Owens DK, et al. Interventions to prevent perinatal depression: US Preventive Services Task Force recommendation statement. *JAMA*. 2019;321(6):580–587. https://doi.org/10.1001/jama.2019.0007
2. Wyckoff AS. Ruling on Medicaid coverage of maternal depression screening a "victory" for children. June 21, 2016. Available at: https://publications.aap.org/aapnews/news/13444/Ruling-on-Medicaid-coverage-of-maternal-depression. Accessed March 12, 2025.
3. Payne JL, Umberson D, Kellogg E. Maternal mental health: where should our research and policy priorities be? *NAM Perspect*. 2020;2020:10.31478/202011g. https://doi.org/10.31478/202011g
4. Screening and diagnosis of mental health conditions during pregnancy and postpartum: ACOG clinical practice guideline no. 4. *Obstet Gynecol*. 2023;141(6):1232–1261. https://doi.org/10.1097/AOG.0000000000005200
5. Byatt N, Masters GA, Twyman J, et al. Building obstetric provider capacity to address perinatal depression through online training. *J Womens Health (Larchmt)*. 2021;30(10):1386–1394. https://doi.org/10.1089/jwh.2020.8843
6. Treatment and management of mental health conditions during pregnancy and postpartum: ACOG clinical practice guideline no. 5. *Obstet Gynecol*. 2023;141(6):1262–1288. https://doi.org/10.1097/AOG.0000000000005202
7. Pearlstein T, Howard M, Salisbury A, Zlotnick C. Postpartum depression. *Am J Obstet Gynecol*. 2009;200(4):357–364. https://doi.org/10.1016/j.ajog.2008.11.033
8. D'souza PC, Rasquinha SL, D'souza TL, Jain A, Kulkarni V, Pai K. Effect of a single-session communication skills training on empathy in medical students. *Acad Psychiatry*. 2020;44(3):289–294. https://doi.org/10.1007/s40596-019-01158-z
9. Paulus CM, Meinken S. The effectiveness of empathy training in health care: a meta-analysis of training content and methods. *Int J Med Educ*. 2022;13:1–9. https://doi.org/10.5116/ijme.61d4.4216
10. US Institute of Medicine Committee on Quality of Health Care in America. *Crossing the Quality Chasm: A New Health System for the 21st Century*. Washington, DC: US National Academies Press; 2001.
11. Nembhard IM, David G, Ezzeddine I, Betts D, Radin J. A systematic review of research on empathy in health care. *Health Serv Res*. 2023;58(2):250–263. https://doi.org/10.1111/1475-6773.14016
12. Nash KA, Perdomo J, Hsu HE. Health equity rounds—root-cause and solutions-oriented discussions of medical racism. *N Engl J Med*. 2024;391(19):1763–1765. https://doi.org/10.1056/NEJMp2410910

# Beyond Boundaries: Navigating Challenges and Charting the Future of Reproductive Health Care in the Post-*Roe* Landscape

*Tuyet Mai Ha Hoang, PhD, MS, Radia DeLuna, MA, Elise Albertson, BS, Ainslee Wong, BS, Aaron Santoyo, and Victoria Ferrara*

We explored the challenges facing abortion providers after *Dobbs v Jackson Women's Health Organization* was decided in 2022. We conducted six focus groups with 26 abortion providers between October 2023 and April 2024. Two themes emerged: (1) there was a lack of comprehensive patient care, and (2) we must forge a collective future for reproductive health. Our findings demonstrate that abortion bans contribute directly to the increasing burden on providers and to diminishing resources. We identify recommendations and multilevel solutions from stakeholders to address care coordination challenges. (*Am J Public Health*. 2025;115(7):1037–1041. https://doi.org/10.2105/AJPH.2025.308084)

AJPH July 2025, Vol. 115, No. 7

In 2022, when the landmark *Roe v Wade* (410 US 113 [1973]) decision was overturned, 13 states sought to criminalize all abortions through trigger bans. Legislators expected these bans to drastically reduce the number of abortions. However, that is not what happened. The abortion bans did not prevent people from seeking care but, rather, forced individuals, including those with limited resources, to travel farther to receive care.[1–3] The lack of access to abortion providers is a growing concern. States where abortion is legal are increasingly challenged as they balance resources and support providers, and providers face increased demands and higher levels of stress.[3,4]

## STUDY OBJECTIVE

To understand this tension and explore remedies, our objectives were twofold: (1) to explore the experiences of abortion providers and how they navigate difficulties, and (2) to offer recommendations based on stakeholders' experiences.

## PARTICIPANTS, SAMPLE, GEOGRAPHIC LOCATION, SETTING, AND YEAR OF STUDY

We conducted six virtual focus groups with 26 abortion providers between October 2023 and April 2024. The age of the participants ranged from 26 to 35 years, and most provided care in a Northeastern or Northwestern state. Most identified as non-Hispanic White and female (see supplemental material, available as a supplement to the online version of this article at http://www.ajph.org).

## METHODS

We used a semistructured interview protocol and conducted a reflexive thematic analysis (supplemental material).[5]

## KEY FINDINGS

We identified two themes: (1) there is a lack of comprehensive patient care, and (2) it is essential to forge a collective future for reproductive health.

### Lack of Comprehensive Patient Care

Providers reported consistent challenges in their attempts to deliver practical and logistical support to their patients. Four subthemes demonstrate these challenges.

*Breakdown of logistical support.* Providers shared their stories of struggling to continue care as logistical barriers, such as funding and travel support for patients, have increased. By law, federal funding cannot be used to provide abortion. Therefore, abortion clinics rely primarily on state-level aid and donations to provide abortion care.[6] Seventeen states stipulate that Medicaid must cover all abortions deemed necessary to protect the woman's health.[7] For individuals seeking care who do not qualify for Medicaid, donations and grants are necessary to alleviate financial burdens. Because donations and grants have dwindled over time since *Dobbs v Jackson Women's Health Organization* (597 US 215 [2022]) was decided, providers reported that their patients need more support and resources to pay for care, travel, lodging, and childcare.[8,9] One provider said:

> So many people are having to travel much further . . . and needing to take time off of work, and needing childcare, and needing help with transportation. And for every patient that we do see here in Washington [who] are [sic] able to travel from whatever state they're from, I know there's so many other patients who have not been able to come here . . . and are essentially forced to continue unwanted pregnancy.

*Psychosocial costs to providers and their patients.* Providers expressed intense feelings, such as guilt and anger. Some who moved from restricted states to abortion-access states reported feeling that they had "abandoned" their former communities and patients. They also described overwhelming feelings of sadness and anxiety at the growing number of patients coming into their clinics from up to 2000 miles away. Feelings of dread and anxiety reflected fear of harm or retribution for providing this necessary health care as well as looming burnout[10–12]:

> I do feel much more stress and, sort of, obligation to bring everything I have to work and to, sort of, just exhaust all of my personal resources and I always feel like I am not quite doing enough.

Providers emphasized that their patients also felt compounding stressors, such as expending limited resources to access health care.[13]:

> People have used so much of their coping mechanisms. . . . And then, by the time they get to the facility, they really need so much more support because they're sort of out of coping mechanisms . . . [and] are a lot more stressed.

*Lack of updated information among stakeholders.* Providers highlighted a lack of updated information and guidance available on health care protocols. Given the ever-changing political landscape, policies related to abortion care are constantly in flux. Consequently, to ensure their own and their communities' safety and well-being, providers may have to maintain an encyclopedia of policies. Many providers expressed a need for regularly updated educational and informational resources to empower them and their patients. One medical fellow recalled:

> It was . . . kind of a sudden sense of fear of like, "Oh, the trigger laws that we had were very unclearly written. So, can I say this? Can we do this? How do we document our options counseling?"

*Burden of care.* Providers also reported skyrocketing patient caseloads along with more complex patient needs. With the increased barriers, many patients cannot access care until later in their pregnancies. As a result, providers disclosed increasing morbidities alongside the increasing gestational ages among patients. Furthermore, providers face medical complexities and unclear management protocols. Concerningly, many providers said that the idea of best practice had been compromised, given the volatile state of abortion legislation. For some, this meant providing otherwise contraindicated care to patients who needed an abortion in hostile states. One provider and organizer stated:

> And it's so [sad] to think that there is no one standard anymore. . . . In Texas, it's a public health emergency. It's harm reduction. . . . You know, they [abortion seekers] would still be better off not pregnant than pregnant, but would you [provide care] differently in Illinois or in California? And so it's interesting how we can't even come up with that basic best practices standard of care anymore.

## Forging a Collective Future for Reproductive Health

Although feelings of anxiety and anger were clearly present, providers also reported hope and optimism for change. Three subthemes emerged.

*Sense of purpose.* Against seemingly insurmountable odds, providers noted that they found glimmers of positivity and optimism in the work they do. Many providers, such as this family planning fellow, reported feeling a sense of community as they worked toward a shared goal:

> I love my job. I feel so lucky to be doing this work. I feel so much

gratitude from our patients, like way more than I ever do from our [obstetric] patients and doing deliveries and things like that. So, I feel very lucky and I hope people keep feeling inspired to do this [work].

*Hope.* Hope was a sentiment the providers shared throughout their stories. Providers described cultivating hope through organizing and improving training for future providers. They noted that being able to connect to people with similar experiences had been helpful in building hope for a better reproductive future:

I also feel like so many people I know say when Trump was elected in 2016, [they] felt so much distress. "What can I do? What is this? The world is falling apart." And I felt like I go to work every day with lots of fabulous people and do something really important that changes lives every day. And that is really fulfilling. . . . At least my job, my life, and what I've dedicated my career to is part of the solution.

*Activism and community.* Providers emphasized the range of systems and degrees of resistance they encountered in policies and in their institutions. From national legislation to local organizing, providers noted that community and activism were key to their work and hope for a better future. The grief and anger shared motivated their organizing efforts. During the focus groups, many providers advocated seeking community members' support to work together at local and national levels. A medical fellow said:

My residency state, as well, was very much a small but mighty community of a handful of advocacy- and repro-oriented folks from across the state. That had, kind of, been working together on various projects for a bit but really channeled a lot of that anger and energy into trying to at least put some safeguards in place. . . . So even though it's pretty spread out, that community was still really helpful.

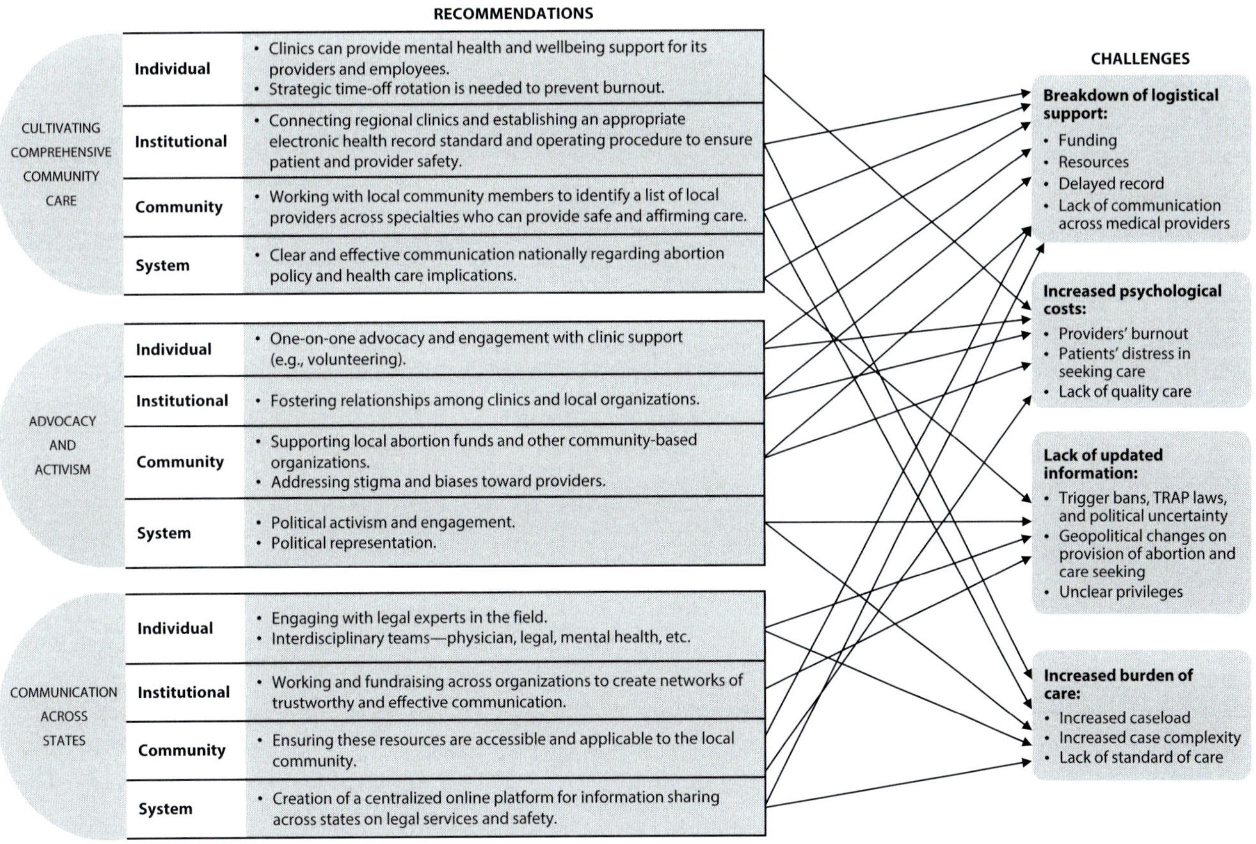


**FIGURE 1— Themes of and Provider-Informed Recommendations for Addressing Reproductive Health Care Challenges**

*Note.* TRAP = targeted regulation of abortion providers.

## Summary

For recommendations we developed during this study, see Figure 1. Although we saw increasing burdens and fragmented logistical coordination with psychological costs and increased barriers for everyone, we also found an unexpected sustaining hope and an increased sense of purpose among providers.

## EVALUATION, TRANSFERABILITY, AND ADVERSE EFFECTS

The study answers our research objective and our findings are transferable to other legally precocious and stigmatized medical practices (e.g., gender-affirming care, harm-reduction services).

## SCALABILITY

The study is transferable to other sexual and reproductive health providers. The study is scalable to a larger sample.

## PUBLIC HEALTH SIGNIFICANCE

Abortion restrictions have long-term consequences that reduce access and quality of care nationwide.[11,12,14] Our participants, particularly those in residency training, discussed moving to different types of practice and different locations, where they would have more comprehensive training opportunities and could practice their specialization without criminalization. They also discussed the risk of burnout owing to isolation and a heightened level of stress in navigating the laws and safety; similar experiences have been documented among providers in restrictive states.[11,15] In the long term, the current abortion restrictions can delay both patients' access to providers and lack of quality of care across all types of medical service, increasing US medical costs for delayed, untreated conditions. AJPH

## ABOUT THE AUTHORS

Tuyet Mai Ha Hoang and Victoria Ferrara are with the School of Social Work, University of Illinois Urbana-Champaign, Urbana. Radia DeLuna is with the Department of Educational Psychology, University of Illinois Urbana-Champaign. Elise Albertson is with the University of Illinois College of Medicine, Chicago. Ainslee Wong is with Department of Health and Kinesiology, University of Illinois Urbana-Champaign. Aaron Santoyo is with the School of Molecular and Cellular Biology, University of Illinois Urbana-Champaign.

## CORRESPONDENCE

Correspondence should be sent to Tuyet Mai H. Hoang, School of Social Work, University of Illinois at Urbana-Campaign, 1010 W. Nevada, M/C 082, Room 2040, Urbana, IL 61801 (e-mail: Thhoang3@illinois.edu). Reprints can be ordered at https://www.ajph.org by clicking the "Reprints" link.

## PUBLICATION INFORMATION

Full Citation: Hoang TMH, DeLuna R, Albertson E, Wong A, Santoyo A, Ferrara V. Beyond boundaries: navigating challenges and charting the future of reproductive health care in the post-*Roe* landscape. *Am J Public Health*. 2025;115(7):1037–1041.

Acceptance Date: February 16, 2025.

DOI: https://doi.org/10.2105/AJPH.2025.308084

ORCID iDs:

Tuyet Mai Ha Hoang https://orcid.org/0000-0001-7565-4373

Radia DeLuna https://orcid.org/0009-0000-9097-5095

Ainslee Wong https://orcid.org/0000-0003-1884-7472

Aaron Santoyo https://orcid.org/0009-0009-1664-5771

Victoria Ferrara https://orcid.org/0009-0007-6350-4686

## CONTRIBUTORS

T. M. H. Hoang conceptualized the study. T. M. H. Hoang and R. DeLuna wrote the article. T. M. H. Hoang, R. DeLuna, A. Wong, and A. Santoyo analyzed the data. All authors acquired the data and approved the final version of the article.

## CONFLICTS OF INTEREST

The authors have no conflicts of interest to disclose.

## HUMAN PARTICIPANT PROTECTION

This study received institutional review board approval from the University of Illinois Urbana-Champaign (protocol 24050).

## REFERENCES

1. Rader B, Upadhyay UD, Sehgal NKR, Reis BY, Brownstein JS, Hswen Y. Estimated travel time and spatial access to abortion facilities in the US before and after the *Dobbs v Jackson Women's Health* decision. *JAMA*. 2022;328(20):2041–2047. https://doi.org/10.1001/jama.2022.20424
2. Maddow-Zimet I, Gibson C. Despite bans, number of abortions in the United States increased in 2023. May 10, 2024. Available at: https://www.guttmacher.org/2024/03/despite-bans-number-abortions-united-states-increased-2023. Accessed April 2, 2025.
3. Smith MH, McGowan ML, Kerestes C, Bessett D, Norris AH. Longitudinal impact of *Dobbs v Jackson Women's Health Organization* on abortion service delivery in Ohio, 2022–2023. *Am J Public Health*. 2024;114(10):1034–1042. https://doi.org/10.2105/AJPH.2024.307775
4. Declercq E, Barnard-Mayers R, Zephyrin LC, Johnson K. The US maternal health divide: the limited maternal health services and worse outcomes of states proposing new abortion restrictions. December 14, 2022. Available at: https://www.commonwealthfund.org/publications/issue-briefs/2022/dec/us-maternal-health-divide-limited-services-worse-outcomes. Accessed April 2, 2025.
5. Braun V, Clarke V. One size fits all? What counts as quality practice in (reflexive) thematic analysis? *Qual Res Psychol*. 2021;18(3):328–352. https://doi.org/10.1080/14780887.2020.1769238
6. Ely GE, Hales T, Jackson DL, Maguin E, Hamilton G. The undue burden of paying for abortion: an exploration of abortion fund cases. *Soc Work Health Care*. 2017;56(2):99–114. https://doi.org/10.1080/00981389.2016.1263270
7. Guttmacher Institute. State funding of abortion under Medicaid. March 6, 2025. Available at: https://www.guttmacher.org/state-policy/explore/state-funding-abortion-under-medicaid. Accessed February 11, 2025.
8. Snyder J, Grewal A. Abortion-related crowdfunding post-*Dobbs*. *Perspect Sex Reprod Health*. 2024;56(3):228–234. https://doi.org/10.1111/psrh.12249
9. Sherman C. As funding dries up, private abortion clinics across the US are closing. *The Guardian*. December 11, 2024. Available at: https://www.theguardian.com/us-news/2024/dec/11/abortion-clinics-closing#:~:text=In%20total%2C%2076%20independent%20abortion,to%20states%20with%20restrictive%20laws. Accessed April 3, 2025.
10. Keegan G, Francis M, Chalmers K, et al. Trauma of abortion restrictions and forced pregnancy: urgent implications for acute care surgeons. *Trauma Surg Acute Care Open*. 2023;8(1):e001067. https://doi.org/10.1136/tsaco-2022-001067
11. Chowdhary P, Newton-Levinson A, Rochat R. "No one does this for the money or lifestyle": abortion providers' perspectives on factors affecting workforce recruitment and retention in the Southern United States. *Matern Child Health J*. 2022;26(6):1350–1357. https://doi.org/10.1007/s10995-021-03338-6

12. Sagar K, Rego E, Malhotra R, Lacue A, Brandi KM. Abortion providers in the United States: expanding beyond obstetrics and gynecology. *AJOG Glob Rep*. 2023;3(2):100186. https://doi.org/10.1016/j.xagr.2023.100186
13. Kimport K. Reducing the burdens of forced abortion travel: referrals, financial and emotional support, and opportunities for positive experiences in traveling for third-trimester abortion care. *Soc Sci Med*. 2022;293:114667. https://doi.org/10.1016/j.socscimed.2021.114667
14. Wetsman N, Brownstein J, Rader B. Maternal care deserts overlap with lack of abortion access, analysis shows. August 1, 2023. Available at: https://abcnews.go.com/Health/abortion-access-restrictions-affect-maternity-care-access-research/story?id=101770115. Accessed April 2, 2025.
15. Dempsey B, Callaghan S, Higgins MF. Providers' experiences with abortion care: a scoping review. *PLoS One*. 2024;19(7):e0303601. https://doi.org/10.1371/journal.pone.0303601

# Conflict and the Environment: The Tragic Example of Gaza

Jonathan M. Samet, MD, MS

**ABOUT THE AUTHOR**

*Jonathan M. Samet is with the Colorado School of Public Health, Aurora, CO.*

**See also Conflict and the Environment: The Tragic Example of Gaza, pp. 1044–1061.**

As I write this commentary in April 2025, the Global Conflict Tracker of the Council on Foreign Relations lists more than 25 conflicts, some armed and others not (https://bit.ly/3ETkGaA). We learn about them as they flare, human casualties rise, and notable destruction occurs. We infrequently hear about the environmental consequences of conflict, even though they may be devastating and leave uninhabitable lands. For general background on conflict and the environment, Meaza et al. review 193 publications on the topic between 1914 and 2023, and Levy's book, *From Horror to Hope*, provides a public health framing of the consequences of war.[1,2] The evidence is clear: conflict does create public health crises.

## ENVIRONMENTAL DAMAGE IN GAZA

In this issue of *AJPH*, a team of authors from the United States, the United Kingdom, and Palestine provides a snapshot of one ongoing crisis: the environmental damage in Gaza from the conflict with Israel and its impact on public health (Abuawad et al., p. 1053). They catalog devastation of the water supply, sanitation facilities, waste management, agricultural lands, and the electric power grid. The housing stock and other buildings have been destroyed, leaving an estimated 40 million tons of debris to clear. The conflict generates noise and air pollution and has contaminated the ground and the water supply with chemicals. The inhabitants of Gaza face inadequate amounts of food and water and the threat of infection from microbial contamination of what they eat and drink. For public health, the article's title tells the story: "The Ongoing Environmental Destruction and Degradation of Gaza: The Resulting Public Health Crisis."

How did Abuawad et al. obtain this powerful information in the conflict setting? They cite existing sources, including reports from nonaligned international agencies (e.g., the United Nations Environment Program [UNEP]; https://bit.ly/3EHw49s) and the peer-reviewed literature.[3] Also, they have done some work on microbial contamination of water. Other summaries in the peer-reviewed literature have provided similar compilations.[3] The June 2024 UNEP report, carried out at the request of the State of Palestine, is the most comprehensive survey of environmental damage and is heavily cited by Abuawad et al. Its sources include damage assessments carried out by the United Nations and other agencies, remote sensing, on-the-ground observations, previous studies in Gaza, and the general peer-reviewed literature. UNEP's methods were pragmatic, scouring all available resources, because a systematic environmental assessment with on-the-ground surveys could not be undertaken.

## USING REMOTE SENSING TO TRACK CONFLICT AND ITS CONSEQUENCES

Remote sensing has proved to be a powerful tool that has been applied to Gaza and elsewhere to track conflict itself, such as the dramatic images of the invasion of Ukraine by Russia, and damage to structures and the environment. Sticher et al. review the literature on the topic and propose enhanced utilization of satellite imagery by using artificial intelligence tools to advance analysis of the enormous data sets available as images are collected over time.[4] In a recent commentary, Bennett et al. call for infrastructure to support remote monitoring of armed conflicts.[5] Remote imaging has been applied to the conflict in Gaza, providing a picture of the massive destruction of structures; the loss of water, sanitation, and hygiene facilities; and the damage to agricultural land. The September 24, 2024, report from United Nations Satellite Centre provides a count of 163 778 damaged structures in Gaza, corresponding to approximately 66% of the total structures and an estimated 227 591 damaged housing units (https://bit.ly/3GJiXFh). Perlman et al. chart the fate of 239 water, sanitation, and hygiene sites, finding that almost half were already damaged by February 2024,[6] and Yin et al. documented the devastation of agricultural land and greenhouses.[7] Similarly, satellite imaging showed that conflict had reversed progress in landscape restoration in Tigray, Ethiopia (https://bit.ly/4m2aQDR).

Turning back to the paper by Abuawad et al., of course, the root cause of the public health crisis they document is the conflict between Israel and Palestine. The public health consequences are currently acute but will stay in play for decades across the life courses of the inhabitants of Gaza. Numerous pathways could be diagrammed for how the health of individuals and of the population has been and will be adversely affected. That exercise could be useful for setting priorities and strategic planning. For now, Abuawad et al. document the enormity of the damage to Gaza and its inhabitants and foreshadow the necessity and the challenge of restoring a habitable and healthy Gaza.

## IF GAZA WERE A SUPERFUND SITE

The Superfund process of the US Environmental Protection Agency (EPA) offers a framework for considering the restoration of Gaza to being habitable.[8] Per the EPA, the goal of the Superfund is "to make sure site cleanup is consistent with the likely future use of a site." For Gaza, the goal would be the restoration of the homeland for 2 million people. The Superfund process proceeds from a site assessment through reuse and redevelopment with community engagement throughout. Notably, EPA makes efforts through various procedures for the "polluter to pay."

Extending this framework to Gaza identifies the challenges to come: What entity would plan and lead the cleanup effort? Who would pay for the cleanup, which will have an enormous cost? What level of residual risk would be acceptable after the cleanup? The Superfund framework, which emphasizes mitigation of harmful environmental exposures, does not cover much of what will need to be done to protect the health of Gaza's residents. As described by Abuawad et al., critical public health and environmental infrastructure has been destroyed. Sanitation and a safe water supply must be restored and agriculture reimplemented on lands that are free of contamination.

And, how will a homeland be restored when the majority of structures, including homes, have been damaged? The authors offer the compelling story of the cultural and family implications of losing olive trees as a reminder of what has been lost. Restoration of olive trees is not within frameworks for environmental remediation, and generations may pass before the trauma of their loss fades.

I began by noting how many conflicts are in progress, some undoubtedly leading to harm to the environment. For Ukraine as a current example, the *New York Times* recently reported on widespread environmental damage in the country from the conflict with Russia, using the term "ecocide" (https://bit.ly/3GFrhWy). The tragic body counts receive media attention, as they should. The toll of conflict on the environment, a silent victim, should also be tracked, anticipating the restoration effort to come. The report by Abuawad et al. shows that a picture of environmental damage can be obtained, even in the setting of active combat, and provides warning of the scope of the restoration to come for Gaza. AJPH

## CORRESPONDENCE

Correspondence should be sent to Jonathan M. Samet, 13001 E 17th Place, Aurora, CO 80045 (e-mail: jon.samet@cuanschutz.edu). Reprints can be ordered at https://ajph.org by clicking the "Reprints" link.

## PUBLICATION INFORMATION

Full Citation: Samet JM. Conflict and the environment: the tragic example of Gaza. *Am J Public Health*. 2025;115(7):1042–1043.

Acceptance Date: April 16, 2025.

DOI: https://doi.org/10.2105/AJPH.2025.308168

ORCID iD:

Jonathan M. Samet https://orcid.org/0000-0001-5676-9175

## CONFLICTS OF INTEREST

The author has no conflicts of interest to declare.

## REFERENCES

1. Meaza H, Ghebreyohannes T, Nyssen J, et al. Managing the environmental impacts of war: what can be learned from conflict-vulnerable communities? *Sci Total Environ*. 2024;927:171974. https://doi.org/10.1016/j.scitotenv.2024.171974
2. Levy BS. *From Horror to Hope: Recognizing and Preventing the Health Impacts of War*. New York, NY: Oxford University Press; 2022.
3. Dardona Z, Amane M, Dardona A, Boussaa S. Health and environmental impacts of Gaza conflict (2023–2024): a review. *One Health Bulletin*. 2025;5(1):1–12. https://doi.org/10.4103/ohbl.ohbl_42_24
4. Sticher V, Wegner JD, Pfeifle B. Toward the remote monitoring of armed conflicts. *PNAS Nexus*. 2023;2(6):pgad181. https://doi.org/10.1093/pnasnexus/pgad181
5. Bennett M, Van Den Hoek J, Zhao B, Prishchepov A. Improving satellite monitoring of armed conflicts. *Earth's Future*. 2022;10(9):e2022EF002904. https://doi.org/10.1029/2022EF002904
6. Perlman B, Collins SM, Van Den Hoek J. Public health implications of satellite-detected widespread damage to WASH infrastructure in the Gaza Strip. *PLOS Glob Public Health*. 2025;5(2):e0004221. https://doi.org/10.1371/journal.pgph.0004221
7. Yin H, Eklund L, Habash D, Qumsiyeh MB, Van Den Hoek J. Evaluating war-induced damage to agricultural land in the Gaza Strip since October 2023 using PlanetScope and SkySat imagery. *Science of Remote Sensing*. 2025;11:100199. https://doi.org/10.1016/j.srs.2025.100199
8. US Environmental Protection Agency. About the Superfund cleanup process. October 9, 2024. Available at: https://www.epa.gov/superfund/superfund-cleanup-process. Accessed April 11, 2025.

# Personal Reflections on the Environmental Destruction and Degradation of Gaza: A Maelstrom of Misfortune

Lawrence O. Gostin, JD

**ABOUT THE AUTHOR**

*Lawrence O. Gostin is Distinguished University Professor at Georgetown University, Washington, DC, and directs the World Health Organization Center on Global Health Law.*

**See also Conflict and the Environment: The Tragic Example of Gaza, pp. 1042–1061.**

AJPH July 2025, Vol. 115, No. 7

In reading this deeply moving, yet disturbing, article about the ongoing environmental destruction of Gaza, I could easily catalog all the violations of international human rights and humanitarian law—sacred and binding norms applicable to every nation: The human rights to health, a clean environment, and to life itself. The Geneva Conventions prohibit the targeting of civilians and their essential infrastructures, as well as health personnel and facilities. But those norms have been cited and discussed throughout the Gaza war, to no avail.[1] (To assist *AJPH* readers, see (Box 1 on international law.)

The more fundamental point is the moral one: That the children of Gaza, their parents, and the community all have dreams for healthy and safe lives. Those dreams are universal, desired more than anything else in every corner of the globe.

## THIS IS WHAT I DREAM FOR EVERY CHILD ON EARTH

Every child deserves to fall asleep in a warm, safe home. When she wakes up, she will go to the bathroom, and there will be clean, potable water and flushable toilets. When she goes to the kitchen table, she will eat nutritious and wholesome food. When she leaves home, the air will be clean and breathable. She will not be exposed to chemical or other toxins, raw sewage, or rats or vermin. She will not be traumatized by guns and bombs or hear the terrifying sounds of artillery. She will have the joy of walking, biking, or recreating on clean, safe streets, with parks and playgrounds. And if she falls ill, there will be nurturing health professionals to care for her, and affordable vaccines and medicines to keep her healthy.

Is that too much to ask for a child living anywhere in the world? Safe environmental conditions are simply taken for granted among most of the populations in high-income countries like the United States. No parent anywhere tolerates having his or her child growing up without the bare necessities of life. Then why do we accept it for the children of the world, from sub-Saharan Africa and Latin America to Southeast Asia? In Gaza, the children are experiencing a maelstrom of hardship. Even before the war, many Gazan children were food insecure and lacked basic infrastructure, sanitation, and environmental conditions needed to ensure a healthy lifespan. But during the war, health security has simply vanished, both physical and emotional.

## THE PUBLIC HEALTH APPROACH FOR HUMANITY

Let us dig a bit deeper into what I call the public health approach to the human experience. It is a belief that government's highest calling is to create the basic conditions for people to be healthy and safe. Yes, it requires medical care like childhood immunizations, primary care, and specialist care—what the World Health Organization calls universal health coverage. But we in public health focus mostly on prevention rather than treatment, and whole populations rather than individuals.

The public health approach recognizes that all human beings have the best chance of thriving if they live in a healthful, wholesome built and natural environment. That means clean air and water, hygiene and sanitation, vector control (e.g., mosquitoes, ticks, flies, and fleas), prevention of violence and injuries (e.g., firearms, motor vehicles, safe workplaces), and tobacco and alcohol control. It means readily accessible, affordable, and nutritious foods. It means green spaces for walking, biking, playing, and recreating.

Of course, I realize that many children lack these basic conditions for health, especially in resource-constrained countries, and countries experiencing natural emergencies or intense armed conflict—in Sudan, Democratic Republic of Congo, and

## BOX 1— Gaza Environmental Destruction and the Rule of International Law

Attacks on the environment are a frontal assault on human rights and violations of international humanitarian law. Destruction of water and sanitation infrastructure undermines people's right to clean water and sanitation, among the underlying determinants of health and a right that the UN General Assembly recognized in 2010 as a freestanding human right. The extensive destruction of agricultural land undermines the right to adequate food and to be free from hunger, especially when combined with the restrictions, at times complete, on humanitarian aid, including food, entering Gaza. And given the link between the environment and culture, particularly the importance of olive trees to Palestinian culture, the widespread uprooting of olive trees in Gaza undermines Palestinians' right to take part in cultural life.

Beyond these violations of human rights that date back to the foundational instruments of the human rights regime is the right to a clean environment itself, which has a history dating back at least to the 1972 Stockholm Conference's Declaration of the United Nations Conference on the Human Environment. Nearly half a century later, in 2021, the UN Human Rights Council recognized the right to a clean, healthy, and sustainable environment—a step that the UN General Assembly itself took the following year.

Methods of warfare that harm the environment can also be war crimes. The first Additional Protocol to the Geneva Conventions of 1949 prohibits intentionally attacking or otherwise rendering useless civilian objects necessary for the survival of the population (art. 54). That instrument also prohibits using methods of warfare that are intended or expected to cause "widespread, long-term and severe damage" to the natural environment, linking such harm to the population's health and survival (art. 55).

Ukraine, to name a few. But to witness such wholesale environmental destruction in Gaza in ways that sometimes seem purposeful is agonizing.

And that is why I want to end this editorial with my own personal reflections—speaking as a first-generation American whose mother, aunts, and uncles fled Warsaw during the rise of Nazism, and where many of my family who remained in Europe died in concentration camps. My family history is etched in Ellis Island, and my life in America has been teaching at our great universities. That is why I take offense at President Trump's attacks on universities and the press in the name of antisemitism.[2] Most assuredly, there is prejudice against Jewish people, but it has nothing to do with programs designed to advance diversity, equity, and inclusion. And quelling free speech on campuses will not remove that antisemitism.

In my bones, I yearn for Israel to be safe and secure. My heart simply broke when Hamas fighters killed and abducted children, women, and men on October 7, 2023, including brutal rapes.

And yet, as a Jew, I hold Israel to a higher moral standard. We as a people know what it is like to be persecuted, attacked, and killed. We know more than any peoples of the evils of hate, retribution, vengeance, and prejudice. How, then, is it possible to justify the utter destruction of all the conditions in which people can be happy and healthy? Children have the human right to grow up healthy and safe. It really is that simple.

For a moment, forget geopolitics and the acrimonious history of the Middle East. Forget "them" and "us." Forget endless excuses: About Hamas fighters embedding themselves in schools, hospitals, and mosques (they do). About why United Nations aid workers are a threat (they are not). Or why cutting off humanitarian aid is justified (it never is). For a moment, focus on that little girl who has no home, no food, no health care, and, for many, no parents to nurture her. As Jew—especially as a Jew—and as a person who believes in the human right to health, I cannot accept these deep moral wounds. AJPH

### CORRESPONDENCE

Correspondence should be sent to Lawrence O. Gostin, Georgetown University Law Center, 600 New Jersey Ave NW, Washington, DC 20001 (e-mail: gostin@georgetown.edu). Reprints can be ordered at https://www.ajph.org by clicking the "Reprints" link.

### PUBLICATION INFORMATION

Full Citation: Gostin LO. Personal reflections on the environmental destruction and degradation of Gaza: a maelstrom of misfortune. *Am J Public Health*. 2025;115(7):1044–1045.

Acceptance Date: April 18, 2025.

DOI: https://doi.org/10.2105/AJPH.2025.308176

### CONFLICTS OF INTEREST

The author declares no conflicts of interest.

### REFERENCES

1. Gostin LO, Goodwin MB. Wars in Gaza and beyond: why protecting the sacredness of health matters. *JAMA*. 2024;331(3):191–192. doi:10.1001/jama.2023.26391.
2. Roth MS. Trump is selling Jews a dangerous lie. *New York Times*. Opinion section. April 7, 2025. Available at: https://www.nytimes.com/2025/04/07/opinion/trump-jewish-antisemitism-wesleyan.html. Accessed April 16, 2025.

# Israel and Gaza: Keeping Room for Hope Based on Past Cooperation in Public Health

*Theodore H. Tulchinsky, MD, MPH, Aron M. Troen, DPhil, Dorit Nitzan, MD, RD, MPH, Ron Lobel, MD, and Gordon DeFriese, PhD*

**ABOUT THE AUTHORS**

*Theodore H. Tulchinsky is with the Faculty of Medicine, Hebrew University–Hadassah Braun School of Public Health and Community Medicine, Jerusalem, Israel. Aron M. Troen is with the Institute of Biochemistry Food and Nutrition Science, Robert H. Smith Faculty of Agriculture Food and Environment, Hebrew University of Jerusalem, Israel. Dorit Nitzan is with the Faculty of Health Sciences, School of Public Health, Ben Gurion University of the Negev, Be'er Sheva, Israel. Ron Lobel is with the Department of Emergency Medicine, Barzilai University Medical Center, Ashkelon, Israel. Gordon DeFriese is with the Department of Social Medicine, School of Medicine, University of North Carolina, Chapel Hill.*

**See also Conflict and the Environment: The Tragic Example of Gaza, pp. 1042–1061.**

From 1967 until the mid-1990s, civilian health care in the Gaza Strip was administered by the Israel Defense Forces' Civil Administration, under the direction of the Israeli Ministry of Health. During this period, the Palestinian population of Gaza, along with the United Nations Relief and Works Agency, partnered with Israeli health experts in a series of initiatives that achieved dramatic gains in immunization coverage, mother–child care, and disease surveillance.[1–4] One of the authors (T. H.T.) served as coordinator of health in Gaza and the West Bank (1978–1994; Appendix Figure A, available as a supplement to the online version of this article at https://www.ajph.org), and another (R. L.), who served as Israeli chief physician in Gaza, was tasked with improving the health of the Palestinian population as rapidly as possible within the limits of available resources.

It is crucial to remember such collaboration, which has yielded significant benefits for both sides. Current reporting on the 2023 to 2025 war between Israel and Hamas ignores this important historical record, and extremist rejection of cooperation and "normalization" between Palestinians and Israelis endangers the necessary revival of joint efforts for the benefit of both. Public health in the region has long been a two-way street, as when vaccination policies pioneered in Gaza in the 1970s were later adopted widely across the region, including by Israel. This shared past is important. The examples we present underscore that Israeli–Palestinian public health cooperation could be revived—even before the current crisis subsides—with significant, reciprocal benefits.

## RIFT VALLEY FEVER: A MODEL OF REGIONAL PREVENTION

From 1977 to 1978, a major outbreak of Rift Valley fever spread through Egypt, threatening Gaza, Israel, and the West Bank.[5] Rift Valley fever is a mosquito-borne virus that affects wild and domestic animals and can infect humans. It is also a potential biological warfare agent. In a massive joint effort, approximately 1.5 million domestic animals were immunized throughout the region. This cross-border collaboration, including coordinated monitoring of human cases, successfully prevented Rift Valley fever's spread beyond Egypt and protected all populations.[5]

## CONTROLLING POLIO

Between 1977 and 1978, polio surged in Gaza, with more than 70 clinical cases annually.[6] After a team of Palestinian and Israeli public health staff, joined by a World Health Organization consultant from Baylor College, implemented a new policy combining oral Sabin and inactivated Salk vaccines, polio cases dropped swiftly and sharply (Figure 1). This dual oral Sabin–inactivated Salk vaccine strategy became an international standard for eradicating polio.[6,7]

That Gaza reported no polio cases for the next 25 years is evidence of the long-term efficacy of earlier collaborative gains.[4] However, in the early 2020s, vaccine-derived poliovirus reemerged in Gaza. When the 2023 to 2025 Israeli–Hamas war began, officials discovered a clinical case of polio in a child and multiple sewage samples testing positive for vaccine-derived poliovirus. A polio vaccination campaign was immediately mounted and prevented a broad outbreak.[8,9]

## MEASLES VACCINATION

By 1973, Gaza had begun administering measles vaccines, achieving coverage of

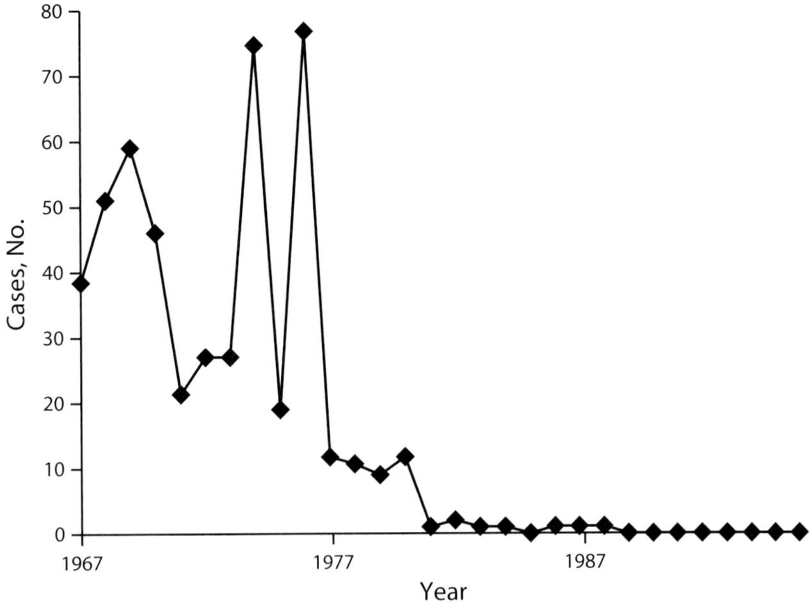


**FIGURE 1— Poliomyelitis Cases in Gaza, 1967–1996**

*Source.* Theodore H. Tulchinsky, personal archive.

AJPH July 2025, Vol. 115, No. 7

about 75% in the late 1970s. In 1983, authorities introduced a two-dose measles control program: a measles vaccine alone at aged nine months to protect infants was followed by a second dose of the measles, mumps, and rubella vaccine, pushing coverage above 90%, achieving control of measles transmission, and reducing deaths, especially of younger children.[4] Israel retained a single-dose schedule for about a decade longer and experienced multiple measles outbreaks, albeit with relatively low mortality rates.

## MOTHER–CHILD HEALTH AND TRAINING

By adopting Israeli models integrated with local expertise, mother–child health centers in Gaza increased from merely three in 1976 to 29 by 1994.[1,3] This contributed to a dramatic drop in infant mortality, from roughly 76 per 1000 live births in 1978 to 40 by 1991, and even lower rates in subsequent decades.[4] Enhanced training programs followed this success. In the 1970s alone, 25 physicians from Gaza and the West Bank undertook 30-month residencies in Israeli hospitals, specializing in anesthesiology, and through 2005, multiple Palestinian physicians, nurses, and technicians participated in specialty training and study days in other fields in Israel.[1,3,5]

## CROSS-BORDER HEALTH MONITORING

Founded in 2003, the Middle East Consortium on Infectious Diseases Surveillance fosters joint epidemic intelligence by establishing standardized laboratory procedures and enabling rapid outbreak responses across Israel, Jordan, and the Palestinian territories.[10] These professional relationships remained resilient even during periods of political tension, as demonstrated during the 2006 avian influenza outbreak and the COVID-19 pandemic.

## ENVIRONMENTAL HEALTH AND NUTRITION

Collaborative conferences and publications have advanced nutrition science and policy in both communities.[11] They provided the impetus for a Palestinian Authority mandate to iodize salt (in 1996) to prevent thyroid deficiency disorders—including damage to physical and mental development in children—and to fortify flour with iron, folic acid, and other essential micronutrients (in 2006). Israel has yet to implement fortification. Nongovernmental organizations, such as the Canadian-based Rozana, distributed folic acid to pregnant women in remote Gaza villages (E. Abadi, written personal communication, December 1, 2024), addressing micronutrient gaps and reducing preventable cases of neural tube defects, a common birth disorder. A joint study (1996–2000) investigated childhood lead exposure in Gaza, the West Bank, Jordan, and Israel. These examples of successful collaboration highlight the prospective benefits of cooperation in public health for post-conflict reconstruction.[12,13]

## COOPERATION DURING THE CURRENT WAR

Sewage treatment plants and water supplies severely compromised by intense fighting allowed the reemergence of a circulating poliovirus (i.e., circulating vaccine-derived poliovirus type 2, mutated [cVDPV2m]) that threatened communities in Gaza, Israel, and neighboring areas. The vaccination program conducted by Palestinian, Israeli, and international health agencies in 2024 reached approximately 560 000 children, or 95% of its target population, despite the ongoing war.[8,9]

Israeli and Palestinian researchers and public health practitioners have jointly called for enhanced water, sanitation, and hygiene measures and for cease-fire to restore—and improve—basic infrastructure in Gaza. Moreover, cooperation is essential in managing wastewater to address shared water scarcity and safeguard fresh produce from contaminants that pose health risks to all.

In other words, Israelis and Palestinians inhabit an interlinked ecosystem. Unified health and environmental frameworks to protect citizens make cooperation a necessity. Despite severe challenges to maintaining the provision of health care, Palestinian and Israeli clinicians have published firsthand accounts of providing aid to victims on both sides.[14]

Contemporary perspectives on food security; water, sanitation, and hygiene intervention; trust-building clinical work; and polio eradication efforts confirm that collaborative health strategies are effective and necessary. They can contribute to rebuilding health systems and reestablishing cooperation essential for the future.

## WHY THIS MATTERS NOW

Severe disruption to hospitals, water systems, and vaccine supply chains in the ongoing Hamas–Israel conflict threatens to unravel gains made over decades. The global media and, most importantly, current scientific literature have a role to play in restoring positive attention to public health. They could make a significant contribution by highlighting that until about a generation ago, Israeli–Palestinian health collaborations thrived and directly benefited all populations.

Cooperation between Israeli and Palestinian public health professionals was crucial. It improved access to primary care, disease control, and staff professional development. It strengthened health systems through shared responsibility for health development. Well-governed joint efforts are crucial now for rebuilding postconflict cooperation. Gaza's people urgently need the reconstruction of their devastated health infrastructure. The region's public health needs, including Israel's, must be met. The enlightened self-interest of all parties requires resuming and expanding such cooperative undertakings. They have benefited so many. They can and must do so again. AJPH

### CORRESPONDENCE

Correspondence should be sent to Aron M. Troen, DPhil, Robert H. Smith Faculty of Agriculture Food and Environment, The Hebrew University of Jerusalem, Rehovot, 7610001, Israel (e-mail: aron.troen@mail.huji.ac.il). Reprints can be ordered at https://www.ajph.org by clicking the "Reprints" link.

### PUBLICATION INFORMATION

Full Citation: Tulchinsky TH, Troen AM, Nitzan D, Lobel R, DeFriese G. Israel and Gaza: keeping room for hope based on past cooperation in public health. *Am J Public Health*. 2025;115(7):1046–1049.

Acceptance Date: May 2, 2025.

DOI: https://doi.org/10.2105/AJPH.2025.308190

ORCID iDs:

Aron M. Troen https://orcid.org/0000-0001-9738-2524

Dorit Nitzan https://orcid.org/0000-0002-4280-2939

### CONTRIBUTORS

T. H. Tulchinski conceptualized and wrote the first draft of the editorial. All other authors revised the editorial.

### CONFLICTS OF INTEREST

The authors have no conflicts of interest to report.

### REFERENCES

1. World Health Organization. Health in Judea/Samaria and Gaza: 1967–1994. 1995. Available at: https://iris.who.int/bitstream/handle/10665/177366/WHA47_Inf.Doc-5_eng.pdf?sequence=1&isAllowed=y. Accessed April 16, 2023.
2. World Health Organization. Health conditions in the occupied Palestinian territory, including east Jerusalem, and in the occupied Syrian Golan. May 17, 2023. Available at: https://apps.who.int/gb/ebwha/pdf_files/WHA76/A76_15-en.pdf. Accessed April 16, 2023.
3. Lasch EE, Abed Y, Goldberg J, el Shawa R. Child health services in Gaza—an experiment in integration. *Public Health Rev.* 1984;12(3–4):370–372.
4. Shani M, Tulchinsky TH. Health in Gaza. *BMJ.* 1993;307(6902):509. https://doi.org/10.1136/bmj.307.6902.509
5. Shimshony A, Orlag U, Peleg BA, et al. Evaluation of knowledge concerning the pathogenicity and transmission of Rift Valley Fever during the period 1978–1980 and its contributions to epidemiology and biostatistics. In: Proceedings of a Workshop on Rift Valley Fever, Herzlia, Israel, March 18–21, 1980. Vol. 3 Basel, Switzerland: Karger; 1980. https://doi.org/10.13140/2.1.1813.0563
6. Tulchinsky T, Abed Y, Shaheen S, et al. A ten-year experience in control of poliomyelitis through a combination of live and killed vaccines in two developing areas. *Am J Public Health.* 1989;79(12):1648–1652. https://doi.org/10.2105/ajph.79.12.1648
7. Tulchinsky TH, Ramlawi A, Abdeen Z, et al. Polio lessons. 2013: Israel, the West Bank, and Gaza. *Lancet.* 2013;382(9905):1611–1612. https://doi.org/10.1016/S0140-6736(13)62331
8. World Health Organization. Second round of polio campaign in Gaza completed amid ongoing conflict and attacks: UNICEF and WHO. November 6, 2024. Available at: https://www.who.int/news/item/06-11-2024-second-round-of-polio-campaign-in-gaza-completed-amid-ongoing-

conflict-and-attacks–unicef-and-who. Accessed April 16, 2025.

9. Grotto I, Agha H, Abu Al-Halaweh A, Davidovitch N, McKee M, Nitzan D. Public health, war and cross-border challenges: the recent cVDPV2 polio outbreak in Gaza. *EClinicalMedicine*. 2025; 81:103136. https://doi.org/10.1016/j.eclinm.2025.103136
10. Leventhal A, Ramlawi A, Belbiesi A, et al. Enhanced surveillance for detection and management of infectious diseases: regional collaboration in the Middle East. *Emerg Health Threats J*. 2013;6. https://doi.org/10.3402/ehtj.v6i0.19955
11. Troen AM, Fraser D, Abdeen Z, Rosenberg IH. Child nutrition initiative in Israel and Palestine: status of food security, micronutrient malnutrition, and behavioural change and communication programs. *Food Nutr Bull*. 2006;27(2):180–185. https://doi.org/10.1177/156482650602700209
12. Skinner H, Abdeen Z, Abdeen H, et al. Promoting Arab and Israeli cooperation: peacebuilding through health initiatives. *Lancet*. 2005;365(9466): 1274–1277. https://doi.org/10.1016/S0140-6736(05)74817-0. PMID: 15811462
13. Landesman LY, Rubinstein RA, Englander BS. Peacebuilding through cooperation in health care and public health between Israel and Palestine. *J Public Health Manag Pract*. 2024;30(3):315–318. https://doi.org/10.1097/PHH.0000000000001919. PMID: 38603739
14. Abu Fraiha Y, Ahmed A, Alon N, Halperin A. Health care bridges—pathways toward trust in Gaza and beyond. *N Engl J Med*. 2025;392(12): 1145–1147. https://doi.org/10.1056/NEJMp2416553

# Destruction of Public Health and the Environment in Wars in Gaza and Beyond: What Must be Done

*Leonard Rubenstein, JD, LLM*

**ABOUT THE AUTHOR**

*Leonard Rubenstein is Distinguished Professor of the Practice at the Johns Hopkins Bloomberg School of Health, Baltimore, MD, and author of* Perilous Medicine: The Struggle to Protect Health Care From the Violence of War.

**See also Conflict and the Environment: The Tragic Example of Gaza, pp. 1042–1061.**

AJPH July 2025, Vol. 115, No. 7

In 1862, Henri Dunant, a Swiss philanthropist and pacifist, published an account of the aftermath of a major battle in northern Italy in 1859 where thousands of wounded soldiers lay unattended on the field, desperate for water and in agony from their injuries. In what became a European best-seller, *A Memory of Solferino,* Dunant famously wrote, "In an age when we hear so much of progress and civilization, is it not a matter of urgency, since unhappily we cannot always avoid wars, to press forward in a human and truly civilized spirit to attempt to prevent, or at least alleviate, the horrors of war?"[1(p127)]

## POWERFUL LAWS BUT PERSISTENTLY FLOUTED

So began the effort to protect health care and civilians in war. Dunant cofounded the International Committee of the Red Cross and drove the adoption of the 1864 Geneva Convention, which obliged signatories to collect and care for wounded soldiers and refrain from attacking them, their caregivers, and the facilities where they are treated. Over time, and especially in the last three quarters of a century, the law evolved to protect civilians as well as soldiers and to impose affirmative obligations on fighting forces to take precautions in military operations to avoid, or at least minimize, harm. It also forbids punishment of health providers for adhering to medical ethics, such as duties of impartiality and medical independence, and the use of means or methods of war that are intended or expected to cause widespread, long-term, and severe damage to the natural environment. These provisions are binding on all combatants as customary law.[2] Intentional breaches of these laws can amount to war crimes.

Yet, combatants in contemporary wars largely act with indifference toward and even contempt for the law and commit violations with impunity. Until recently, moreover, the impact of violence against health in war received little attention from United Nations (UN) agencies, nongovernmental organizations, or academia. In the past decade, however, scholars, human rights organizations, and UN agencies have increasingly collected data and published studies that reveal staggering levels of mortality, morbidity, health systems breakdown, degradation of water and sanitation infrastructure, and environmental damage as a product of disregard for the law.

The paper by Abuawad et al. in this issue (p. 1053) brings together data, mostly collected by UN agencies operating in Gaza, as well as the Ministry of Health, on the catastrophic health and environmental impacts of the war. Ministry figures show that more than 50 000 people have been killed, among them hundreds of health and humanitarian workers and thousands of children, by bombs, artillery, tanks, missiles, and drones (the Ministry does not distinguish between civilians and combatants). Israel has repeatedly launched explosive weapons against hospitals, often followed by detention of health workers. Water and sanitation systems have been disabled by both ordnance and cut-offs of electricity and fuel. More than 90% of Gaza's physical infrastructure, including housing, has been severely damaged or destroyed. Restrictions on humanitarian aid have led to widespread hunger and famine, as well as desperate shortages of medical supplies and medication. Gaza's agricultural land has been significantly contaminated from ordnance. The authors also alert us to the potential for future harms from exposure to unexploded ordnance and white phosphorus, the burning of substitute fuels, and deep psychological trauma. Though not the subject of the article, the war has also brought widespread psychological trauma to Israelis stemming from Hamas's killing of more than 1200 Israeli civilians on October 7, 2023, and its taking and continued holding and abuse of hostages.

The scale and intensity of the destruction and suffering in Gaza is in many ways unique, characterized by massive use of explosive weapons in densely populated areas, multiple forced displacements of the population, lack of safe areas, and the inability of Gaza residents to flee. Yet, violence inflicted on the population, health facilities, and the environment in Gaza is all too typical of many contemporary wars. In 2024, the Safeguarding Health in Conflict Coalition and Insecurity Insight found more than 3600 acts of violence inflicted on health workers and facilities; the cumulative number of attacks on health care in major wars in the past three years includes almost 2000 in Ukraine, more than 1500 in Myanmar, and more than 500 in Sudan.[3]

In Gaza, as elsewhere, dedicated health workers have persevered, often heroically, to keep services going, but recovery from the systemic impacts of the violence will take years, even decades. In Syria, where hospitals were bombed or subjected to missile attacks 600 times, repeated targeting over years led to severe weakening of the health system as a result of loss of essential infrastructure and human resources, especially among the most experienced clinicians, and governance mechanisms.[4] The Tigray region of Ethiopia faces similar challenges as a result of the damage and destruction to 80% of its hospitals and clinics during the war from 2020 to 2022. The economic cost of the violence against health facilities and their administration is estimated at almost $4 billion.[5]

The enormous scale and long-term effects of environmental degradation from war are increasingly understood. In Ukraine, damage from the contamination of air, soil, and water, including the toxic residue of heavy metals ordnance, the legacy of millions of landmines, and destruction of forests and wildlife, is estimated at more than $50 billion. Future environmental calamity could also strike as a result of Russian assaults on the Zaporizhzhia Nuclear Power Plant and the Nova Kakhovka Dam.[6] In the war in Yemen, between 2015 and 2017, 74 Saudi airstrikes on water-related infrastructure led to a major cholera epidemic.[7]

## ABDICATION OF RESPONSIBILITY

Abuawad et al. rightly call for more research and, more urgently, an end to the war in Gaza. More broadly, the best way to end the suffering of populations, the destruction of health systems, and the impairment of ecosystems exposed to contemporary war is to end war. But as long as war continues, Dunant's admonition to alleviate war's horrors must guide us as well. To date, it has not. The international community has abdicated its responsibilities, ignoring a 2016 UN Security Council resolution setting a pathway to protecting health care in war and ending impunity for perpetrators.[8] (There has been no equivalent resolution on protection of the environment in war.) The health professions have largely declined to demand action or show solidarity with colleagues who suffer through the violations. In some cases, including in the war in Gaza, pressures have been in the other direction, toward self-censorship. And the appetite for providing resources to support rebuilding and attending to the enormous trauma people living in war have experienced is declining.

There are opportunities for action, though. A report from the World Health Organization and the Qatar Foundation's World Innovation Summit on Health Foundation urged a new alliance of states, UN agencies, and nongovernmental organizations to press for prevention and an end to impunity.[9] Leaders in public health, including from the APHA, have called for health professional groups to fulfill their duty to promote public health by overcoming reluctance to engage in political action toward the protection of health in conflict. That includes demanding the cessation of arms transfers to perpetrators of attack and justice for those who commit crimes of war.[10] International and national prosecutors are investigating almost 250 cases of environmental destruction in Ukraine.[11]

The urgency of such initiatives is as great, and perhaps even greater, than it was in 1862. AJPH

### CORRESPONDENCE

Correspondence should be sent to Leonard Rubenstein, Johns Hopkins Bloomberg School of Public Health, 615 N Wolfe St, E7158, Baltimore, MD 21205 (e-mail: lrubenstein@jhu.edu). Reprints can be ordered at https://ajph.org by clicking the "Reprints" link.

### PUBLICATION INFORMATION

Full Citation: Rubenstein L. Destruction of public health and the environment in wars in Gaza and beyond: what must be done. *Am J Public Health*. 2025;115(7):1050–1052.

Acceptance Date: April 17, 2025.

DOI: https://doi.org/10.2105/AJPH.2025.308175

### ACKNOWLEDGMENTS

The author's work on violence against health care in conflict is supported by the UK Foreign, Commonwealth, and Development Office, via a subgrant from the University of Manchester, and an anonymous family foundation.

### CONFLICTS OF INTEREST

The author is chair of the Safeguarding Health in Conflict Coalition.

## REFERENCES

1. Dunant H. *A Memory of Solferino*. Geneva, Switzerland: International Committee of the Red Cross; 1959.
2. International Committee of the Red Cross. International Humanitarian Law Databases, Customary IHL. Available at: https://ihl-databases.icrc.org/en/customary-ihl/v1. Accessed April 15, 2025.
3. Insecurity Insight, Safeguarding Health in Conflict Coalition, MAP Action. Attacked and threatened: health care at risk. Available at: https://mapaction-maps.herokuapp.com/health. Accessed April 16, 2025.
4. Haar R, Rayes D, Tappis H, Rubenstein L, et al. The cascading impacts of attacks on health in Syria: a qualitative study of health system and community impacts. *PLOS Global Health*. 2023; 4(6):e0002967. https://doi.org/10.1371/journal.pgph.0002967.
5. Gufue ZH, Haftu HK, Alemayehu Y, et al. Damage to the public health system caused by war-related looting or vandalism in the Tigray region of Northern Ethiopia. *Front Public Health*. 2024;12(12): 1271028. https://doi.org/10.3389/fpubh.2024.1271028.
6. Hryhorczuk D, Levy BS, Prodanchuk M, et al. The environmental health impacts of Russia's war on Ukraine. *J Occup Med Toxicol*. 2024;19(1):1. https://doi.org/10.1186/s12995-023-00398-y.
7. Spiegel P, Ratnayake R, Hellman N, et al. Responding to epidemics in large-scale humanitarian crises: a case study of the cholera response in Yemen, 2016–2018. *BMJ Glob Health*. 2019;4(4): e001709. https://doi.org/10.1136/bmjgh-2019-001709.
8. United Nations Security Council. Resolution 2286, S/RES/2286, 2016. Available at: https://www.securitycouncilreport.org/atf/cf/%7B65BFCF9B-6D27-4E9C-8CD3-CF6E4FF96FF9%7D/s_res_2286.pdf. Accessed April 15, 2025.
9. Brennan R, Martinez E, Rubenstein L, Kim HJ, et al. In the line of fire: protecting health in armed conflict. World Innovation Summit on Health and World Health Organization. 2024. Available at: https://cdn.who.int/media/docs/default-source/health-workforce/hwp/in-the-line-of-fire-(1).pdf. Accessed April 15, 2025.
10. Hoffman B, Riabenko J. How Ukraine's environment became a casualty of Russia's war. *New York Times*. April 2, 2025. Available at: https://www.nytimes.com/interactive/2025/04/02/world/europe/ukraine-russia-war-environment.html. Accessed April 14, 2025.
11. Chalfie M, Rubenstein L, Alqodmani L, et al. Mobilizing the health community to protect health care from attack. *Lancet*. 2024; 404(10470):2399–2402. https://doi.org/10.1016/S0140-6736(24)02421-8.

# The Ongoing Environmental Destruction and Degradation of Gaza: The Resulting Public Health Crisis

Ahlam Abuawad, PhD, Mark Griffiths, PhD, Graham H. Edwards, PhD, Adan Eftekhari, Mohammed Al-Ebweini, PhD, Husam Al-Najar, PhD, Abeer Butmeh, MA, Rasha Abu Dayyeh, BSc, Mohamed El-Shewy, PhD, and Amira Aker, PhD

**See also Conflict and the Environment: The Tragic Example of Gaza, pp. 1042–1052.**

This essay examines the resulting environmental health conditions in Gaza since October 2023. Evidence is drawn from international agency reports and peer-reviewed literature to document destruction and public health impacts over 18 months. Key themes include water, sanitation, contamination, noise and air pollution, food insecurity, susceptible populations, health system collapse, and trauma.

Palestinians are beset with a public health crisis resulting from targeted environmental destruction. Water shortages and sewage contamination increase dehydration, famine, and disease. Air pollution from explosives and waste burning exposes residents to toxins. Waste management has collapsed, heightening disease outbreaks, including polio. Agricultural land is devastated, and food security is threatened with the aid blockade. Power grid destruction has crippled essential services. The health care system's collapse further exacerbates risks, especially for susceptible populations. In addition to mental and physical trauma, cultural and identity loss are immeasurable.

The crisis in Gaza has severe and lasting consequences for health, the environment, and regional stability. An end to the bombardment, along with urgent humanitarian aid, release of all hostages, infrastructure rebuilding, and environmental remediation, are essential to mitigate long-term impacts.
(*Am J Public Health*. 2025;115(7):1053–1061. https://doi.org/10.2105/AJPH.2025.308140)

AJPH July 2025, Vol. 115, No. 7

There is growing concern surrounding the environmental impacts of modern military warfare, including deforestation, soil erosion, wildlife loss, waste generation, and pollution,[1] with studies documenting and calling for an end to military-driven environmental destruction taking place worldwide, including in Ethiopia[1] and Ukraine.[2] Our essay focuses on an evidence-based summary of Gaza's current environmental conditions resulting from Israeli bombardment and occupation, which present significant threats to the short- and long-term health of its population. We integrate existing sources on issues concerning

1. water, wastewater, and hygiene;
2. chemical and debris contamination from bombings;
3. noise pollution;
4. food insecurity;
5. environmental health impacts on susceptible populations;
6. destruction of health systems and lack of access to care, and
7. traumatic impacts of targeted environmental destruction.

We focused on reports from nonaligned international agencies (e.g., the United Nations [UN], Amnesty International, and Human Rights Watch) and peer-reviewed literature. We also refer to preliminary results from analyses conducted in Gaza by coauthors of this essay (M. G., M. A., H. A., A. B., R. A. D., M. E.). While we focus on the most recent conditions, the state of the environment was already dire before the latest war that began in October 2023. We highlight these past conditions to provide context where necessary.

## WATER, WASTEWATER, AND HYGIENE

By the end of August 2024, the average amount of drinking water entering Gaza had been reduced to a quarter of what was available in August 2023.[3] By December 2023, displaced children in southern Gaza had access to only 1.5 to 2.0 liters per day of total water use, less than the 3.0 liters of drinking water per day required for basic survival, and far below the minimum requirement of 15.0 liters of total water in emergency situations.[4] Restrictions on drinking water access combined with the destruction of 88% of Gaza's water wells and all of its desalination plants have resulted in a 94% decrease in the total water volume compared with the previous year.[5] As a consequence, up to 70% of Gaza's population reported consuming salinized or contaminated water,[6] posing severe risks of dehydration and the spread of infectious diseases—evidence of which is widespread.[7] Conditions have further deteriorated since then, exacerbated by the destruction of electricity and water infrastructure, as well as shortages of fuel, repair and spare parts, or chlorine.[8,9] The entry of aid, water, and electricity into Gaza was blocked once again in March 2025, intensifying fears of dehydration and disease among Palestinians in Gaza.[10,11]

Even before 2023, Palestinians in Gaza were restricted to water consumption levels well below the recommended minimum. The World Health Organization (WHO) recommends 100 liters of water per day per person, yet, before the most recent war, Palestinians in Gaza had access to only 83 liters per day because of the occupation-driven lack of control over their own water resources.[5]

While sample collection and testing has been limited because of ongoing bombardment and destruction of laboratories, from February to August 2024, the Palestinian Environmental NGOs Network (PENGON) and researchers at Newcastle University measured contamination of solid waste landfills with total and fecal coliform bacteria, confirming the presence of untreated sewage water and toxic leachate in the groundwater reservoir.[12]

Similarly, solid and hazardous waste are piling up throughout Gaza. Bombardment destroyed approximately 70% of all sewage pumps and wastewater treatment plants in Gaza.[5,8] These pumps require electricity or diesel to function, leaving most of the remaining pumps nonoperational. Solid waste management was already a concern before the recent attacks, with landfill sites exceeding capacity and municipalities resorting to burning waste. According to the UN Environment Programme (UNEP), almost 40 million tons of debris have been generated between October 2023 and May 2024, equating to 107 kilograms of debris per square meter in Gaza, alongside an almost complete destruction of solid waste management systems.[13] In addition to the solid waste generated from everyday usage, the tons of debris in Gaza are composed of building materials, asbestos, and human remains. The volumes of waste create a breeding ground for disease-carrying vectors (e.g., insects), increasing infectious disease risk.[14]

The destruction of homes, water, and waste infrastructure has led to a disintegration of sanitation and hygiene infrastructures. According to the UN Children's Fund (UNICEF), as of March 2024, an average of 340 individuals were forced to share a single toilet, and 1290 persons shared 1 shower.[15] Hygiene products, including soap, are unavailable or prohibitively expensive,[16] and the more than 690 000 girls and women of childbearing age are forced to use scrap material as menstrual products.[17] The impacts have led to an increase in communicable diseases; the WHO reports increases in acute respiratory infections, scabies, lice, and jaundice, with cases of diarrhea more than 25 times pre–October 2023 levels.[13] There was a 99% polio vaccination coverage in 2022; however, vaccine-derived poliovirus type-2 was detected in wastewater samples across the region in June 2024.[18] In the first case in 25 years, a 10-month-old infant was infected with polio and became paralyzed.[19] Despite the attempts to obstruct a UN convoy's vaccination team and bomb vaccination-designated areas,[20] UN agencies managed to vaccinate approximately 560 000 Palestinian children by September 2024.[21] A second dose was required to effectively contain the spread; however, because of the Israeli siege of northern Gaza, extreme bombardment and escalated mass displacement, the final phase of the campaign was postponed in October 2024.[22] In November 2024, children were killed at a health center in northern Gaza while attempting to get vaccinated hours after the WHO campaign was reinitiated.[23]

## CHEMICAL AND DEBRIS CONTAMINATION FROM BOMBINGS

A major source of direct and indirect environmental exposures is the Israeli bombardment of Gaza. We describe the air and soil pollution in greater detail.

## Air Pollution

A major source of contamination in Gaza is the destruction of buildings, roads, and infrastructure attributed to bombardment. To quote the 2024 UNEP report,

> The debris situation in Gaza is unprecedented in several ways including: i) the extent of damage to the housing stock; ii) its geographic spread and spatial density across almost the entire territory of the Gaza Strip; iii) the quantity of debris generated; iv) the rate at which debris is being generated; and v) the expected extremely high levels of UXO [unexploded ordnance, i.e., military ammunition or explosive that failed to explode] contamination.[13(p23)]

UNEP estimates that the approximately 40 million tons of debris will take 15 years to clear, based on the assumptions that the military blockade is lifted and 105 trucks with 12-cubic-meter or 19-ton capacity operating in 8-hour shifts for 30 days per month are available to carry the debris.[13] To further demonstrate the extent of debris in Gaza, UN-HABITAT and UNEP estimated that the amount of debris is more than 14 times the combined total debris from all global conflicts over the past 16 years.[24] The potential health impacts of this debris are immense. For example, individuals involved in cleanup efforts after the events of 9/11 experienced elevated rates of respiratory diseases and cancer.[25] Particulate matter from the destruction can spread over long distances, contaminating air, water, and soil, with long-term health consequences for people in the wider region.[26] Damaged fibers of asbestos are estimated to contaminate approximately 800 000 tons of the debris, and should be treated as hazardous waste.[13] However, because of the constant displacement of Palestinians and their struggle to find shelter, widespread asbestos exposure is likely, with hard-to-document long-term public health repercussions because of long latency periods (> 10 years).[27]

With 90% of Palestinians in Gaza internally displaced (some displaced 10 or more times within a year),[13] burning materials for cooking or warmth and open-air waste burning are commonplace[13]—worsening air quality and heightening the risk of respiratory diseases, adverse birth outcomes, neurodevelopmental disorders, and other diseases. Fires ignited by explosives further contribute to this risk, releasing volatile organic compounds and building materials into the air, which will likely have long-term health impacts for those who survive the bombings. The Gaza Power Plant was bombed in January 2024, and the damages related to the fires of the diesel-powered plant are unknown.[13] Between October 2023 and January 2024, 165 fires were captured by NASA's open-source Fire Information for Resource Management System, likely a significant underestimate because of low temporal resolution.[13] In October 2024, *Médecins Sans Frontières*–supported Al-Aqsa Hospital was struck by Israel, leading to fires that burned several people alive, including patients.[28]

More than 29 000 bombs have been dropped on Gaza.[29] This estimate includes the regular use of 2000-pound bombs, where 84% of hospitals in Gaza were within the damage range of 800 meters.[29] Between 5% and 10% of weapons fired into Gaza have not detonated.[30] Following a pattern of previous use, including Operation Cast Lead (2008–2009), there are also reports of the use of "unconventional weapons" in Gaza (and South Lebanon), such as white phosphorus.[31] The constitutive chemical of white phosphorous is prevalent in high concentrations in the northern part of Gaza, and scientists warn it could "destroy the natural ecosystem of animals and plants and contaminate agricultural products through the food chain . . . caus[ing] health problems especially among children and the elderly."[32] White phosphorus exposure can lead to birth defects, as detected in Gaza before October 2023.[33] Surviving Palestinians in Gaza are likely to suffer from these long-term health and environmental consequences.

Although there are no air quality measures available for Gaza since October 2023, particulate matter was measured at higher concentrations at nearby Israeli air quality monitoring sites.[13] A multiyear study is currently underway by coauthors of this essay to examine the air quality in Gaza more comprehensively. In addition, the first 3 months alone of emissions from bombardment since October 2023 are estimated to exceed the annual emissions of 26 countries and territories (> 400–600 kilotons carbon dioxide–equivalent emissions).[34] Though difficult to quantify, military conflicts significantly contribute to global greenhouse gas emissions through various processes,[35] and these global carbon budget perturbations have widespread climatic and environmental impacts.

## Soil Contamination

Although the heavy metal, chemical, and radioactive contamination of Gaza's soil is unknown because of laboratory functionality in Gaza, previous attacks involving munitions containing heavy metals, asbestos, and other hazardous materials have already contaminated the soil with high concentrations of cobalt and other metals.[36] The bombing and use of bulldozers disrupted soil layers and burned (with temperatures of explosions as high as 2000°C), deteriorated, scattered, or completely destroyed the soil (including soil microorganisms). This exacerbated the already severe food insecurity, with trees and other crops killed or rendered fruitless as a result.[12]

UNEP reported, "soil was significantly contaminated with Total Petroleum Hydrocarbons (TPHs) and aliphatic hydrocarbons, levels which surpassed the threshold requiring intervention."[13(p30)] Solar panels (initially installed to reduce dependency on Israel for electricity) were also destroyed by bombardment and may contaminate the soil through the leaching of cadmium and lead. From here, we can confidently speculate 2 important aftermaths of this war for Gaza: (1) crop yields are likely to be greatly reduced, exacerbating issues of food security for the (remaining) population of Gaza, and (2) crops that are yielded will be susceptible to levels of toxicity potentially damaging to human health, like the effects documented in Iraq after the US-led invasion of 2003.[37]

## NOISE POLLUTION

Since 1997, studies have shown that more than 90% of Palestinians in Gaza were affected by noise pollution.[38] Today, as noise pollution is at an all-time high with an average of 1 bomb dropped every 10 minutes in Gaza, "continuous drone and jet flights, rockets, bombardment from tanks and ships, and other military activities was noted to result in more than double the allowable limit [of 75 A-weighted decibels; dBA[39]] (the allowable limit is for short periods [of 8 hours] not for months as in this case)."[40(p8)] To put that into perspective, 75 dBA is equivalent to a vacuum cleaner, and double that would be equivalent to a jackhammer.[39] Chronic exposure to noise pollution is linked to adverse mental and physical health outcomes, including, but not limited to, sleep disruption, hearing loss, cardiovascular disease, negative social behavior, and absenteeism.[41] A review identified psychological and mental impacts in children and youths living in Gaza from hearing shelling and drones.[42] Among preschool-aged children, noise exposures were linked with anxiety disorders, phobias, and posttraumatic stress disorder,[43] highlighting the psychological toll of drone warfare and shelling in Gaza.

## FOOD INSECURITY

Following Israel's 2005 internal withdrawal from Gaza and its subsequent military blockade, food supplies entering the region were heavily restricted. The quantity of food permitted was determined by a report from the Israeli Ministry of Health entitled "The Red Lines Document." This report relied on several assumptions, including estimates of the population size, food production within Gaza at the time, and Israeli dietary habits. However, the report failed to consider key factors, such as the ways in which food would be transported into Gaza and the closing of borders, such as the Rafah crossing between Egypt and Gaza, preventing goods from entering.[44,45] Before the current war, 63% of households were already experiencing moderate to severe food insecurity, equating to more than 990 000 Palestinians in Gaza (about 50% of the total population of approximately 2 million people) experiencing food insecurity.

According to an Integrated Food Security Phase Classification (IPC) report published in November 2024, the entire population of Gaza contends with emergency levels of food insecurity (IPC phase 4 classification), of which 345 000 people are expected to experience catastrophic levels of food insecurity (IPC phase 5 classification) through April 2025.[46] The IPC phase 4 classification[47] indicates that the entire population is suffering from severe food shortages, acute malnutrition, and a high risk of starvation-related deaths. An independent commission to the Human Rights Council found that starvation most severely impacts infants, children, and pregnant and lactating women,[48] leading to child and infant deaths from malnutrition and dehydration.[49] Oxfam International reports that people in northern Gaza were forced to survive on 245 calories per day,[50] less than 12% of the IPC's minimum required daily requirement of 2100 calories for an average adult.[51] Unsurprisingly, in 2024, Gaza was seeing the worst level of child malnutrition anywhere in the world.[49]

As a direct result of the destruction and ruination of 68% of all agricultural lands and 33% of greenhouses,[52] which Palestinians have historically relied on for food before the current crisis, and the reinitiation of the aid and food blockade during the month of Ramadan, Palestinians are dealing with a human-made high risk of famine.[11,53] Most of Gaza's remaining trees, including olive, pomegranate, and citrus orchards—essential not only for food and income but also for air purification and shade—were completely uprooted.[54] As of May 2024, the UN's Food and Agricultural Organization estimated that every governorate had 36% or more of its agricultural wells damaged, with the Khan Younis region experiencing 56% of its 410 wells damaged or destroyed.[52] As a result, groundwater overpumping has led to a sharp increase in water salinity from 1800 to 4000 milligrams per liter, resulting in newly planted olive trees drying out in the nursery stage.[12]

## IMPACTS ON SUSCEPTIBLE POPULATIONS

Pregnant people, children, infants, the elderly, and disabled Palestinians in Gaza are highly susceptible to bombardment and are directly targeted.[48,55,56] From October 2023 to April 2024, the largest percentage of Palestinians killed were aged 5 to 9 years, followed by children aged 10 to 14 years and 0 to 4 years.[57] In May 2024, an estimated 183 women were giving birth in Gaza each day without pain medication or anesthetics; miscarriages increased by 300%; and 95% of pregnant and nursing people were severely food insecure.[58] With a lack of or limited access to health care facilities and decreasing sanitation, many women are giving birth in high-risk environments such as tents, on streets amid the rubble, or in overcrowded, partially functioning health care facilities.[59]

This has important adverse health implications for children and infants, who are not only more susceptible to the devastating conditions but are also exposed during critical developmental periods with potential lifelong impacts. In utero and early life exposures to contaminants in Gaza from previous Israeli bombardments are linked to various adverse birth and health outcomes.[60,61] In addition, malnutrition and dehydration increase the risk of fetal and infant morbidity and mortality. Nine of every 10 families in Gaza were displaced, and at least 19 000 children were forced to fend for themselves because of being separated from or being the only survivors in their families. The acronym, WCNSF (wounded children, no surviving family), was coined in Gaza because of the frequency of these cases.[62] This does not account for the cumulative effects of being born and surviving in Gaza: a 16-year-old child has lived through 6 separate wars. Gaza is now home to the largest number of child amputees worldwide,[63] all of whom have an exacerbated risk of infection because of open and untreated wounds.

Many Palestinian elderly have been forcefully displaced multiple times over the past 77 years.[64] With 70% of elderly Palestinians suffering from chronic illnesses, their frailty and comorbidities make them particularly susceptible to environmental exposures.[65] For both the elderly and amputees requiring wheelchairs or crutches, navigating through the rubble is nearly impossible, leaving them highly susceptible to malnutrition, dehydration, injuries, and illnesses. Without access to adequate health care, the deaths of susceptible populations will continue to rise.

Palestinians have been experiencing a combination of high environmental exposures, war-related trauma, chronic stress, mass displacement, and famine, with predictable systemic health effects likely lasting decades according to the developmental origins of disease.[66] In addition, a serious epidemic of poverty is unfolding, with more than 60% of Palestinians now estimated to experience poverty.[67]

## DESTRUCTION OF HEALTH SYSTEMS AND LACK OF ACCESS TO CARE

In addition to the severe impacts on public health systems described thus far, the resources available to provide care have been decimated, with the entire health system on the "brink of collapse,"[68] exacerbating the health effects of Palestinians. As of February 2025, 18 of Gaza's 36 hospitals remain operational, all of which are only partially accessible and functioning.[69] The lack of fuel and critical shortage of medicine, essential medical supplies, and blood units severely threaten the functionality of the health care system. Between October 2023 and July 2024, 498 strikes on health care facilities were documented by the UN Independent International Commission of Inquiry on the Occupied Palestinian Territories, including in East Jerusalem and Israel.[70] More than 700 Palestinians were killed in those attacks, with hundreds more injured since. The WHO representative for the West Bank and Gaza stated, "it would take five to ten years to evacuate all these critically ill patients [in Gaza]."[68] The UN Commission also reported violence against medical personnel.[70] The future of Palestinians is also under attack, with the destruction of the largest fertility clinic in Gaza, which housed 4000 embryos.[48]

## IMPACTS OF TARGETED ENVIRONMENTAL DESTRUCTION

We have detailed the impacts of this war on the environment and human physiology in a traditional Western sense. However, institutions often fail to highlight the mental and psychological damage, cultural cost, and loss of identity from the destruction of the Palestinian environment and the uprooting of wildlife, orchards, and farms. Historic Palestinian lands are home to olive, fig, pomegranate, and citrus trees, as well as wild herbs and plants used for cooking and medicinal purposes, such as zaatar (wild oregano), sage, chamomile, orchids, and chard. The olive tree is symbolic to Palestinians, not only as an important source of economic livelihood but also because of its representation of connection to the land.[71,72] An olive tree in historic Palestine can take 10 to 12 years to bear fruit, and orchards are often passed down through generations, making them a symbol of heritage and continued connection to land.[72]

A thematic analysis revealed 3 main key elements regarding how Palestinians view olive trees in their communities: *sutra* (securing sustenance for a family), *a'wna* (collaboration and family solidarity), and *sumud* (perseverance, steadfastness, and connection to community).[73] The occupation has uprooted or burned olive trees for decades, some of which were thousands of years old.[71,73,74] Nonetheless, while harvesting amid the bombs, Palestinians feel that "Olive trees are like us: resilient and with deep roots in this land."[75] Olive harvesting was historically viewed as a time of community and joy; however, it has been transformed into a time of tension, as olives need to be harvested quickly to avoid destruction and death.[54,74,75] This is comparable to the buffalo slaughter in North America, severely impacting populations' reliance on and connection to their land.[76] This loss of connection to land and previous and future generations through olive trees is a traumatic experience, expressed heavily in various Palestinian literature and art forms.[77] For example, Khaled Baraka, a 65-year-old Palestinian who was forced to flee his home, shared his anguish: "These trees lived through my moments of joy and sadness. They know my secrets. When I was sad and worried, I would talk to the trees, take care of them . . . but the war killed those trees."[78]

## CONCLUSION

Our essay does not describe the full magnitude of the devastating environmental and health impacts of the bombardment and occupation of Palestinians. More research and practical knowledge are urgently needed by the global scientific community to protect Indigenous communities and the environments they reside in from further harm. In all that we have highlighted thus far, we have not touched on the destruction of 80% of schools or the destruction of every university in Gaza.[79] As of February 2024, at least 95 professors have been killed.[80] Palestinians, who have one of the highest literacy rates in the world and deeply value education, are facing an attack on their future.[81] We write this as Palestinians in Gaza no longer have space to bury their dead (an estimated at least 186 000 deaths[82] and an estimated 41% of mortality being underreported[83]—with only approximately 40 000 deaths having been reported since June 2024). On March 2, 2025, the Israeli authorities announced a halt to humanitarian aid entering the Gaza Strip, including fuel.[84,85]

The 1-year mark has been surpassed of what the International Court of Justice labeled a "plausible" genocide[86]; what Amnesty International,[14] Human Rights Watch,[8] and the UN Special Committee[87] labeled consistent with genocide; and what journalistic investigations have labeled an ecocide.[54,88,89] UNEP called the environmental impacts of Israeli bombardment in Gaza "unprecedented,"[13] as "Water and sanitation have collapsed. Critical infrastructure continues to be decimated. Coastal areas, soil and ecosystems have been severely impacted." Palestinian human rights organizations (including Al Haq and Al Mezan Center for Human Rights) and groups in Israel (including B'Tselem and Yesh Din), have called for preventing the crimes of starvation and forcible transfer, which are leading to the liquidation of northern Gaza.[90]

Despite overwhelming evidence objectively gathered by many well-respected organizations of violations of international law, the situation has not improved for Palestinians. The crisis in Gaza has severe and lasting consequences for human health, the environment, and regional stability that can only be mitigated by an end to the bombardment and occupation, urgent humanitarian aid, release of all hostages, infrastructure rebuilding, and environmental remediation. The critical air, water, and food quality contamination in Gaza must be acknowledged and addressed immediately for the health of Palestinians now and future generations to come. AJPH

### ABOUT THE AUTHORS

Ahlam Abuawad is with the Department of Epidemiology, Geisel School of Medicine at Dartmouth, Hanover, NH. Mark Griffiths and Mohamed El-Shewy are with the School of Geography, Politics and Sociology, Newcastle University, Newcastle, UK. Graham H. Edwards is with the Earth and Environmental Geosciences, Trinity University, San Antonio, TX. Adan Eftekhari is with Harvard University, Cambridge, MA. Mohammed Al-Ebweini is with the Coastal Municipalities Water Utility, Gaza Strip in Palestine. Husam Al-Najar is with Islamic University of Gaza, Gaza Strip in Palestine. Abeer Butmeh and Rasha Abu Dayyeh are with the Palestinian Environmental NGOs Network in Palestine. Amira Aker is with the School of Public Health, Boston University, Boston, MA.

### CORRESPONDENCE

Correspondence should be sent to Amira Aker, Department of Epidemiology, Boston University School of Public Health, 715 Albany St, Boston, MA 02118 (e-mail: amaker@bu.edu). Reprints can be ordered at https://www.ajph.org by clicking the "Reprints" link.

## PUBLICATION INFORMATION

Full Citation: Abuawad A, Griffiths M, Edwards GH, et al. The ongoing environmental destruction and degradation of Gaza: the resulting public health crisis. *Am J Public Health*. 2025;115(7):1053–1061.

Acceptance Date: March 26, 2025.

DOI: https://doi.org/10.2105/AJPH.2025.308140

ORCID iDs:
Ahlam Abuawad https://orcid.org/0000-0002-7241-4574

Mark Griffiths https://orcid.org/0000-0002-2284-4533

Graham H. Edwards https://orcid.org/0000-0002-3285-4858

Adan Eftekhari https://orcid.org/0009-0005-0713-5818

Mohamed El-Shewy https://orcid.org/0009-0008-0353-6528

Amira Aker https://orcid.org/0000-0002-0063-7955

## CONTRIBUTORS

A. Abuawad provided substantial contributions to the conceptualization or design of the work and the analysis and interpretation of data for the work, and wrote and edited the manuscript for important intellectual content. M. Griffiths provided the acquisition, analysis, and interpretation of data for the work and wrote and edited the work for important intellectual content. G.H. Edwards provided the analysis and interpretation of data for the work and wrote and edited the work for important intellectual content. A. Eftekhari provided the interpretation of data for the work and wrote and edited the work for important intellectual content. M. Al-Ebweini, H. Al-Najar, A. Butmeh, R. Abu Dayyeh, and M. El-Shewy provided the acquisition, analysis, and interpretation of data for the work and helped draft portions of the work. A. Aker provided substantial contributions to the conceptualization or design of the work and the analysis and interpretation of data for the work, wrote and edited the work for important intellectual content, and provided final approval of the version to be published. All authors critically reviewed and approved the final manuscript.

## ACKNOWLEDGMENTS

This work received no funding from any agency. However, the data being collected by some coauthors and referred to in the article (albeit not shared in detail) was conducted as part of the following project based at Newcastle University: "War and Geos: The Environmental Legacies of Militarism" (United Kingdom Research and Innovation Horizon Europe grant EP/X042642/1 [awarded as a European Research Council Starting Grant]; El-Shewy and Griffiths).

We acknowledge the hardships and sacrifices made by the hundreds of humanitarian workers, without whom this work would not be possible. We also acknowledge the health care workers who remain steadfast in their mission to protect their patients, the journalists who continue to document, and the people of the region (men, women, and children) who continue to teach us life, no matter the personal cost.

## CONFLICTS OF INTEREST

The authors have no conflicts of interest to declare.

## HUMAN PARTICIPANT PROTECTION

No approval was required because the essay did not involve human participants.

## REFERENCES

1. Meaza H, Ghebreyohannes T, Nyssen J, et al. Managing the environmental impacts of war: what can be learned from conflict-vulnerable communities? *Sci Total Environ*. 2024;927:171974. https://doi.org/10.1016/j.scitotenv.2024.171974
2. Sousa R, da Silva JP, Douda K, Mammola S. The cost of war for biodiversity: a potential ecocide in Ukraine. *Front Ecol Environ*. 2022;20(7):394–396. https://doi.org/10.1002/fee.2548
3. United Nations Office for the Coordination of Humanitarian Affairs. Gaza humanitarian response update, 19 August–1 September 2024. September 4, 2024. Available at: https://www.unocha.org/publications/report/occupied-palestinian-territory/gaza-humanitarian-response-update-19-august-1-september-2024. Accessed October 4, 2024.
4. United Nations Children's Fund. 'Barely a drop to drink': children in the Gaza Strip do not access 90 per cent of their normal water use. December 20, 2023. Available at: https://www.unicef.org/press-releases/barely-drop-drink-children-gaza-strip-do-not-access-90-cent-their-normal-water-use. Accessed October 4, 2024.
5. Abdul Samad L, Butcher M, Khalidi B, Oxfam International. Water War Crimes: How Israel Has Weaponised Water in Its Military Campaign in Gaza. Oxfam International. 2024. Available at: https://oxfamilibrary.openrepository.com/bitstream/handle/10546/621609/bp-water-war-crimes-180724-en.pdf;jsessionid=7CC44290BE07A7E503547DA95CAEC8E1?sequence=1. Accessed October 4, 2024.
6. United Nations Office of the High Commissioner for Human Rights. Israel must stop using water as a weapon of war: UN expert. November 17, 2023. Available at: https://www.ohchr.org/en/press-releases/2023/11/israel-must-stop-using-water-weapon-war-un-expert. Accessed October 7, 2024.
7. Abuzerr S, Zinszer K, Mahmoud H. Healthcare collapse and disease spread: a qualitative study of challenges in Gaza strip. *BMC Public Health*. 2025;25(1):589. https://doi.org/10.1186/s12889-025-21817-1
8. Human Rights Watch. Extermination and acts of genocide: Israel deliberately depriving Palestinians in Gaza of water. December 19, 2024. Available at: https://www.hrw.org/report/2024/12/19/extermination-and-acts-genocide/israel-deliberately-depriving-palestinians-gaza. Accessed January 7, 2025.
9. United Nations Children's Fund. UNICEF and partners distribute clean water to children and families in dire need of this resource. September 20, 2024. Available at: https://www.unicef.org/sop/stories/unicef-and-partners-distribute-clean-water-children-and-families-dire-need-resource. Accessed October 7, 2024.
10. Amnesty International. Israel's decision to cut off electricity supply to Gaza desalination plant cruel and unlawful. March 10, 2025. Available at: https://www.amnesty.org/en/latest/news/2025/03/israels-decision-to-cut-off-electricity-supply-to-gaza-desalination-plant-cruel-and-unlawful. Accessed March 12, 2025.
11. Jafarnia N. Israel again blocks Gaza aid. Further risking lives: Palestinians deliberately deprived of food, water, and other necessities. Human Rights Watch. 2025. Available at: https://www.hrw.org/news/2025/03/05/israel-again-blocks-gaza-aid-further-risking-lives. Accessed March 12, 2025.
12. Palestinian Environmental NGOs Network. Ecocide in Gaza: the environmental impact of Israel. PENGON - Friends of the Earth Palestine, Newcastle University. 2024. Available at: https://www.pengon.org/articles/view/170/en. Accessed October 15, 2024.
13. United Nations Environment Programme. *Environmental Impact of the Conflict in Gaza: Preliminary Assessment of Environmental Impacts*. 2024. Available at: https://wedocs.unep.org/20.500.11822/45739. Accessed October 8, 2024.
14. Amnesty International. 'You feel like you are subhuman': Israel's genocide against Palestinians in Gaza. 2024. Available at: https://www.amnesty.org/en/documents/mde15/8668/2024/en. Accessed January 7, 2025.
15. United Nations Children's Fund. UNICEF in the State of Palestine escalation humanitarian situation report no. 19. 2024. Available at: https://www.unicef.org/sop/reports/unicef-state-palestine-escalation-humanitarian-situation-report-no19. Accessed October 7, 2024.
16. Water, Sanitation and Hygiene Cluster. Urgent hygiene crisis: combatting diarrhea and skin infections in Gaza. World Health Organization. 2024. Available at: https://healthcluster.who.int/publications/m/item/urgent-hygiene-crisis-combatting-diarrhea-and-skin-infections-in-gaza. Accessed October 7, 2024.
17. United Nations Women Regional Office for the Arab States. Scarcity and Fear: A Gender Analysis of the Impact of the War in Gaza on Vital Services Essential to Women's and Girls' Health, Safety, and Dignity—Water, Sanitation and Hygiene (WASH). United Nations Women. 2024. Available at: https://www.un.org/unispal/wp-content/uploads/2024/04/gender-alert-gender-analysis-of-the-impact-of-the-war-in-gaza-on-vital-services-essential-to-womens-and-girls-health-safety-en.pdf. Accessed October 7, 2024.
18. World Health Organization, Regional Office for the Eastern Mediterranean. Variant type 2 poliovirus isolated from sewage samples in Gaza. July 19, 2024. Available at: http://www.emro.who.int/opt/news/variant-type-2-poliovirus-isolated-from-sewage-samples-in-gaza.html. Accessed March 5, 2025.
19. Sherry L. How did polio reemerge in Gaza after a quarter of a century? Q&A with a virologist. *The Conversation*. September 3, 2024. http://theconversation.com/how-did-polio-reemerge-in-gaza-after-a-quarter-of-a-century-qanda-with-a-virologist-238015. Accessed October 8, 2024.

20. Euro-Med Monitor. Israel obstructs polio vaccination campaign in Gaza with its military attacks, detention of UN convoy. September 10, 2024. Available at: https://reliefweb.int/report/occupied-palestinian-territory/israel-obstructs-polio-vaccination-campaign-gaza-its-military-attacks-detention-un-convoy-enar. Accessed October 8, 2024.
21. World Health Organization. Around 560 000 children vaccinated in first round of polio campaign in Gaza. 2024. Available at: https://www.who.int/news/item/13-09-2024-around-560-000-children-vaccinated-in-first-round-of-polio-campaign-in-gaza. Accessed October 8, 2024.
22. United Nations. Gaza: Israeli strikes delay polio vaccine campaign in the north. *UN News: Global Perspective Human Stories*. October 23, 2024. Available at: https://news.un.org/en/story/2024/10/1156011. Accessed October 23, 2024.
23. United Nations. Gaza: Strike hits health centre as polio vaccine campaign resumes in ravaged north. *UN News: Global Perspective Human Stories*. November 2, 2024. Available at: https://news.un.org/en/story/2024/11/1156441. Accessed November 4, 2024.
24. United Nations Institute for Training and Research. Gaza: debris generated by the current conflict is 14 times more than the combined sum of all debris generated by other conflicts since 2008. August 1, 2024. Available at: https://unitar.org/about/news-stories/news/gaza-debris-generated-current-conflict-14-times-more-combined-sum-all-debris-generated-other. Accessed October 2, 2024.
25. Rahim S, Grist. Israel's war in Gaza is creating enormous hidden health problems. *Scientific American*. January 19, 2024. Available at: https://www.scientificamerican.com/article/israels-war-in-gaza-is-creating-enormous-hidden-health-problems. Accessed October 8, 2024.
26. Griffiths M, Redwood H. Late modern war and the geos. *Int Polit Sociol.* 2024;18(2):olae011. https://doi.org/10.20935/AcadBiol6035
27. Frost G. The latency period of mesothelioma among a cohort of British asbestos workers (1978–2005). *Br J Cancer.* 2013;109(7):1965–1973. https://doi.org/10.1038/bjc.2013.514
28. Médecins Sans Frontières. Gaza: MSF treats victims of Israeli strike on Al-Aqsa Hospital compound. October 14, 2024. Available at: https://reliefweb.int/report/occupied-palestinian-territory/gaza-msf-treats-victims-israeli-strike-al-aqsa-hospital-compound. Accessed October 16, 2024.
29. Kunichoff D, Mills D, Asi Y, et al. Are hospitals collateral damage? Assessing geospatial proximity of 2000 lb bomb detonations to hospital facilities in the Gaza Strip from October 7 to November 17, 2023. *PLOS Glob Public Health.* 2024;4(10):e0003178. https://doi.org/10.1371/journal.pgph.0003178
30. United Nations. Aid efforts in Gaza escalate, as risk from deadly unexploded ordnance grows. *UN News: Global Perspective Human Stories*. January 29, 2025. Available at: https://news.un.org/en/story/2025/01/1159571. Accessed March 4, 2025.
31. Human Rights Watch. Israel: white phosphorus used in Gaza, Lebanon. October 12, 2023. Available at: https://www.hrw.org/news/2023/10/12/israel-white-phosphorus-used-gaza-lebanon. Accessed March 4, 2025.
32. Hamada MS, Aish A, Shahwan M. Potential of phosphorus pollution in the soil of the Northern Gaza Strip, Palestine. *AGRIVITA J Agric Sci.* 2011; 33(3):297. https://doi.org/10.17503/agrivita.v33i3.87
33. Naim A, Al Dalies H, El Balawi M, et al. Birth defects in Gaza: prevalence, types, familiarity and correlation with environmental factors. *Int J Environ Res Public Health.* 2012;9(5):1732–1747. https://doi.org/10.3390/ijerph9051732
34. Otu-Larbi F, Neimark B, Bigger P, Cottrell L, Larbi R. A multitemporal snapshot of greenhouse gas emissions from the Israel-Gaza conflict. Preprint. Published online June 6, 2024. SSRN 4855947. https://doi.org/10.2139/ssrn.4855947
35. Bun R, Marland G, Oda T, et al. Tracking unaccounted greenhouse gas emissions due to the war in Ukraine since 2022. *Sci Total Environ.* 2024;914:169879. https://doi.org/10.1016/j.scitotenv.2024.169879
36. Safi AS. 2014 War on Gaza Strip: Participatory Environmental Impact Assessment. Palestinian Environmental NGOs Network – Friends of the Earth Palestine. October 2015. Available at: https://ps.boell.org/sites/default/files/uploads/2015/12/wareia_report_final.pdf. Accessed October 8, 2024.
37. Gibson GR, Campbell JB, Wynne RH. Three decades of war and food insecurity in Iraq. *Photogramm Eng Remote Sensing.* 2012;78(8): 885–895. https://doi.org/10.14358/PERS.78.8.895
38. Al-Agha MR. Environmental management in the Gaza Strip. *Environ Impact Assess Rev.* 1997; 17(1):65–76. https://doi.org/10.1016/S0195-9255(96)00072-8
39. RPF Environmental Testing & Consulting Services. Acceptable noise level: What decibel levels can cause hearing loss? May 27, 2023. Available at: https://www.airpf.com/acceptable-noise-level-what-decibel-levels-can-cause-hearing-loss. Accessed March 5, 2025.
40. Qumsiyeh MB. Impact of the Israeli military activities on the environment. *Int J Environ Stud.* 2024; 81(2):977–992. https://doi.org/10.1080/00207233.2024.2323365
41. Jariwala H, Syed H, Pandya M, Gajera Y. Noise pollution & human health: A review. Presented at: Noise and Air Pollution: Challenges and Opportunities. March 17, 2017. Available at: https://www.researchgate.net/publication/319329633_Noise_Pollution_Human_Health_A_Review. Accessed March 5, 2025.
42. Abudayya A, Bruaset GTF, Nyhus HB, Aburukba R, Tofthagen R. Consequences of war-related traumatic stress among Palestinian young people in the Gaza Strip: a scoping review. *Ment Health Prev.* 2023;32:200305. https://doi.org/10.1016/j.mhp.2023.200305
43. Al Ghalayini H, Thabet A. The relationship between war trauma and anxiety and posttraumatic stress disorder among preschool children in the Gaza Strip. *Arab J Psychiatry*. Published online May 2017. Available at: https://hdl.handle.net/10315/42032. Accessed October 16, 2024.
44. State of Israel, Ministry of Defense. Food consumption in the Gaza Strip—Red Lines. Gisha. January 1, 2008. Available at: https://www.gisha.org/UserFiles/File/publications/redlines/red-lines-presentation-eng.pdf. Accessed October 4, 2024.
45. Israel Gaza blockade study calculated Palestinians' calories. *Reuters*. October 17, 2012. Available at: https://www.reuters.com/article/world/israel-gaza-blockade-study-calculated-palestinians-calories-idUSBRE89G0NM. Accessed October 7, 2024.
46. Integrated Food Security Phase Classification. Gaza Strip: IPC acute food insecurity analysis, September 2024–April 2025. November 8, 2024. Available at: https://www.ipcinfo.org/fileadmin/user_upload/ipcinfo/docs/IPC_Gaza_Strip_Acute_Food_Insecurity_Malnutrition_Sept2024_Aug2025_Special_Brief.pdf. Accessed March 5, 2025.
47. Integrated Food Security Phase Classification. IPC overview and classification system. 2024. Available at: https://www.ipcinfo.org/ipcinfo-website/ipc-overview-and-classification-system/en. Accessed March 5, 2025.
48. UN Independent International Commission of Inquiry on the Occupied Palestinian Territory, including East Jerusalem, and Israel. "More than a human can bear": Israel's systematic use of sexual, reproductive and other forms of gender-based violence since 7 October 2023. United Nations Human Rights Council. March 13, 2025. Available at: https://www.ohchr.org/en/press-releases/2025/03/more-human-can-bear-israels-systematic-use-sexual-reproductive-and-other. Accessed March 25, 2025.
49. United Nations Office for the Coordination of Humanitarian Affairs. Today's top news: Occupied Palestinian Territory. February 28, 2024. Available at: https://www.unocha.org/news/todays-top-news-occupied-palestinian-territory-9. Accessed October 15, 2024.
50. Oxfam International. People in northern Gaza forced to survive on 245 calories a day, less than a can of beans – Oxfam. April 3, 2024. Available at: https://www.oxfam.org/en/press-releases/people-northern-gaza-forced-survive-245-calories-day-less-can-beans-oxfam. Accessed September 25, 2024.
51. Integrated Food Security Phase Classification Global Partners. *Integrated Food Security Phase Classification Technical Manual: Version 1.1*. 2008. Available at: https://www.fao.org/4/i0275e/i0275e.pdf. Accessed October 11, 2024.
52. Agricultural Damage Assessment in the Gaza Strip from October 7th 2023 to September 1st 2024. Food and Agriculture Organization of the United Nations and United Nations Satellite Centre. 2024. Available at: https://openknowledge.fao.org/server/api/core/bitstreams/669e3b2a-d8d8-45de-b64f-056f997ea793/content. Accessed October 8, 2024.
53. Relief Web. Israel's immoral and illegal decision to block all aid into Gaza will be fatal. Occupied Palestinian Territory. March 3, 2025. Available at: https://reliefweb.int/report/occupied-palestinian-territory/israels-immoral-and-illegal-decision-block-all-aid-gaza-will-be-fatal. Accessed March 5, 2025.
54. Forensic Architecture. 'No traces of life': Israel's ecocide in Gaza 2023–2024. March 29, 2024. Available at: https://forensic-architecture.org/investigation/ecocide-in-gaza. Accessed October 8, 2024.
55. Euro-Med Human Rights Monitor. Gaza: About 4 percent of victims of Israel's genocide are elderly; numerous cases of execution are well-documented. September 1, 2024. Available at: https://euromedmonitor.org/en/article/6455/Gaza:-About-4-percent-of-victims-of-Israel%E2%80%99s-genocide-are-elderly;-numerous-cases-of-execution-are-well-documented. Accessed October 16, 2024.
56. Oxfam International. More women and children killed in Gaza by Israeli military than any other recent conflict in a single year. September 30, 2024. Available at: https://www.oxfam.org/en/press-releases/more-women-and-children-killed-gaza-israeli-military-any-other-recent-conflict. Accessed October 16, 2024.
57. Office of the United Nations High Commissioner for Human Rights. Six-month update report on

the human rights situation in Gaza: 1 November 2023 to 30 April 2024 – OHCHR. November 8, 2024. Available at: https://www.un.org/unispal/document/update-report-08nov24. Accessed November 13, 2024.

58. Office of the United Nations High Commissioner for Human Rights. Onslaught of violence against women and children in Gaza unacceptable: UN experts. May 6, 2024. Available at: https://www.ohchr.org/en/press-releases/2024/05/onslaught-violence-against-women-and-children-gaza-unacceptable-un-experts. Accessed October 15, 2024.
59. World Health Organization. Women and newborns bearing the brunt of the conflict in Gaza, UN agencies warn. November 3, 2023. Available at: https://www.who.int/news/item/03-11-2023-women-and-newborns-bearing-the-brunt-of-the-conflict-in-gaza-un-agencies-warn. Accessed October 15, 2024.
60. Manduca P, Al Baraquni N, Parodi S. Long term risks to neonatal health from exposure to war-9 years long survey of reproductive health and contamination by weapon-delivered heavy metals in Gaza, Palestine. *Int J Environ Res Public Health.* 2020;17(7):2538. https://doi.org/10.3390/ijerph17072538
61. Vänskä M, Diab SY, Perko K, et al. Toxic environment of war: Maternal prenatal heavy metal load predicts infant emotional development. *Infant Behav Dev.* 2019;55:1–9. https://doi.org/10.1016/j.infbeh.2019.01.002
62. Nichols M. MSF slams US on Gaza at UN, says children as young as 5 want to die. *Reuters.* February 22, 2024. Available at: https://www.reuters.com/world/middle-east/msf-slams-us-gaza-un-says-children-young-5-want-die-2024-02-22. Accessed October 15, 2024.
63. United Nations. Israeli efforts to dismantle Palestinian refugee agency's life-saving operations in Gaza would be disastrous, senior officials, speakers warn security council. Available at: https://press.un.org/en/2024/sc15849.doc.htm. Accessed October 15, 2024.
64. Pappé I. The 1948 ethnic cleansing of Palestine. *Journal of Palestine Studies.* 2006;(141). Available at: https://ciaotest.cc.columbia.edu/olj/jps/vol36-141/vol36-141_b.pdf. Accessed March 5, 2025.
65. Euro-Med Human Rights Monitor. Death rate of elderly people in northern Gaza Strip soars due to bombing, starvation, dehydration, and lack of healthcare. March 10, 2024. Available at: https://euromedmonitor.org/en/article/6218/Death-rate-of-elderly-people-in-northern-Gaza-Strip-soars-due-to-bombing,-starvation,-dehydration,-and-lack-of-healthcare. Accessed March 11, 2025.
66. Roseboom T, de Rooij S, Painter R. The Dutch famine and its long-term consequences for adult health. *Early Hum Dev.* 2006;82(8):485–491. https://doi.org/10.1016/j.earlhumdev.2006.07.001
67. United Nations Development Programme, United Nations Economic and Social Commission for Western Asia. Gaza War: expected socio-economic impacts on the State of Palestine update. May 2, 2024. Available at: https://www.undp.org/arab-states/publications/gaza-war-expected-socio-economic-impacts-state-palestine-0. Accessed ?show $6#?>October 23, 2024.
68. United Nations. 'Hospitals have become battlegrounds': Gaza's health system on brink of collapse. *UN News: Global Perspective Human Stories.* January 3, 2025. Available at: https://news.un.org/en/story/2025/01/1158741. Accessed January 7, 2025.
69. United Nations. WHO oPt Emergency Situation Update 55 (7 Oct 2023 – 14 Feb 2025). The Question of Palestine. February 22, 2025. Available at: https://www.un.org/unispal/document/who-opt-emergency-situation-update-55-7-oct-2023-14-feb-2025. Accessed March 11, 2025.
70. United Nations Human Rights Council. Report of the Independent International Commission of Inquiry on the Occupied Palestinian Territory, Including East Jerusalem, and Israel. 2024. Available at: https://documents.un.org/doc/undoc/gen/n24/262/79/pdf/n2426279.pdf. Accessed October 11, 2024.
71. Karkar S. The olive trees of Palestine weep. In: Cook WA, ed. *The Plight of the Palestinians: A Long History of Destruction.* New York, NY: Palgrave Macmillan US; 2010:51–53. https://doi.org/10.1057/9780230107922
72. Sharkawi M. *Introducing Olive Oil Culture in Palestine.* PhD Dissertation. University of Lorraine–Nancy; 2019. Available at: https://www.researchgate.net/profile/Maissoun-Sharkawi-2/publication/340096699_INTRODUCING_OLIVE_CULTURE_IN_PALESTINE/links/5e78a0f592851cf271a0cc0b/INTRODUCING-OLIVE-CULTURE-IN-PALESTINE.pdf. Accessed October 15, 2024.
73. Simaan J. Olive growing in Palestine: A decolonial ethnographic study of collective daily-forms-of-resistance. *J Occup Sci.* 2017;24(4):510–523. https://doi.org/10.1080/14427591.2017.1378119
74. United Nations. UN calls for protection of olive trees and of Palestinian farmers amidst escalating Israeli settler violence—World Olive Tree Day 2023. November 26, 2023. Available at: https://palestine.un.org/en/253865-un-calls-protection-olive-trees-and-palestinian-farmers-amidst-escalating-israeli-settler. Accessed October 15, 2024.
75. United Nations Office for the Coordination of Humanitarian Affairs. Olive harvest 2023: hindered access afflicts Palestinian farmers in the West Bank. Occupied Palestinian Territory. February 22, 2024. Available at: https://www.ochaopt.org/content/olive-harvest-2023-hindered-access-afflicts-palestinian-farmers-west-bank. Accessed March 11, 2025.
76. Clark C. Buffalo slaughter left lasting impact on Indigenous peoples. *Emory News.* August 23, 2023. Available at: https://news.emory.edu/stories/2023/08/esc_bison_impact_24-08-2023/story.html. Accessed October 16, 2024.
77. Gandolfo KL. Representations of conflict: images of war, resistance, and identity in Palestinian Art. *Radic Hist Rev.* 2010;2010(106):47–69. https://doi.org/10.1215/01636545-2009-020
78. Amer R. The olive tree, symbol of Palestine and mute victim of Israel's war on Gaza. *Al Jazeera.* January 22, 2024. Available at: https://www.aljazeera.com/features/2024/1/22/the-olive-tree-symbol-of-palestine-and-mute-victim-of-israels-war-on-gaza. Accessed October 16, 2024.
79. United Nations Office of the High Commissioner for Human Rights. UN experts deeply concerned over 'scholasticide' in Gaza. Special Procedures. April 18, 2024. Available at: https://www.ohchr.org/en/press-releases/2024/04/un-experts-deeply-concerned-over-scholasticide-gaza. Accessed March 14, 2025.
80. London L, Watterson A, Mergler D, et al. A call from 40 public health scientists for an end to the continuing humanitarian and environmental catastrophe in Gaza. *Environ Health.* 2024;23(1):59. https://doi.org/10.1186/s12940-024-01097-9
81. Irfan A. Why Palestinians are known as the world's "best educated refugees." Columbia University Press Blog. August 23, 2023. Available at: https://cupblog.org/2023/08/23/why-palestinians-are-known-as-the-worlds-best-educated-refugeesanne-irfan. Accessed March 14, 2025.
82. Khatib R, McKee M, Yusuf S. Counting the dead in Gaza: difficult but essential. *Lancet.* 2024;404(10449):237–238. https://doi.org/10.1016/S0140-6736(24)01169-3
83. Jamaluddine Z, Abukmail H, Aly S, Campbell OMR, Checchi F. Traumatic injury mortality in the Gaza Strip from Oct 7, 2023, to June 30, 2024: a capture–recapture analysis. *Lancet.* 2025;405(10477):469–477. https://doi.org/10.1016/S0140-6736(24)02678-3
84. United Nations. Gaza power cut impacts safe water access for hundreds of thousands. *UN News: Global Perspective Human Stories.* March 10, 2025. Available at: https://news.un.org/en/story/2025/03/1160961. Accessed March 11, 2025.
85. United Nations Relief and Works Agency for Palestine Refugees in the Near East. UNRWA situation report #162 on the humanitarian crisis in the Gaza Strip and the West Bank, including East Jerusalem. March 9, 2025. Available at: https://www.unrwa.org/resources/reports/unrwa-situation-report-162-humanitarian-crisis-gaza-strip-and-west-bank-including. Accessed March 11, 2025.
86. United Nations Office of the High Commissioner for Human Rights. Gaza: ICJ ruling offers hope for protection of civilians enduring apocalyptic conditions, say UN experts. Special Procedures. January 31, 2024. Available at: https://www.ohchr.org/en/press-releases/2024/01/gaza-icj-ruling-offers-hope-protection-civilians-enduring-apocalyptic. Accessed January 7, 2025.
87. United Nations. Report of the Special Committee to Investigate Israeli Practices Affecting the Human Rights of the Palestinian People and Other Arabs of the Occupied Territories. Special Committee to Investigate Israeli Practices. 2024. Available at: https://documents.un.org/doc/undoc/gen/n24/271/19/pdf/n2427119.pdf. Accessed March 14, 2025.
88. Ahmed K, Gayle D, Mousa A. 'Ecocide in Gaza': does scale of environmental destruction amount to a war crime? *The Guardian.* March 29, 2024. Available at: https://www.theguardian.com/environment/2024/mar/29/gaza-israel-palestinian-war-ecocide-environmental-destruction-pollution-rome-statute-war-crimes-aoe. Accessed October 17, 2024.
89. Younes L. Israel's campaign in Gaza is fueling demands to make 'ecocide' an international crime. *Grist.* February 26, 2024. Available at: https://grist.org/international/israel-gaza-demands-ecocide-international-law. Accessed October 17, 2024.
90. B'Tselem. Israeli NGOs warn international community it will be complicit if Israel forcibly transfers the population of Northern Gaza. October 14, 2024. Available at: http://www.btselem.org/press_releases/20241014_international_community_will_be_complicit_if_Israel_forcibly_transfers_the_population_of_northern_gaza. Accessed March 25, 2025.

# A Flexible Framework for Urgent Public Health Climate Action

Heather A. Joseph, MPH, Stephenie C. Lemon, PhD, Karin Valentine Goins, MPH, Semra A. Aytur, PhD, MPH, Sara Zimmerman, JD, Edward Alexander, MPH, Claudia Brown, MDP, Shubhayu Saha, PhD, MA, and Paul J. Schramm, MS, MPH

Climate change poses profound threats to human safety, health, and well-being. Public health agencies, especially state, territorial, local, and Tribal health departments, can play an essential role in climate change adaptation and mitigation. Public health climate action can protect health, promote health equity, and increase climate change resilience.

The Centers for Disease Control and Prevention has updated its original climate and health framework for practitioners and expanded its utility by developing practical guidance. The revised framework, Building Resilience Against Climate Effects, supports health departments and their partners by providing an accessible approach that can be tailored to different contexts.

The framework has been updated to center justice, equity, and belonging; integrate climate change mitigation or reduction of greenhouse gas emissions that cause climate change; and address agency capacity. The Building Resilience Against Climate Effects framework also emphasizes collaboration, especially cross-sectoral and community partnerships, communication, and evaluation. Framework elements, key tactics, and guiding principles are presented in a pragmatic, step-by-step implementation guide. The implementation guide can be used by state, territorial, local, and Tribal health departments to galvanize or expand their engagement with public health climate action, which grows more urgent each year. (*Am J Public Health*. 2025;115(7):1062–1073. https://doi.org/10.2105/AJPH.2025.308061)

AJPH July 2025, Vol. 115, No. 7

Climate change is threatening the foundations of human health and well-being.[1–3] Human-generated greenhouse gas emissions cause large-scale changes, including rapid warming, rising seas and acidification, changing rainfall patterns, and shifts in seasonal events.[4] Across the United States, impacts of extreme weather are expanding, with more intense heat waves, costlier storms, longer droughts, and larger and more severe wildfires.[4] Weather-related billion-dollar disaster events have increased more than 8-fold since the 1980s.[5]

The profound health-related effects include displacement, disruptions in access to health care and other critical systems, heat-related morbidity and mortality, worsening mental health, increases in the geographic range of some infectious disease agents and vectors, exposure to poor air quality, adverse birth outcomes, and increases in pulmonary, neurologic, and cardiovascular diseases.[1,3,6,7] Likely to become more frequent with continued climate change, compound climate events result from the cooccurrence of multiple climate drivers or hazards that can have greater effects than isolated hazards.[8] As examples, the 2020 to 2021 episodes of heat and drought caused concurrent wildfires across multiple Western US states, causing millions of people to be exposed to wildfire air pollutants.[8] Power failures during heat waves are also expected to amplify heat-related morbidity and mortality.[9,10] Reducing the use of fossil fuels could, over the next 50 years, prevent approximately 4.5 million premature deaths, 1.4 million hospitalizations and emergency department visits, 300 million lost workdays, and 1.7 million incidences of dementia in the United States alone.[11]

Communities overburdened by the cumulative effects of adverse environmental, health, economic, and social conditions and by ongoing systemic discrimination and disinvestment experience disproportionate harms. Climate change worsens long-standing inequities and perpetuates a cycle of vulnerability and health disparities.[4] For example, owing in part to historical discriminatory housing policies, Black Americans are more likely to live in housing with greater exposure to extreme heat, poor air quality, and flooding.[12–15] Increasing climate change resilience—the capacity of communities and their interconnected social, economic, and ecological systems to cope with and respond to climate disruption in ways that yield overall improvements in well-being—can minimize the harms and inequities associated with climate change.

State, territorial, local and Tribal (STLT) health departments can support this work. Many public health agencies are broadening their scope to address the health effects of climate change and promote climate change resilience in 2 essential areas. First, public health agencies can promote adaptation, the process of adjusting to the effects of the changing climate to mitigate harm. Second, health departments can support climate change mitigation as a primary prevention. Mitigation refers to measures to reduce future climate change by decreasing emissions of heat-trapping gases or removing carbon dioxide from the atmosphere. Public health agencies recognize that there are limits to adaptation.[16] Mitigation can often have immediate and localized ancillary health benefits.[17–20] Consequently, practitioners are increasingly looking for "triple win" opportunities that reduce emissions, prepare for climate impacts, and advance health and equity outcomes.[21]

The Centers for Disease Control and Prevention's (CDC's) Climate and Health Program launched the BRACE (Building Resilience Against Climate Effects) framework in 2011 to support STLT health departments in using the best available science to project regional climate change health effects and prioritize, implement, and evaluate interventions.[22] Since its launch, BRACE has been used by STLT health department grant recipients of the CDC's Climate Ready States and Cities Initiative. Guidance documents, evaluations, and reports have continued to inform framework-guided practice.[23–27]

Grant recipients report that BRACE has increased public engagement, helped mainstream climate and health, and offered structure and direction for climate activities. Gaps and limitations of the original framework have also surfaced, such as requirements for technical skills; lack of tailoring to capacity; and the need for additional practical guidance on BRACE steps, cross-sector partnership development, authentic community engagement, communication, and navigating political contexts.[28] The Climate and Health Program has also observed that grant recipients are increasingly supporting jurisdictional mitigation efforts and that state and local climate action plans are increasingly likely to feature health outcomes as ancillary community benefits.

## REVISION PROCESS

In 2022, the Climate and Health Program undertook a BRACE revision to (1) center the role of justice, equity, and belonging; (2) provide step-by-step practical guidance that can be tailored to different types of health departments and contexts; and (3) incorporate climate change mitigation along with adaptation to climate action.[28] Like the original framework, the revised BRACE supports STLT health departments in selecting, implementing, and evaluating up-to-date, evidence-based climate action that will benefit public health.

The revision was conducted through a cooperative agreement with the Prevention Research Center at the University of Massachusetts Chan Medical School, which brought together a multidisciplinary leadership team, including contributors from the Climate Equity Policy Center, Health Resources in Action, the Public Health Institute, the American Public Health Association, the University of New Hampshire, and George Washington University.

The methods are described in detail elsewhere.[28] Briefly, the team first drafted the framework and the implementation guide based on a review of the scientific literature, practice briefs from professional organizations, and other climate action frameworks, particularly the National Oceanic and Atmospheric Administration's Steps to Resilience.[29] A 32-member expert panel participated in a modified Delphi approach of multiple rounds of discussion, feedback, and input on concepts and draft materials.[30] The expert panel represented STLT health departments, Tribal or community organizations focused on climate justice or equity more broadly, federal agencies, and academic organizations. Panelists represented 19 US states and the District of Columbia.

## FRAMEWORK OVERVIEW

The revised BRACE framework is intended to support STLT health departments as they undertake public health climate action.

## Essential Concepts

Several key ideas informed the BRACE revision.

Climate action must center justice, equity, and belonging to address widening disparities in climate change harms and achieve resilience. The principle of justice is defined as fairness in the treatment of people and groups, and it includes the following: a fair distribution of benefits and burdens; fair access to rights, resources, opportunities, and power; and remedy of past harms. Achieving justice involves dismantling systems of oppression and privilege that create systemic disadvantages and barriers for certain individuals and groups.[31] Equity is framed as the consistent and systematic fair and just treatment of all individuals and groups, with particular attention to race, ethnicity, ability status, gender identity, sexual orientation, and income status. Achieving equity involves recognizing that individuals and groups have different circumstances and needs, often owing to systems of oppression, and providing resources and opportunities to address those needs. Last, climate equity is the goal of recognizing and addressing the unequal burdens made worse by climate change, while ensuring that all people share the benefits of climate protection efforts.[32] In BRACE, belonging is the fundamental human need for deep connection with others, which is achieved when all people are treated like and feel like full members of the overall community.

Working toward justice, equity, and belonging requires that BRACE practitioners engage and partner with the people most affected by climate change and the organizations that serve them. Community engagement is the process of working collaboratively with groups of people affiliated by geographic proximity, particular interests, or similar situations to address issues affecting the well-being of those people.[33] BRACE prioritizes actions that are community driven and integrate the voices and experiences of community members, particularly those who have historically been left out of decision-making. Climate justice involves recognizing, valuing, and incorporating local and Indigenous knowledges. Experts in their own experiences, people living in the areas most affected by climate change are deeply aware of the outcomes, obstacles, and necessary changes for their well-being.[34]

Building and sustaining partnerships facilitate processes and outcomes associated with transformational resilience and adaptation—a state in which governments and communities work together to create more sustainable systems by addressing the root causes of climate vulnerability so that people will thrive despite change and uncertainty.[35]

BRACE encourages a holistic framing of health and well-being. The Vital Conditions framework reframes the concept of social determinants of health by identifying the core elements needed to create thriving communities instead of factors that lead to vulnerabilities and inequities.[36] Vital Conditions reminds practitioners that health is just 1 part of well-being. BRACE encourages health departments to work across sectors and disciplines to increase climate action impact. Sectors such as land use, housing, natural resources, transportation, emergency preparedness, and energy agencies may already have established goals, strategies, mandates, and funding for climate change resilience. Bidirectional exchange is ideal: public health professionals can bring a health equity perspective, specialized skill sets and data, new interest holders and existing community relationships, and credibility to other sector efforts and learn from those who are more experienced or advanced in climate action or who bring different and complementary perspectives.

## Key Principles

The essential concepts were synthesized with expert panel feedback into 10 user-friendly key principles that informed the BRACE elements (Box 1). Users can use these principles as the foundation of their climate and health work and decision-making or as a springboard for tailoring their own guiding principles.

## The Six Elements of Action

To help users implement the BRACE framework, a process is set out through 6 elements: get ready, stay ready; partner; listen and assess; investigate options; prioritize and plan; and take action. Three key activities are essential across each element: collaboration, communication, and evaluation (Figure A, available as a supplement to the online version of this article at http://www.ajph.org).

The elements are likely to work best when implemented in the suggested order. However, the framework was designed to be flexible and practical and can be used in alignment with a health department's circumstances. Each element includes 3 to 6 key tactics, specific actions that can be taken to accomplish the element's goals. The BRACE implementation guide, expected to be published in 2025, describes the framework and tactics in greater detail and includes examples, case studies,

## BOX 1— Building Resilience Against Climate Effects (BRACE) Principles

| | |
|---|---|
| Take timely, evidence-informed action | Respond to the urgency of climate change by acting quickly, sustaining efforts, and using the best available evidence to prevent further climate change and minimize its harmful effects on human health and well-being. Ensure that resilience efforts are responsive to acute disruptions and disasters, slower onset threats, and cascading and compounding effects of climate change. |
| Prioritize community experience | Climate action can focus on community-level experience by seeking input and engagement, especially from representatives of the communities most affected. Bolster community resilience by fostering trust, building on existing strengths and resources, coimplementing programs, and sharing decision-making. |
| Understand injustice and work toward justice | To ensure that everyone reaps the benefits for health and well-being of BRACE programming, public health climate action must acknowledge the historical and contemporary contexts that create ongoing systems of injustice based on race, gender, class, locality, and other identities. |
| Promote climate, justice, and health in all policies | Integrate climate, justice, and health considerations into policymaking, policy revision, and associated activities in health and nonhealth sectors. |
| Work across sectors to increase impact | Health departments can collaborate across sectors (i.e., outside public health) and partner with interest holders such as community organizations, grassroots coalitions, Tribes, academia, government agencies, and the private sector. |
| Address the causes of climate change | Appreciate the limits to adaptation and promote climate change mitigation. Initiate and support actions, policies, and partnerships that prevent climate change by reducing use of fossil fuels and lowering generated greenhouse gas emissions. |
| Prioritize inclusive and sustainable nature-based solutions | Act and think holistically, recognizing that humans are a part of nature and healthy ecosystems have benefits for human health. Support actions that protect, sustainably manage, or restore ecosystems in ways that promote nature, biodiversity, and human well-being. |
| Minimize harms | Consider a range of possible outcomes of actions and work to prevent negative effects, particularly those with justice consequences. |
| Emphasize multiple benefits | Design public health climate actions to address multiple problems. Communicate the range of health and societal benefits of climate change mitigation and adaptation strategies across sectors to increase partnerships and support. |
| Promote a culture of learning | Acknowledge uncertainty and the dynamic aspects of climate change and continuously integrate emerging evidence, programmatic observations, evaluation results, and community insights to iterate and make decisions. Share results and lessons learned. |

prompts for reflection, worksheets, and resources. Various options are presented for STLT health departments with low, medium, or high capacity.

*Get ready, stay ready.* This element recognizes that health departments and the communities they serves are unique, thus different combinations of barriers and facilitators to BRACE implementation will emerge. A starting place is to understand current capacity in terms of staff expertise, staff availability, administrative and leadership support, and financial resources.[37] BRACE suggests that users informally classify their agency as high, medium, or low capacity in each of these 4 domains and consider how this might affect options moving forward. This is framed not as a 1-time exercise but as a process to be revisited over time.

Practitioners can build capacity through leadership support, engaging internal collaborators, hiring, and establishing capacity-building infrastructure for staff such as training and networking. There is no single right way to structure climate and health activities in a health department. However, because climate change affects virtually all aspects of health, there are benefits to integrating climate perspectives across programmatic areas, as siloing could lead to competition for scarce resources. BRACE encourages practitioners to consult the *Guide to Climate and Health Programs* developed by the National Association of County and City Health Officials for ways to conceptualize and organize climate and health efforts.[38]

Practitioners also begin exploring community history and local perspectives on climate change and other environmental or social issues. BRACE encourages practitioners to think broadly about potential opportunities and partnerships, which serve as the foundation for the partner element. This can be done through partner mapping that identifies community-based organizations and coalitions that have deep connections with community members; institutions that provide services, such as health care agencies and faith-based groups; other municipal, regional, Tribal, and state government agencies; or institutions that can bring technical expertise, such as universities.

Health departments also develop overarching climate and health vision, values, and goals for the community or jurisdiction, including collaborative identification of values or principles to be used to guide the approach to climate and health equity. This element plants the seeds of adaptive management, an iterative, learning-based approach to designing, implementing, and evaluating strategies in complex systems that is particularly helpful in the continuously changing area of climate and health.[22]

*Partner.* This element establishes partnerships that will guide the entire BRACE process. Although the cross-cutting activity recognizes that partnership is a continuous process, this element has specific activities to initiate and nurture partnerships.

BRACE encourages practitioners to engage new and existing cross-sector partners because the highest impact climate action—transformative strategies that addresses root causes of climate vulnerability—requires multisector approaches and, ideally, those that integrate interest holders from both the public and private sectors. Multisectoral engagement is inherent in both the Vital Conditions framework and systems thinking.

The priorities and lived experience of the people most affected by climate change are central to effective public health climate action.[4] BRACE encourages reflection on health departments' history and capacity for facilitating this process. Practitioners can also work with partners to develop an inclusive and collaborative approach that details leadership structure, principles, and decision-making processes and authority. It is important to consistently assess the effectiveness of partnerships over time and identify potential improvements. It is also critical to provide partners with resources, such as financial support and technical assistance, and to compensate community members for their time.[39,40]

*Listen and assess.* The goal of this element is to gather, synthesize, and interpret the best available data and information. Information includes traditional public health data and the lived experiences of communities disproportionately affected by climate change.

This element begins with listening to community members and partners to understand their priorities, concerns, hopes, and experiences related to climate and health. Recognizing and amplifying community assets and strengths are essential for understanding community resilience as well as climate vulnerability. Developing community visions for the future can help to identify mitigation and adaptation solutions that the community will support. Participatory information-gathering approaches can amplify community and partner voices and center justice, equity, and belonging; generate local, place-based information; and contextualize quantitative data.[41]

Next, BRACE guides practitioners to empirically assess climate hazards, health and health equity consequences, and resilience, typically using existing data. The BRACE implementation guide includes a data guide and a listing of data sets and portals that will be continually updated.

Users identify relevant climate hazards and their effects and delineate the pathways through which health is affected. Next, they identify the population or groups who are most exposed, are most sensitive to given climate hazards, and have lower capacities to adapt or respond to these exposures. Users can also characterize community strengths and assets that buffer the negative health effects of climate change. To develop an integrated understanding of vulnerability and resilience, BRACE recommends employing general approaches such as mapping and geospatial techniques, indices, and matrices. Systems thinking–based participatory diagrams, such as rich pictures and causal loop diagrams, can be used to engage a variety of audiences and clarify relationships and boundaries.[42]

BRACE encourages users to explore mitigation-related data. Users may assess health harms and inequitable fossil fuel and copollutant impacts, identify emission-reduction opportunities, and identify data and resources to illuminate equity, health, and other benefits of mitigation at the jurisdiction level. Health benefits can stem from a range of mitigation efforts, such as improved outdoor air quality from reduced use of fuel combustion vehicles, improved physical fitness from active transportation, improved nutrition from shifting from animal-based to plant-based foods, and improved indoor air quality from electrification and home weatherization.[17–19,43,44]

Last, practitioners can collaborate with partners and communities to cointerpret data and codevelop integrated data stories. Data storytelling combines quantitative and qualitative data with visualizations (e.g., graphs, maps) and narrative.[45] Beyond simply sharing information, data storytelling attempts to use data in an intentional way that blends data analytics and communication principles to inform action and facilitate change. Whereas traditional data presentations rely on sharing data as facts and appeal to logic, data stories foreground human experience and insights in a visually appealing way to help data resonate with the audience.

*Investigate options.* In the investigate options element, users create a list of strategies to address the identified climate threats and consequences.

Developing options begins with the outputs developed in the previous elements (e.g., partner maps, documented community priorities and concerns, vulnerability and resilience data and visual outputs, mitigation-related data, data story outputs). BRACE recommends a systems thinking approach to help focus solutions on underlying causes, moving beyond reacting to acute (e.g., heat wave, hurricane) or chronic (e.g., prolonged drought) events. Systems thinking encourages users to look below the surface of events and identify opportunities for transformative adaptation and mitigation responses, moving toward changes that are structural or that alter underlying mindsets, values, and beliefs.[35]

BRACE provides multiple sources of options and resources, including a synopsis of strategies and actions across a range of mitigation and adaptation areas that previous CDC and partner grantees have implemented and reported in the literature.

BRACE recommends that users reflect on potential solutions that do the following:

1. Address both adaptation and mitigation. For example, expanding green infrastructure provides multiple benefits by cooling urban heat islands, reducing flood runoff, providing amenities for physical activity, and sequestering carbon.
2. Protect nature. Inclusive and sustainable nature-based solutions are actions that protect, sustainably manage, or restore ecosystems in ways that promote nature, biodiversity, Indigenous sovereignty, and human well-being. Although not historically viewed through a public health lens, nature-based solutions can support public health and well-being, improve biodiversity and ecosystem services, and provide a range of other benefits that greatly expand the range of possible partnerships.[46–49] Nature-based solutions with health benefits include greenways, street trees, urban forests, green roofs, urban agriculture, and wetland protection.[50,51]
3. Promote climate mainstreaming. Mainstreaming embeds climate change into the core structure, funding, and decision-making of a health department.[52] This approach can also integrate health and climate across sectors, agencies, policies, and actions, rather than addressing them only through an isolated set of specific activities.

Box 2 lists adaptation and mitigation strategies that health departments have undertaken for public health benefits. There are several publicly available inventories of solutions, including the Climate Adaptation Knowledge Exchange,[53] the Environmental Protection Agency's Public Health Adaptation Strategies for Climate Change,[54] the CDC's Climate and Health Intervention Assessment,[55] and the American Public Health Association's Center for Climate, Health, and Equity[56] webpages.

Once a list of potential strategies has been identified, the next step is to systematically investigate each. Activities include assessing the evidence base, articulating the potential health and health equity benefits of strategies, incorporating partner perspectives, and considering capacity, feasibility, resource requirements, and time frames. The aim is to generate enough information to support the final selection process in the next element.

*Prioritize and plan.* This element involves collectively setting prioritization criteria, selecting action strategies, and developing action plans. Building directly from the products of investigate options, a prioritization process to decide on 1 or more climate action strategies is identified. This involves deciding on an intentional and collaborative prioritization process, setting out explicit criteria and ranking procedures, and making a final determination.

Practitioners are then guided through developing action, communication, and monitoring and evaluation plans. Central to this process, users are advised to create a theory of change, a visual representation of how and why a desired change is expected to happen in a particular context as a result of the specified strategy. It focuses on the "missing middle" between what an initiative does (i.e., its activities or interventions) and its desired goals, filling in how the actions will achieve the desired outcomes.[57] Other elements of planning include objectives, timelines, resources, and staffing; partner and community engagement; and implementation.

Optimal action planning addresses potential maladaptation: unintended consequences of climate action that increase the risk of adverse climate-related outcomes. Maladaptation can include increased greenhouse gas emissions, reinforced or redistributed vulnerability, introductions of new risks and sources of vulnerability, inequitable outcomes, or diminished health or well-being now or in the future.[35,58] Maladaptation is more likely when drivers of vulnerability are poorly understood or not considered, often because of the incomplete engagement of all interest holders, particularly with residents of affected communities, or a

## BOX 2— Examples of Adaptation and Mitigation Strategies That Health Departments (HD) Could Lead or Support

| Category | Strategy | Focus Level/Group[a] | Example Substrategies/Actions |
|---|---|---|---|
| HD Capacity Building | Conduct HD climate and health planning | HDs/community | Develop climate and health plan for health department; develop planning, surveillance, and decision support tools for climate and health topics |
| | Create subgrant program for local HDs or other local partners | Local HDs/partners | Build capacity through training, funding, and technical assistance; provide training and technical assistance to support priority community-level actions |
| Forecasting and Data | Develop forecasting, early warning, alerts, and monitoring systems for health practitioners and the public | HDs/community | Develop forecasting, early warning, and monitoring systems for health practitioners and the public; develop and maintain alert systems for health practitioners and the public |
| | Develop climate and health data collection and surveillance system | HDs/practitioners | Collect and disseminate climate and health data for decision-making and awareness; conduct, expand, or enhance syndromic surveillance to monitor climate-sensitive health outcomes |
| Planning | Bring health perspective to jurisdiction-level planning | Jurisdiction/community | Develop/contribute health perspective to comprehensive jurisdictional climate and health plans |
| | | Jurisdiction/community | Develop jurisdictional hazard and emergency response plans |
| | | Health services/health needs population | Enhance access to health services in disasters and emergencies, especially for populations with existing health needs |
| | Develop institutional emergency response plans | Specific institutions | Develop institutional or organizational response plans (e.g., heat, wildfire, flooding, and extreme precipitation response plans) for places such as hospitals, schools, workplaces, small businesses, and incarceration centers |
| Program, Policy or Intervention Implementation | Advance building decarbonization | Community | Educate the public about rebates and health benefits of indoor appliance electrification; provide information about the health benefits of indoor appliance electrification, especially for indoor air quality |
| | | Decision-makers | Provide information about the health benefits of green building codes and standards |
| | | Contractors | Train contractors on health benefits of green building and appliances |
| | Protect community and vulnerable groups from extreme heat and other extreme weather events | Employers of outdoor workers | Provide information about the health benefits of workplace policies that protect outdoor workers from weather extremes (e.g., employers providing shade and hydration, adjusting work/rest schedules during temperature extremes, or providing personal protective equipment for cooling) |
| | | Workplace and schools | Advise and support policies that regulate safe indoor temperatures and air quality for schools, offices, and congregate settings |
| | | Community/community organizations | Increase access to in-home cooling and heating; promote social connectedness and cohesion to foster community climate change resilience, disaster preparedness, and readiness for action |
| | Support transition to clean, renewable power | Jurisdiction/community/utilities | Conduct community education about health benefits of renewables compared with fossil fuel power; provide information about the health benefits of clean renewable energy |
| | Advance waste reduction, circular economy, extended producer responsibility | Jurisdiction/community | Educate decision-makers on benefits of reducing single-use plastics; assist programs that facilitate local food production, distribution, and purchasing to reduce distance between consumption and production (e.g., community gardens) |

*Continued*

## BOX 2— Continued

| Category | Strategy | Focus Level/Group[a] | Example Substrategies/Actions |
|---|---|---|---|
| | Support community greening, urban greening, nature-based solutions | Jurisdiction | Provide information about the health benefits of green spaces, blue spaces, and trees to reduce heat islands; provide information about the health benefits and trade-offs of climate-resilience initiatives regarding trees and bushes |
| | | Community/community organizations | Assist programs that seek to expand the health benefits of community gardening |
| | | Jurisdiction/contractors | Provide information about the health benefits of smart surfaces, such as light-colored reflective pavement or roofs, to reduce ambient temperatures |
| | Reduce emissions from transportation and land use | Transportation agencies | Provide information about the health benefits of options that shift from vehicular-based highways to active transportation infrastructure |
| | | Children and youths | Provide information about the health benefits of safe routes to school programs for elementary, middle, and high schools |
| | | Children and youths | Provide information about the health benefits of expanding access to public transportation |
| | | Community/jurisdiction | Provide information about the health benefits of zoning and street design standards to encourage more density and walkable communities |
| | | Community | Provide information about the health benefits of vehicle electrification |
| | | Jurisdiction | Provide information about the health benefits of high-quality vehicle charging in zoning and building standards for multifamily housing |
| | Support green and climate resilient health care | Health care | Evaluate and enhance health care facilities to ensure that they can withstand extreme weather events; support emergency planning to ensure that generators are located in areas not vulnerable to floodwaters, especially in relation to health care facilities |
| | | | Assist in efforts to decarbonize health care, with attention to efficiency, power, anesthetic practices, and transportation |
| | Support resilience and decarbonization in select sectors | Workforce | Provide technical assistance and training on special climate and health topics to improve skills and capacity |
| | | School-based partners | Promote climate action in schools, including food procurement, solar panels, curriculum, resilience, and active transportation |
| | Reduce emissions from food | Jurisdiction/staff | Work with agency staff and other interest holders to update food procurement and food service guidelines to increase climate-friendly food, including plant-based diets, and local produce |
| | | Community | Educate the public on health and climate benefits of a plant-based diet |

*Note*. Examples are from several sources, including the Building Resilience Against Climate Effects expert panel, peer review literature, annual progress reports performance measures, and anecdotal information from the Centers for Disease Control and Prevention's Climate and Health Program grant recipients. Inclusion in this table is not a Centers for Disease Control and Prevention endorsement.
[a]Focus level or group refers to the population addressed or the level of the strategy in terms of geographical area that may be involved.

scope that is too narrow in terms of time and space.[59,60] Effective action planning includes awareness of potential maladaptation and plans to identify and minimize these outcomes.

A communication plan is an essential part of implementation. Sharing information about a project helps build sustained buy-in from community members and partners and improves the collective understanding of best practices for others seeking to do similar work.

Developing the monitoring and evaluation plan early allows users to prioritize feasibility, address the questions and issues partners and interest holders may bring up, and refine a strategy before implementation. Well-constructed and transparent monitoring and evaluation will also foster buy-in and trust with partners and communities and can assess the justice, equity, and belonging outcomes of the strategy.

***Take action.*** The last element of BRACE supports implementing selected actions, monitoring progress, measuring effectiveness, and adjusting actions as needed. Practitioners are encouraged to share findings and lessons learned.

As noted, BRACE recommends adaptive management, which recognizes that practitioners have incomplete knowledge and that strategies should be updated regularly as new understanding is gained and circumstances change.[29] BRACE prompts practitioners to incorporate feedback into management and implementation. Ways to regularly incorporate learning to improve implementation and outcomes include using monitoring and evaluation to watch for suboptimal results and address problems as they appear; anticipating challenges (e.g., changes in staffing, leadership, prioritization, budget, and partner or community buy-in); and establishing certain events, thresholds, or longer-term trends as triggers for iteration or change.

Effective communication should highlight the many potential benefits of public health climate action. These include better health, increased social cohesion, cleaner air and water, and improved ecosystem services.[3] This is particularly relevant for nature-based solutions, such as greening gray surfaces and ecosystem restoration, where the nonhealth benefits may be more immediate and tangible.[47] Emphasizing these many benefits helps make the case for environmental health and sustained investment and prioritization.

## Cross-Cutting Activities

Three key activities are essential across each BRACE element: collaboration, communication, and evaluation.

Collaboration entails working with a wide range of partners to identify goals, codesign approaches and actions, and achieve common aims and equitable, community-driven outcomes. This will involve collaborating with community organizations, governmental agencies, private organizations, and community members.

Communication involves routinely sharing and discussing progress, strategies, successes, and challenges with partners and constituents. Poor communication can lead to a lack of commitment, a misunderstanding of expectations, misaligned definitions of success, and conflict.

Evaluation is the ongoing process of systematically assessing the effectiveness of efforts, identifying successes and opportunities for improvement, distilling lessons, and incorporating best practices and improvements into ongoing and new efforts. Lack of evaluative thinking can lead to unmet community needs, continued harm, and unachieved goals.

## CONCLUSIONS

Public health climate action faces significant challenges: lack of adequate, dedicated, stable funding; lack of staff capability and capacity; low prioritization in agencies; low political will; and competing public health emergencies.[26,61–63] Other challenges are lack of certainty about climate change effects, limited scientific literature on effective climate and health interventions, the complexity of social and ecological systems, and political polarization.[26,61]

The revised BRACE framework is intended to support health departments in addressing these challenges by providing practical, flexible, context-specific guidance to engage in public health climate action. It centers community input and lived experience and features multisectoral partnerships as important facilitators to success. The framework can serve as the foundation for health departments seeking to use available opportunities to grow their climate and health efforts, including opportunities listed through the Department of Health and Human Services Office of Climate Change and Health Equity's Quickfinder for Leveraging the Inflation Reduction Act for the Health Sector[64] and the National Oceanic and Atmospheric Administration's climate change resilience toolkit, which provides a compilation of funding opportunities, resources, and technical assistance from across the federal government.[65]

Climate change threatens human health and well-being, and the risks are intensifying over time. Health departments can use their roles, skills, and strengths to promote health in this complex and evolving landscape. The BRACE framework has been designed to support this transformation in public health practice and inspire health departments to work collaboratively to realize these tremendous opportunities for promoting human health and well-being. AJPH

### ABOUT THE AUTHORS

At the time of writing, Heather A Joseph, Claudia Brown, Shubhayu Saha, and Paul J. Schramm were with the Climate and Health Program,

Division of Environmental Health Science and Practice, Centers for Disease Control and Prevention, Atlanta, GA. Stephenie C. Lemon and Karin Valentine Goins are with the Department of Population and Quantitative Health Sciences, University of Massachusetts Chan Medical School, Worcester. Semra A. Aytur is with the Department of Health Management and Policy, University of New Hampshire, Durham. Sara Zimmerman is with the Climate Equity Policy Center, Berkeley, CA. Edward Alexander is with Health Resources in Action, Boston, MA.

## CORRESPONDENCE

Correspondence should be sent to Stephenie C. Lemon, University of Massachusetts Medical School, 55 Lake Ave North, AS8-2071, Worcester, MA 01655 (e-mail: stephenie.lemon@umassmed.edu). Reprints can be ordered at https://www.ajph.org by clicking the "Reprints" link.

## PUBLICATION INFORMATION

Full Citation: Joseph HA, Lemon SC, Goins KV, et al. A flexible framework for urgent public health climate action. *Am J Public Health*. 2025;115(7): 1062–1073.

Acceptance Date: February 3, 2025.

DOI: https://doi.org/10.2105/AJPH.2025.308061

ORCID iDs:

Heather A. Joseph https://orcid.org/0000-0003-0470-6759

Sara Zimmerman https://orcid.org/0009-0008-2858-7700

Edward Alexander https://orcid.org/0009-0009-6475-1173

Claudia Brown https://orcid.org/0000-0001-6776-1566

## CONTRIBUTORS

H. A. Joseph and S. C. Lemon wrote the essay. H. A. Joseph, S. C. Lemon, K. V. Goins, C. Brown, S. Saha, and P. J. Schramm planned the project. H. A. Joseph and K. V. Goins participated in developmental methods analysis. H. A. Joseph, S. C. Lemon, K. V. Goins, S. A. Aytur, S. Zimmerman, and E. Alexander created the framework and implementation guide. S. C. Lemon, S. A. Aytur, and S. Zimmerman led developmental methods analysis. S. Zimmerman participated in analysis. C. Brown, S. Saha, and P. J. Schramm informed the framework and implementation guide. All authors reviewed the essay.

## ACKNOWLEDGMENTS

The Building Resilience Against Climate Effects framework was supported by the Centers for Disease Control and Prevention (CDC), Prevention Research Center, University of Massachusetts Chan Medical School (cooperative agreement RFA-DP-22-003, U48DP006381).

We are deeply grateful to the many contributors who made this work possible. We thank senior advisors Katherine Catalano (American Public Health Association), Stacey Chacker (Health Resources in Action), Linda Rudolph (Public Health Institute), Sandra Whitehead (Sustainable Urban Planning Program, George Washington University), and Ben Wood (Health Resources in Action). We also thank the expert panelists: Jessica Abbinett Rosane (Harris County Public Health), Sara Arman (GreenRoots), Marnie Boardman (Washington State Department of Health), Kathleen F. Bush (New York State Department of Health Center for Environmental Health), Jamie Donatuto, McKenna Dunbar (Sierra Club), Diana Felton (Hawaii State Department of Health), Howard Frumkin (University of Washington and Trust for Public Land), Shasta Gaughen, (Pala Band of Mission Indians), Solange Gould (Human Impact Partners), Natalie Grant (Office of Human Services Emergency Preparedness and Response, Administration for Children and Families/US Department of Health and Human Services [HHS]), Brendon Haggerty (Multnomah County Health Department), Michael Hansen (Southeast Climate and Energy Network) Julie Henderson (Virginia Department of Health), Jeremy Hess (University of Washington Schools of Medicine and Public Health), Tisha Holmes (Florida State University), Nils Moe (Global Optimism, formerly with Urban Sustainability Directors Network), E. Benjamin Money, Jr., (National Association of Community Health Centers), Angela Mooney D'Arcy (Sacred Places Institute for Indigenous Peoples), Stephanie Moraga-McHaley (New Mexico Department of Health, Environmental Public Health Tracking Program), Surili Sutaria Patel (Metropolitan Group), Dalton Paxman (Office of the Assistant Secretary for Health/US Department of Health and Human Services), Margaret Thelen (Wisconsin Department of Health Services), Nate Wardle (Bureau of Emergency Preparedness and Response, Pennsylvania Department of Health), and Beverly L. Wright (Deep South Center for Environmental Justice). Last, we appreciate the contributions from CDC Climate and Health Program staff (Erik Hummelman, Michele LaLand, Eric Lahr, Evan Mallen, Arie Manangan, Willow Newcomb, Karen Parker, Ana Paula Pohl Duarte, Julia Raymond, Kathryn Sisler, Chloe Svezia, Jacqueline Teed, and Ambarish Vaidyanathan) and our partners with Health Resources in Action (Kelsey McManus, Arielle Wilson-Dodard, and Olga Vanegas).

This work is published by University of Massachusetts Chan Medical School under the title Building Resilience Against Climate Effects (BRACE) (https://www.umassmed.edu/prc/brace).

**Note.** The contents of this article are solely the responsibility of the authors and do not necessarily represent the official views of the CDC, the HHS, or the US federal government.

## CONFLICTS OF INTEREST

The authors have no conflicts of interest to disclose.

## HUMAN PARTICIPANT PROTECTION

No protocol approval was necessary because no human participants were involved in this study.

## REFERENCES

1. Romanello M, Napoli C, Green C, et al. The 2023 report of the Lancet Countdown on health and climate change: the imperative for a health-centred response in a world facing irreversible harms. *Lancet*. 2023;402(10419):2346–2394. https://doi.org/10.1016/S0140-6736(23)01859-7
2. Watts N, Amann M, Arnell N, et al. The 2019 report of the Lancet Countdown on health and climate change: ensuring that the health of a child born today is not defined by a changing climate. *Lancet*. 2019;394(10211):1836–1878. https://doi.org/10.1016/S0140-6736(19)32596-6
3. Hayden MH, Schramm PJ, Beard CB, et al. Human health. In: Crimmins AR, Avery CW, Easterling DR, Kunkel KE, Stewart BC, Maycock TK, eds. *Fifth National Climate Assessment*. Washington, DC: US. Global Change Research Program; 2023:15-1–15-48.
4. Jay AK, Crimmins AR, Avery CW, et al. Overview: understanding risks, impacts, and responses. In: Crimmins AR, Avery CW, Easterling DR, Kunkel KE, Stewart BC, Maycock TK, eds. *Fifth National Climate Assessment*. Washington, DC: US Global Change Research Program; 2023.
5. National Oceanic and Atmospheric Administration. Billion-dollar weather and climate disasters. Available at: https://www.ncei.noaa.gov/access/billions. 2025. Accessed January 8, 2025.
6. Peters A, Schneider A. Cardiovascular risks of climate change. *Nat Rev Cardiol*. 2021;18(1):1–2. https://doi.org/10.1038/s41569-020-00473-5
7. Thompson R, Hornigold R, Page L, Waite T. Associations between high ambient temperatures and heat waves with mental health outcomes: a systematic review. *Public Health*. 2018;161:171–191. https://doi.org/10.1016/j.puhe.2018.06.008
8. Singh D, Crimmins AR, Pflug JM, et al. Focus on compound events. In: Crimmins AR, Avery CW, Easterling DR, Kunkel KE, Stewart BC, Maycock TK, eds. *Fifth National Climate Assessment*. Washington, DC: US Global Change Research Program; 2023: 12-1–12-42.
9. Stone B Jr, Gronlund CJ, Mallen E, et al. How blackouts during heat waves amplify mortality and morbidity risk. *Environ Sci Technol*. 2023; 57(22):8245–8255. https://doi.org/10.1021/acs.est.2c09588
10. Feng K, Ouyang M, Lin N. Tropical cyclone–blackout–heatwave compound hazard resilience in a changing climate. *Nat Commun*. 2022;13(1): 4421. https://doi.org/10.1038/s41467-022-32018-4
11. Shindell D, Ru M, Zhang Y, et al. Temporal and spatial distribution of health, labor, and crop benefits of climate change mitigation in the United States. *Proc Natl Acad Sci U S A*. 2021;118(46): e2104061118. https://doi.org/10.1073/pnas.2104061118
12. Hoffman JS, Shandas V, Pendleton N. The effects of historical housing policies on resident exposure to intra-urban heat: a study of 108 US urban areas. *Climate*. 2020;8(1):12. https://doi.org/10.3390/cli8010012
13. Wilson B. Urban heat management and the legacy of redlining. *J Am Plann Assoc*. 2020;86(4):443–457. https://doi.org/10.1080/01944363.2020.1759127
14. Katz L. A racist past, a flooded future: formerly redlined areas have $107 billion worth of homes facing high flood risk—25% more than non-redlined

areas. Available at: https://www.redfin.com/news/redlining-flood-risk. Accessed January 8, 2025.

15. Napieralski J, Guin A, Sulich C. Buried but not dead: the impact of stream and wetland loss on flood risk in redlined neighborhoods. *Environ Interact.* 2024;21:100134. https://doi.org/10.1016/j.cacint.2023.100134
16. Schaeffer R, Schipper L, Ospina D, et al. 10 new insights in climate science 2024/2025. Available at: https://10insightsclimate.science. Accessed April 17, 2025.
17. Xia T, Zhang Y, Crabb S, Shah P. Cobenefits of replacing car trips with alternative transportation: a review of evidence and methodological issues. *J Environ Public Health.* 2013;2013:797312. https://doi.org/10.1155/2013/797312
18. Smith M, Hosking J, Woodward A, et al. Systematic literature review of built environment effects on physical activity and active transport—an update and new findings on health equity. *Int J Behav Nutr Phys Act.* 2017;14(1):158. https://doi.org/10.1186/s12966-017-0613-9
19. Soret S, Mejia A, Batech M, Jaceldo-Siegl K, Harwatt H, Sabaté J. Climate change mitigation and health effects of varied dietary patterns in real-life settings throughout North America. *Am J Clin Nutr.* 2014;100(suppl 1):490S–495S. https://doi.org/10.3945/ajcn.113.071589
20. Haines A, McMichael AJ, Smith KR, et al. Public health benefits of strategies to reduce greenhouse-gas emissions: overview and implications for policy makers. *Lancet.* 2009;374(9707):2104–2114. https://doi.org/10.1016/S0140-6736(09)61759-1
21. Bell R, Khan M, Romeo-Velilla M, et al. Ten lessons for good practice for the INHERIT triple win: health, equity, and environmental sustainability. *Int J Environ Res Public Health.* 2019;16(22):456. https://doi.org/10.3390/ijerph16224546
22. Marinucci GD, Luber G, Uejio CK, Saha S, Hess JJ. Building resilience against climate effects—a novel framework to facilitate climate readiness in public health agencies. *Int J Environ Res Public Health.* 2014;11(6):6433–6458. https://doi.org/10.3390/ijerph110606433
23. Sheehan MC, Fox MA, Kaye C, Resnick B. Integrating health into local climate response: lessons from the US. CDC Climate-Ready States and Cities Initiative. *Environ Health Perspect.* 2017;125(9):094501. https://doi.org/10.1289/EHP1838
24. Schramm PJ, Brown CL, Saha S, et al. A systematic review of the effects of temperature and precipitation on pollen concentrations and season timing, and implications for human health. *Int J Biometeorol.* 2021;65(10):1615–1628. https://doi.org/10.1007/s00484-021-02128-7
25. Joseph HA, Mallen E, McLaughlin M, et al. Evaluating public health strategies for climate adaptation: challenges and opportunities from the Climate Ready States and Cities Initiative. *PLOS Climate.* 2023;2(3):e0000102. https://doi.org/10.1371/journal.pclm.0000102
26. Mallen E, Joseph HA, McLaughlin M, et al. Overcoming barriers to successful climate and health adaptation practice: notes from the field. *Int J Environ Res Public Health.* 2022;19(12):7169. https://doi.org/10.3390/ijerph19127169
27. American Public Health Association. Climate change and health playbook. Available at: https://www.apha.org/Topics-and-Issues/Climate-Health-and-Equity/JEDI. Accessed April 17, 2025.
28. Lemon SC, Joseph HA, Williams S, et al. Reimagining the role of health departments and their partners in addressing climate change: revising the Building Resilience Against Climate Effects (BRACE) framework. *Int J Environ Res Public Health.* 2023;20(15)6647. https://doi.org/10.3390/ijerph20156447
29. Gardiner N, Hutchins M, Fox J, Patel A, Rhodes K. Implementing the Steps to Resilience: a practitioner's guide. Available at: https://repository.library.noaa.gov/view/noaa/46456. Accessed April 17, 2025.
30. Hsu C, Sandford B. The Delphi technique: making sense of consensus. *Pract Assess Res Eval.* 2007;12(1):10. https://doi.org/10.7275/pdz9-th90
31. Fang C, Hench J, Daniels C, Walton A. Centering equity in climate change resilience planning and action: a practitioner's guide. Available at: https://library.oarcloud.noaa.gov/noaa_documents.lib/OAR/CPO/Climate_Smart_Communities/Vol_03_CSC_CenteringEquity.pdf. Accessed April 17, 2025.
32. US Environmental Protection Agency. Climate equity. Available at: https://www.epa.gov/climateimpacts/climate-equity. Accessed January 9, 2025.
33. Clinical Translational Science Awards Consortium. *Principles of Community Engagement.* Atlanta, GA: US Centers for Disease Control and Prevention; 2011.
34. Chen AT, Smith DO, Ojikutu BO, Auerbach J. The community as a full partner: a new model for public health. *Health Aff (Millwood).* 2024;43(6):805–812. https://doi.org/10.1377/hlthaff.2024.00033
35. Wasley E, Dahl TA, Simpson CF, et al. Adaptation. In: Crimmins AR, Avery CW, Easterling DR, Kunkel KE, Stewart BC, Maycock TK, eds. *Fifth National Climate Assessment.* Washington, DC: U. Global Change Research Program; 2023:15-1–15-48. https://doi.org/10.7930/NCA5.2023.CH31
36. Community Commons. Seven Vital Conditions for Health and Well-Being. Available at: https://www.communitycommons.org/collections/Seven-Vital-Conditions-for-Health-and-Well-Being. Accessed May 8, 2025.
37. Association of State and Territorial Health Officials. Climate and Health Capacity Survey. Available at: https://www.astho.org/globalassets/report/astho-climate-survey.pdf. Accessed January 8, 2025.
38. National Association of County and City Health Officials. A guide to climate and health programs. Available at: https://www.naccho.org/uploads/downloadable-resources/Climate-and-Health-Program-Guide.pdf. Accessed January 8, 2025.
39. Langness M, Morgan JW, Cedano S, Falkenburger E. Equitable compensation for community engagement guidebook. Available at: https://www.urban.org/research/publication/equitable-compensation-community-engagement-guidebook. Accessed January 8, 2025.
40. Spencer A, Jacobs LS. Engaging community members: a guide to equitable compensation. Available at: https://www.chcs.org/media/Engaging-Community-Members-A-Guide-to-Equitable-Compensation_101723.pdf. Accessed January 8, 2025.
41. Fleming PJ, Stone LC, Creary MS, et al. Antiracism and community-based participatory research: synergies, challenges, and opportunities. *Am J Public Health.* 2023;113(1):70–78. https://doi.org/10.2105/AJPH.2022.307114
42. Baugh Littlejohns L, Hill C, Neudorf C. Diverse approaches to creating and using causal loop diagrams in public health research: recommendations from a scoping review. *Public Health Rev.* 2021;42:1604352. https://doi.org/10.3389/phrs.2021.1604352
43. Institute of Medicine. *Climate Change, the Indoor Environment, and Health.* Washington, DC: National Academies Press; 2011.
44. Barron M, Torero M. Household electrification and indoor air pollution. *J Environ Econ Manage.* 2017;86:81–92. https://doi.org/10.1016/j.jeem.2017.07.007
45. Dykes B. *Effective Data Storytelling: How to Drive Change With Data, Narrative and Visuals.* Hoboken, NJ: Wiley; 2019.
46. Seddon N, Smith A, Smith P, et al. Getting the message right on nature-based solutions to climate change. *Glob Chang Biol.* 2021;27(8):1518–1546. https://doi.org/10.1111/gcb.15513
47. Liu H-Y, Jay M, Chen X. The role of nature-based solutions for improving environmental quality, health and well-being. *Sustainability.* 2021;13(19):1–56. https://doi.org/10.3390/su131910950
48. Reed G, Brunet ND, McGregor D, et al. Toward Indigenous visions of nature-based solutions: an exploration into Canadian federal climate policy. *Clim Policy.* 2022;22(4):514–533. https://doi.org/10.1080/14693062.2022.2047585
49. Ferreira V, Barreira AP, Loures L, Antunes D, Panagopoulos T. Stakeholders' engagement on nature-based solutions: a systematic literature review. *Sustainability.* 2020;12(2):1–27. https://doi.org/10.3390/su12020640
50. Chu EK, Fry MM, Chakraborty J, et al. Built environment, urban systems, and cities. In: Crimmins AR, Avery CW, Easterling DR, Kunkel KE, Stewart BC, Maycock TK, eds. *Fifth National Climate Assessment.* Washington, DC: US Global Change Research Program; 2023:12-1–12-42.
51. Intergovernmental Panel on Climate Change. Urban systems and other settlements. July 21, 2023. Available at: https://www.cambridge.org/core/product/F8AEF956B904563A76D7330DCB1D0D1C. Accessed April 17, 2025.
52. Gurung J, Sinha B, Lee B, et al. Basics of mainstreaming gender into climate change and disaster risk reduction policies. Available at: https://wrd.unwomen.org/sites/default/files/2021-11/BASICS~1.PDF. Accessed January 8, 2025.
53. Climate Action Knowledge Exchange. Your online adaptation destination. Available at: https://www.cakex.org. Accessed April 17, 2025.
54. Environmental Protection Agency. Public health adaptation strategies for climate change. Available at: https://www.epa.gov/arc-x/public-health-adaptation-strategies-climate-change. Accessed April 17, 2025.
55. Centers for Disease Control and Prevention. Guidance and trainings. Available at: https://www.cdc.gov/climate-health/php/resources/guidance-trainings.html. Accessed April 17, 2025.
56. American Public Health Association. Climate, health, and equity. Available at: https://www.apha.org/topics-and-issues/climate-health-and-equity. Accessed April 17, 2025.
57. Center for Theory of Change. What is theory of change? Available at: https://www.theoryofchange.org/what-is-theory-of-change. Accessed January 8, 2025.
58. Möller V, van Diemen R, Matthews JBR, et al. Annex II: glossary. In: *Climate Change 2022—Impacts, Adaptation and Vulnerability.* Cambridge, UK: Cambridge University Press; 2023:2897–2930.

59. Eriksen S, Schipper ELF, Scoville-Simonds M, et al. Adaptation interventions and their effect on vulnerability in developing countries: help, hindrance or irrelevance? *World Dev.* 2021;141: 105383–105383. https://doi.org/10.1016/j.worlddev.2020.105383
60. Schipper ELF. Maladaptation: when adaptation to climate change goes very wrong. *One Earth.* 2020;3(4):409–414. https://doi.org/10.1016/j.oneear.2020.09.014
61. Hartwell C, Lovell S, Hess JJ, Dolan K, Vickery J, Errett NA. Barriers and facilitators to state public health agency climate and health action: a qualitative assessment. *BMC Public Health.* 2023;23(1):1–9. https://doi.org/10.1186/s12889-023-14996-2
62. Eidson M, Clancy KA, Birkhead GS. Public health climate change adaptation planning using stakeholder feedback. *J Public Health Manag Pract.* 2016;22(1):E11–E19. https://doi.org/10.1097/PHH.0000000000000243
63. Schramm PJ, Ahmed M, Siegel H, et al. Climate change and health: local solutions to local challenges. *Curr Environ Health Rep.* 2020;7(4):363–370. https://doi.org/10.1007/s40572-020-00294-1
64. Office of Climate Change and Health Equity. Quickfinder for leveraging the Inflation Reduction Act for the health sector. Available at: https://www.hhs.gov/climate-change-health-equity-environmental-justice/climate-change-health-equity/quickfinder-ira/index.html. Accessed January 8, 2025.
65. National Oceanic and Atmospheric Administration. US climate change resilience toolkit funding opportunities. Available at: https://toolkit.climate.gov/content/funding-opportunities. Accessed January 8, 2025.

# History of Risk Assessments of the Organophosphate Pesticide Chlorpyrifos at the US Environmental Protection Agency, 1980–2024

Christopher Sellers, MD, PhD, Ellen Kohl, PhD, Marianne Sullivan, DrPH, MPH, Gretchen Gehrke, PhD, Jessica Varner, PhD, Mark Chambers, PhD, and the Environmental Data and Governance Initiative

AJPH July 2025, Vol. 115, No. 7

This article examines the history of risk assessments of the organophosphate pesticide chlorpyrifos at the US Environmental Protection Agency (EPA), especially after a ban on household uses in 2000. Federal funding enabled more noncorporate and place-based scientific investigations of this pesticide's harms, including child-cohort epidemiology of populations impacted through environmental injustices. This article argues, first, that their findings challenged the thin knowledge base, mostly from corporate-sponsored toxicology, that originally justified chlorpyrifos's continued use. Second, for decades, outside a court-induced interval in 2015–2016, EPA's risk assessments favored "de-placed" toxicological modes and standards of knowledge—forged in the controlled environment of experimental laboratories—while marginalizing science gathered from the actual places and people EPA is supposed to protect. Third, agency officials stuck with a quantifiable, laboratory- and modeling-centered calculus for assessing health risks in part because a united front of corporate and corporate-consultant scientists harped on the uncertainties of newer findings. The article concludes that the agency needs to rethink its risk assessment practices and dependence, as well as more effectively account for financial conflicts of interest in evaluations of policy-relevant science. (*Am J Public Health*. 2025;115(7):1074–1084. https://doi.org/10.2105/AJPH.2025.308073)

In 2006, six years after the US Environmental Protection Agency (EPA) struck a deal with manufacturers to discontinue household uses of the pesticide chlorpyrifos, alarming levels were detected in samples taken outside the homes of two farmworker families in Washington State's Yakima Valley. The Pesticide Action Network North America (PANNA) and the Farmworker Pesticide Project connected these results to chlorpyrifos's agricultural uses and growing scientific findings about its health impacts. "Scores of animal studies have now documented significant neurological changes in the developing fetus" and "new *human* studies provide strong evidence that people are being adversely affected [emphasis in original]."[1(p8)] These studies, mostly federally funded, were toxicological, but also in the field of prospective epidemiology, with little precedent in pesticide science, pairing measured exposures to chlorpyrifos among hundreds of pregnant women with careful years-long monitoring of their offspring.[2–4] That same year, the EPA reregistered chlorpyrifos for usage on farms and orchards. PANNA and the Natural Resources Defense Council (NRDC) then petitioned EPA to revoke this decision and ban chlorpyrifos. It took 14 years for the EPA to cancel chlorpyrifos's agricultural uses in 2021, a move since overturned by a federal appeals court.[5]

Why has a ban on chlorpyrifos's agricultural uses proven so elusive for EPA, despite science demonstrating its human harms? The reasons are multiple, starting with EPA's limited mandate for controlling pesticides, which, unlike those for air pollutants or endangered species, explicitly requires it to balance economic and public health benefits.[6(p312),7] Political shifts also played an important role: reversals in 2017 and

2021 overturned the previous administration's proposed chlorpyrifos rules, although, up to 2015, both Republican and Democratic administrations upheld its continuing use (Box 1). We argue for two additional, intertwined explanations. First, EPA's practices of risk assessment consistently favored toxicology, especially its older variants and conclusions, over newer knowledge, especially from epidemiology. Second, well-organized and -funded interventions of corporate-aligned experts reinforced this inclination. For nearly two decades after its ban on household uses, EPA risk assessments of chlorpyrifos enabled its continuing concentration in the rural homes and communities of Yakima Valley and other farmworkers, hobbling this agency's ability to address this environmental injustice.

## BACKGROUND AND LITERATURE

Chlorpyrifos, first registered with the US Food and Drug Administration (FDA) by Dow Chemical in 1965, was among the organophosphate pesticides that replaced the chlorinated hydrocarbons like DDT (dichlorodiphenyltrichloroethane) that were driven out of the American market by new environmental concerns and laws.[8,9] A broad-spectrum killer of insects and mites, chlorpyrifos, like other organophosphates, had long been known to be dangerous to nontarget animals and people, as well, with effects ranging from headaches and dizziness to seizures, comas, and death.[10,11] It nevertheless escaped the midcentury public scrutiny of many pesticides in the United States that led to the Federal Insecticide, Fungicide, and Rodenticide Act (FIFRA), which tightened their federal oversight. Passed after a long negotiation with agricultural interests, FIFRA explicitly required "balancing" pesticides' public and ecological health impacts with their economic benefits to manufacturers and farmers while removing decisions about registration and residues from the US Department of Agriculture (USDA) and FDA to a newly created EPA.[6(p312),7] Acting quickly and aggressively against DDT

### BOX 1— A Timeline of the Regulation of Chlorpyrifos in the United States

| |
|---|
| 1965—Chlorpyrifos is first registered by Dow Chemical with FDA. |
| 1970—The US EPA is created. |
| 1972—FIFRA transfers pesticide registration to EPA. |
| Late 1970s to mid-1980s—Risk assessment is institutionalized at EPA. |
| 1985—Chlorpyrifos is reregistered for household as well as agricultural uses. |
| 1996—The FQPA is passed by Congress and signed into law. |
| 1998—EPA joins with NIEHS to fund Children's Health Centers, where prospective epidemiological studies of chlorpyrifos begin. |
| 2000—As EPA reevaluates chlorpyrifos health risks using FQPA standards, manufacturers agree to ban household uses. |
| 2003—EPA's health risk reassessment of chlorpyrifos and first cumulative risk assessment (of organophosphate pesticides) support chlorpyrifos's continued agricultural use. |
| 2006—Report is published by FPP and PANNA; EPA approves the reregistration of chlorpyrifos for agriculture. |
| 2007—PANNA and the NRDC petition EPA to revoke this decision. |
| 2008—An EPA SAB, while expressing "concerns," backs chlorpyrifos's reregistration. |
| 2011-NRDC and PANNA take EPA to court, demanding a timely response to their 2007 petition. |
| 2014—EPA's reassessment of chlorpyrifos's health risks settles upon risk calculations similar to those in the early 2000s, sidelining epidemiological data. |
| 2015—After NRDC and PANNA lawsuit leads a federal judge to require EPA response, the agency proposes a ban and begins to fold epidemiological data into its main health risk calculus. |
| 2016—An EPA SAB meeting on chlorpyrifos proposes an alternative usage of epidemiological data; the agency's ban on agricultural uses of chlorpyrifos moves forward. |
| 2017—New EPA administrator Scott Pruitt revokes the proposed ban and moves to reregister agricultural uses of chlorpyrifos. |
| 2021—The EPA reregistration of chlorpyrifos is struck down by federal appeals courts, and new EPA administrator Michael Regan revives and finalizes a chlorpyrifos ban. |
| 2023-2024—EPA's chlorpyrifos ban is overturned by federal court; EPA proposes limited agricultural use. |

*Note.* EPA = Environmental Protection Agency; FDA = Food and Drug Administration; FIFRA = Federal Insecticide, Fungicide, and Rodenticide Act; FPP = Farmworker Pesticide Project; FQPA = Food Quality and Protection Act; NIEHS = National Institute of Environmental Health Sciences; NRDC = Natural Resources Defense Council; PANNA = Pesticide Action Network North America; SAB = Science Advisory Board.

and other chlorinated hydrocarbons, the EPA put off the reregistration decision of less publicly maligned pesticides like chlorpyrifos until the mid-1980s.[12–15]

By the time the EPA began its deliberations over chlorpyrifos reregistration (Box 1), the clinical signs and symptoms of acute poisoning by organophosphates were well-established in the medical literature.[16] The laboratory test clinching diagnosis reflected the known internal mechanism of chlorpyrifos's toxicity in insects and humans: the inhibition of acetylcholinesterase (AChE), which breaks down the neurotransmitter acetylcholine.[17] An important fraction of these pesticides' real-world harm had become recognizable to doctors, mostly in adult workers or inadvertently doused children whose cases had been studied retrospectively via epidemiology.[18,19] But subclinical and chronic effects remained "not well known."[20(p327)]

To navigate these while side-stepping earlier controversies over pesticide decisions, the EPA, by the mid-1980s, formalized a process of risk assessment that privileged toxicology, a science that began in the laboratory.[13] This discipline's modus operandi was to reduce the complexity of real-world human exposures and harms down to single chemicals applied to experimental bodies, animal or human, then carefully monitored for known or suspected pathological effects. We term this style of knowledge "de-placed"—rather than "placeless" or "universal"—to emphasize how reductive and simplified its findings proved in comparison with the more placed knowledge consolidating after 1985, gathered directly from exposure routes and exposed people, many of whom lived in "environmental justice" communities.

The risk assessment leading to EPA's 1985 reregistration reflected a profound ignorance not just about chlorpyrifos's health effects but also about those places and people that were most susceptible to it—similar to recent findings about per- and polyfluoroalkyl substances (PFAS) under the Toxic Substances Control Act.[21] Assessors frankly acknowledged a "moderate mammalian toxicity," confirmed by Dow's tests for acute effects, but deemed this acceptable—a reflection of FIFRA requirements to balance between economic and health benefits—and best dealt with through guidelines for proper usage. Environmental and exposure data remained extremely thin: Dow-measured toxic residues and metabolites on experimentally sprayed crops, along with data just beginning to be collected by USDA on pesticides in some foods. Most other requirements were toxicological: agency-standardized animal tests for the chronic effects of carcinogenicity and reproductive and genetic damages. For neurotoxicity, an animal test as well as a controlled human exposure study on 16 adult volunteers only looked for "delayed acute effects"—nothing chronic.[22] All studies reported no effects, even at the highest exposure levels.

Then and later, the toxicological slant in EPA risk assessments favored another tilt, toward corporate interests.[23] De-placed from real-world exposures, these required toxicology studies were sociologically very much situated: in corporate or corporate-funded laboratories, where profitable products as well as experimenters' jobs were often at stake. Their underlying purposes and sponsorship incentivized product-friendly results and circumscribed inquisitiveness. Few, if any, were peer-reviewed and published, facilitating scientific flaws as significant as those documented in a published 2020 re-examination of Dow's human exposure experiment. It found that company statisticians had simply excluded data showing effects at the middle and lower levels of exposure, coming to erroneous conclusions that nevertheless anchored EPA's risk calculations for chlorpyrifos into the early 2000s.[24,25]

Reregistration of chlorpyrifos in 1985 thus proceeded in the face of deep ignorance of its actual environmental exposures and the subtle, far-reaching damage it turned out to have, especially on children. By the early 1990s, chlorpyrifos was the second-most-widely used pesticide outside agriculture in the United States. Meanwhile, the National Academy of Sciences and National Research Council had begun promoting a better knowledge base for understanding pesticides' health and environmental impacts, and advocacy groups joined these influential scientific institutions in singling out children's special susceptibilities to pesticides.[26] By 1996, a political coalition had formed that was broad enough for legislative action, leading to Congressional passage of the Food Quality and Protection Act (FQPA), which, among other measures, amplified EPA's mandate to protect children from pesticide exposures.[27–29]

Drawing on the FQPA as well as governmental initiatives to encourage more place-based exposure data and health science, the EPA moved to reassess chlorpyrifos's health risks. The biggest change was a FQPA requirement for an additional 10× safety margin to shield unborn or young children, whom new toxicology experiments were beginning to show had greater susceptibility to the pesticide. Environmental measurements also enabled modeling of chlorpyrifos's complex patterns of exposure, including some 56 calculated "scenarios" of exposure. Many residential ones, as well as dietary exposures of children aged 1 to 6 years, surpassed agency "levels of concern," leading the agency toward recommendations for "risk mitigation" and "reduction."[30] In June 2000, Dow Management then voluntarily agreed to end "virtually all non-agricultural uses."[31] What neither party addressed in these deliberations were exposures in homes next to sprayed fields, where many farmworker families lived.

## KEEPING CHLORPYRIFOS ON THE AMERICAN FARM

While chlorpyrifos use plummeted 70% in the years after the ban on household uses, during the 2010s, agricultural uses kept the sales volume stable, sustaining its reputation as the "number one insecticide used in the United States."[9,32(p8),33] More than a decade after the 2006 finding of chlorpyrifos around farmworker homes in Yakima Valley, in 2019, 36% of armband detectors worn by Latina adolescent girls in a California farmworking community detected chlorpyrifos, despite new EPA rules to curb drift.[34] Place-based science of chlorpyrifos's exposure and harms had meanwhile burgeoned, boosted by federal funding. The new scientific work included prospective epidemiological studies highlighting damages on communities with long legacies of environmental racism, which challenged EPA's earlier conclusions about chlorpyrifos based on corporate-sponsored science.

Nevertheless, outside a court-pressured year-and-a-half interval, EPA, in the two decades after 2000, dealt with the growing knowledge of chlorpyrifos's dangers by consistently downplaying the consolidating strength of these studies and the real-world threat to public health they conveyed. It did so largely through risk assessment's preestablished seamless melding of bureaucratic and scientific imperatives. As Demortain has noted, risk assessment over this period became "much less present in the whole of agency discourse,"[13(p273)] but for chlorpyrifos it still functioned, as Boyd has described, as a "political technology to discipline . . . and constrain," imposing an epistemological roadblock to more aggressive agency action.[35(p153)] The EPA's marginalization of epidemiological findings also reflected the strength of a doubt-promoting pressure campaign by corporate-aligned experts.

The upsurge in federal funding for the study of chlorpyrifos from the late 1990s stoked rising debates about chlorpyrifos's uses. With the EPA and the National Institutes of Health awarding more grants for its study (Figure 1), the dominance of corporate laboratories and experts eroded, as expanding ranks of academic researchers addressed new, more varied questions about this pesticide's harms.

Most influential for chlorpyrifos was EPA's collaboration with the National Institute of Environmental Health Sciences (NIEHS) to fund Children's Environmental Health Centers. Here, as elsewhere, EPA supported epidemiology to learn about health impacts on "at risk populations," through collaboration with another agency like NIEHS, with more in-house epidemiological experts.[36(pI-33)] The new funding enabled academic epidemiologists to apply well-honed prospective methods looking forward in time, tallying exposures following health effects that emerged among study cohorts over time, to test for associated and possibly causal effects.[37,38] Three key studies homed in on communities for whom aggravated pesticide exposure was just one of many environmental and socioeconomic burdens they faced. A University of California–Berkeley study followed nearly 400 children of farmworkers in California's Salinas Valley. The Columbia University and Mount Sinai studies began with 658 and 404 pregnant women, respectively, mostly Black or Latina and living in New York City's inner-city neighborhoods, where housing deterioration had led to heavy pesticide applications against insect pests. Enrolling women in the years just before and after chlorpyrifos had been banned for residential use, the Columbia study gained a "natural" control cohort for comparison.

By the mid-2000s, new findings from these epidemiological studies were producing a more complex and troubling portrait of chlorpyrifos's effects on children's health. In utero exposures were followed by low birth weight, lesser length, decreased head circumference, cognitive and psychomotor delays, hyperactivity and attention deficits, and "pervasive developmental disorder."[2,39,40] Longer-term neurotoxic and developmental outcomes, increasingly supported by animal experiments, challenged scientific contentions about the ambit and mechanism of chlorpyrifos's toxicity that had grounded EPA risk assessments in the 1980s and 1990s. Chronic harms, which earlier tests for "acute delayed" neurotoxicity could never capture, often seemed to work independently of AChE, raising questions about whether it was the sole mechanism of toxic action. Questions were raised about whether

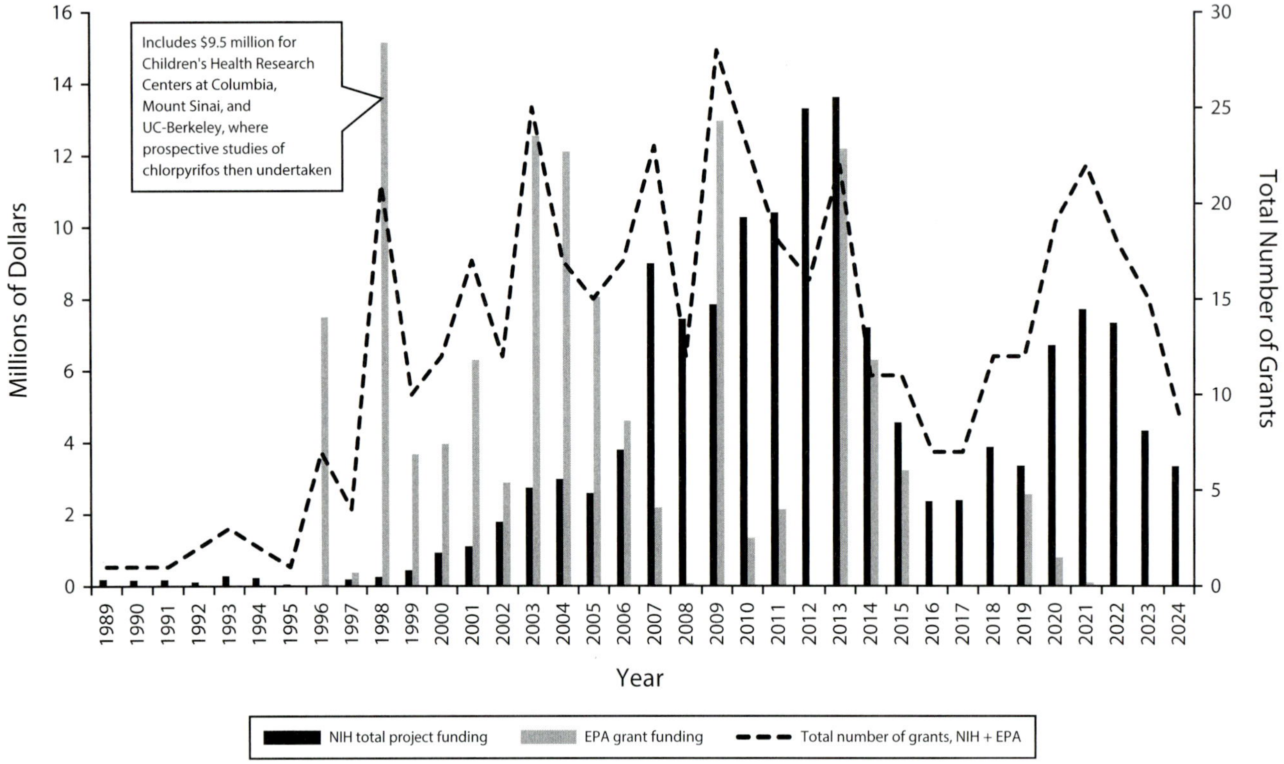


**FIGURE 1— Trends in Federal Grants for Research Involving Chlorpyrifos: United States, 1989-2024**

*Note.* EPA = Environmental Protection Agency; NIH = National Institutes of Health; UC = University of California. EPA database only goes back to 1995.
*Source.* https://cfpub.epa.gov/ncer_abstracts/index.cfm/fuseaction/search.welcome; https://reporter.nih.gov/advanced-search.



chlorpyrifos and other organophosphates had a physiological threshold (deduced from "no-effects" level in experiments), through evidence that it was carcinogenic, which EPA recognized as a non–threshold effect, as well as an endocrine disruptor, a chemical category that the agency did not recognize as without a threshold but many scientists did.[41] Nevertheless, by 2006. the EPA under G. W. Bush moved to reregister chlorpyrifos for agriculture. After PANNA and the NRDC petitioned EPA to revoke this decision, pointing to the newer evidence, EPA turned to its FIFRA Science Advisory Board (SAB) for advice on how to respond.

Dow and its allied manufacturer and consulting firm experts then targeted this meeting as an opportunity to counter the emerging scientific evidence and defend the pesticide's safety, in ways the EPA as well as its science advisors could not ignore. Coordinating testimony from an entire team and including lengthy written reports, they manufactured a formidable front of scientific skepticism. Their public comments outnumbered those by NRDC and academics, who overwhelmingly supported the epidemiological findings and questioned whether chlorpyrifos's toxicity was confined to AChE inhibition (Figure 2 and Table 1).

In 2008, the FIFRA SAB largely backed EPA's reluctance to take further action against chlorpyrifos. It did express concern about "adverse effects . . . below EPA's reference dose" especially given demonstrated neurodevelopmental effects at low levels for "lead, mercury, and PCBs." While split on whether a mechanism other than AChE inhibition might be at work, the SAB ultimately leaned once more on AChE inhibition as the sole mechanism for a "reference dose." It also echoed industry and consultant experts on the "key limitations to the three epidemiological studies." Declaring them "qualitative in nature," the SAB demoted them from EPA's core, de-placed calculus of risk, and relegated them as EPA had only to a preliminary "characterization" or "identification" of the hazard.[42(p43,45)]

During the Obama administration, the EPA struggled with how to handle the increasingly diverse strands of pesticide science in its risk assessments of chlorpyrifos, especially after a 2011 lawsuit brought by NRDC and PANNA demanded a timely response to their 2007 petition. The agency had begun

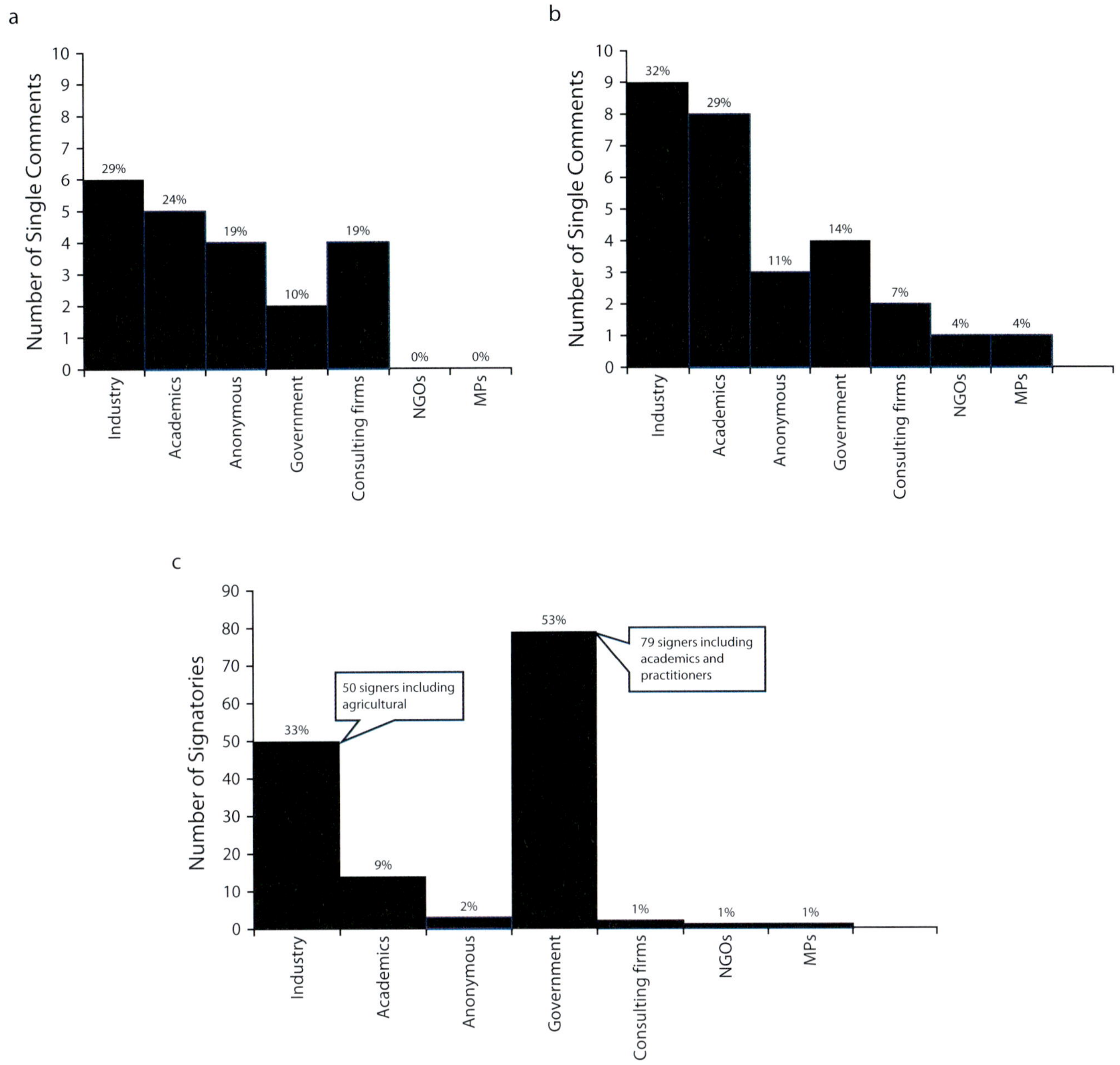


**FIGURE 2— Breakdown of Public Comments/Signatories for Meetings of Environmental Protection Agency's FIFRA Science Advisory Panel Discussing Chlorpyrifos by (a) 2008 Single Comments, (b) 2016 Single Comments, and (c) 2016 Signatories: United States.**

*Note.* FIFRA = Federal Insecticide, Fungicide, and Rodenticide Act; MP = medical practitioner (nonacademic); NGO = nongovernmental organization. Parts a and b enumerate those documents or document sets submitted by single or multiple authors or by a group, counting each as a single comment (n = 21 for 2008 and n = 28 for 2016). For 2008, most comments were signed by one or two individuals, but the total signatories on some 2016 comments were much greater—hence, the separate tally in part c.
*Source.* Docket EPA-HQ-OPP-2008-0274: https://www.regulations.gov/docket/EPA-HQ-OPP-2008-0274.

formally reevaluating the role of epidemiology in its risk assessments, eventually yielding a "framework" that would open the door for using "high quality" studies in risk calculation.[43] But, already by 2014, as officials wrote up another health risk assessment for chlorpyrifos, place-based as well as laboratory studies had proliferated. Just on its longer-term neuro-behavioral effects, they counted "31 papers generated from 14 laboratories" as new data and modeling pinpointed dangers from drinking water and inhalation as well as pesticide drift.[44(p26)]

**TABLE 1—** Breakdown of 2008 and 2016 Public Comments Made by Outside Parties to the Environmental Protection Agency's Federal Insecticide, Fungicide, and Rodenticide Act Science Advisory Board (SAB), by Affiliation and Scientific Positions Taken: United States

| Year of SAB Deliberation and Position Taken in Public Comment | Mechanism of Chlorpyrifos's Toxicity | | | Stance on Epidemiology | | |
|---|---|---|---|---|---|---|
| | Only AChE | Also Other | Position Unclear | Skeptical | Supportive | Unclear |
| 2008 (n = 21) | | | | | | |
| Total comments favoring position | 8 | 4 | 9 | 9 | 4 | 8 |
| Percentage of total comments favoring position | 38 | 19 | 43 | 43 | 19 | 38 |
| Share from industry and consulting firms favoring position | 88 | 0 | 44 | 78 | 0 | 50 |
| Share from NGOs and academics favoring position | 13 | 100 | 11 | 22 | 100 | 0 |
| 2016 (n = 28) | | | | | | |
| Total comments favoring position | 12 | 3 | 13 | 20 | 6 | 2 |
| Percentage of total comments favoring position | 43 | 11 | 46 | 71 | 21 | 7 |
| Share from industry and consulting firms favoring position | 75 | 0 | 62 | 80 | 0 | 50 |
| Share from NGOs and academics favoring position | 8 | 100 | 23 | 10 | 83 | 0 |

*Note.* AChE = acetylcholinesterase; NGO = nongovernmental organization.
*Source.* Docket EPA-HQ-OPP-2008-0274: https://www.regulations.gov/docket/EPA-HQ-OPP-2008-0274; Docket EPA-HQ-OPP-2016-0062: https://www.regulations.gov/docket/EPA-HQ-OPP-2016-0062.

Nevertheless, the 2014 health risk assessment settled upon risk calculations for chlorpyrifos much like those adopted under G. W. Bush. Its risk assessors did differentiate between "two different" pathways of harm: "acetylcholinesterase (AChE) inhibition and potential for neurodevelopmental effects." They acknowledged the consistency with which neurodevelopmental impacts had been found across studies, species, and disciplines. Yet, the lack of consensus about a biological mechanism led them to emphasize the "uncertainties" about this pathway and to urge a continued reliance only on AChE inhibition. Their treatment of the epidemiological findings was similar, pointing to the possible influence of pesticides other than chlorpyrifos on the results, as "preclud[ing] definitive causal inference."[33(p6)] Declaring their own "weight-of-evidence" standard, they framed the epidemiological results as "risk characterization": justifying the full 10× FQPA safety factor to protect children but sidelined in core calculations of risk.[33(p41)] Values of scientific certainty and quantifiable precision downgraded this more placed style of knowledge, thwarting a public health response.

But a courtroom loss led the Obama-era EPA to reverse course. After NRDC and PANNA successfully sued the EPA in 2015 for still not responding to their petition, EPA proposed an order revoking all chlorpyrifos tolerances on food crops—a ban—and then revised its health risk assessment to provide scientific backing for this move.[45] Not only did risk assessors abandon their long-standing reliance on AChE inhibition alone, but they also sought to incorporate data from the Columbia epidemiological study into their core calculations of risk. When the agency asked the FIFRA SAB for input on a proposed use of these data in April 2016, it suggested an alternative—using time-weighted averages or "TWA blood concentration" partly based on Columbia data—that the EPA then adopted. By November of 2016, EPA's revised health risk assessment had more fully embraced epidemiological evidence, which now grounded another new departure for the agency: its proposal for a chlorpyrifos ban.[46(p14)]

While the EPA had shifted course by 2016, public comments for that year's SAB meeting had not. Mirroring the pattern of 2008, industry experts and consulting firms overwhelmingly supported AChE inhibition as the sole mechanism of toxicity and harped on epidemiology's uncertainties, while academic and nongovernmental organization (NGO) experts took opposing stances (Table 1). Now, however, far more people signed some comments (Figure 2, panel C), and, across many, commenters' extrascientific interests and concerns turned more explicit. This time around, NRDC and PANNA culled petition-like signatures from farmworker and environmental justice groups as well as academic health scientists and practitioners. They and their allies wrote about not just the scientific questions but also the people and communities whose health was at stake. An obstetrics/gynecology practitioner in a California agricultural community "respectfully request[ed] that when making recommendations . . . , you will look at it through the lens of a parent, a grandparent, or community member and consider all children to be as precious as your own."[47(p1)] The 69-signature comment by NRDC's Jennifer Sass and Columbia study leader Robin Whyatt urged a ban on agricultural uses of the pesticide to lift the current "toll . . . on farmworkers, their families and their children—born and unborn, on rural and suburban families" residing near sprayed fields, "and on all Americans who consume food that has been treated with chlorpyrifos."[48(p3)] Corporate and consultant commenters, meanwhile, signed on 42 growers' groups to a warning against a "European-style precautionary approach," which would deprive them of "valuable crop protection tools."[49(p1)] Another defended a 40-year tradition of "sound scientific risk assessment" of pesticides, celebrating the thin, de-placed evidence grounding past decision-making while disparaging newer scientific approaches and findings.[50(p1)]

With the Trump presidency, that imagined "tradition" was not just resuscitated but elevated. In March 2017, EPA administrator Scott Pruitt rescinded the pending proposal to ban chlorpyrifos in food crops. EPA's earlier risk assessments supplied him with ample arguments for doing so: in a nutshell, the science on this pesticide's neurobehavioral effects was too "uncertain."[51(p35)] Corporate and consultancy experts, including some from the chlorpyrifos wars, became EPA science advisors; one was even nominated to head its chemicals office.[52] The Trump administration proposed a transparency-in-science rule for EPA risk assessments that targeted child-cohort and other prospective epidemiological studies head-on, essentially barring from policy-making any science that used confidential medical records.[53] Also cutting off funding for chlorpyrifos research (Figure 1), this administration's rhetorical championing of scientific certainty clashed with its clear aversion to improving what was known.

Once Biden replaced Trump in the White House, a federal court of appeals (9th circuit) rejected the Pruitt EPA's revised chlorpyrifos rule. A Michael Regan–led EPA then revived and formalized a chlorpyrifos ban through risk calculations centering on "aggregate exposure data" rather than epidemiological findings.[54] Two years later, another federal appeals court (8th circuit) rescinded this ban, noting how before 2021, "agricultural use of chlorpyrifos had survived multiple safety reviews."[5(p5)] In that courtroom, the agency's long history of poorly informed risk assessments and inaction weighed against the credence of more recent, place-based science, stifling EPA's ability to shield rural and farmworker families from chlorpyrifos.

## CONCLUSION

By the mid-2010s, the soundness of knowledge on chlorpyrifos's exposures and health effects had far outstripped what was available in mid-1980s. As a consequence, by the early 2020s, the European Union and at least 11 other countries, as well as five American states, banned agricultural uses of this pesticide.[55] Exemplifying a larger pattern,[56] the US EPA's reluctance to do so stemmed in important part from epistemological biases in its risk assessment process, which privileged de-placed modes and standards of knowledge from toxicological laboratories over more place-based data and research, especially from epidemiology. Three prospective epidemiological studies of chlorpyrifos had been conducted on hundreds of exposed people, each with peer-reviewed results connecting chlorpyrifos exposure to serious harms. Yet, for many years, EPA risk assessors continued to invoke unmet standards of scientific certainty to blunt their consideration of robust epidemiological evidence, often also to disregard its implied imperative for more protective action. The pattern was the reverse of the public health orientation recommended by Woodruff et al., calling for "swift action . . . to mitigate exposures to hazardous chemicals at the first indication of potential harm."[57]

Another reason for EPA's reluctance lay in the concerted interventions of corporate and consulting experts in the risk assessment process. As federally supported academic investigators undercut their dominance in the scientific study of this pesticide, the latter had carved out a new role: bolstering skepticism of EPA risk assessors toward newer science. Inserting their voices and arguments where they could in EPA's deliberations, they sowed doubts about findings that favored more regulation of a profitable product, much as they have in recent decades in other medical and scientific realms.[58] The uniformity and predictability of their interventions helped drive a growing politicization of risk assessment and the SABs. One remedy may lie in the recommendations of Woodruff et al.: EPA and other agencies need more formal and effective ways of accounting for financial conflicts of interests within their risk assessments.[57]

This history exemplifies how the prioritization of de-placed over placed knowledge in EPA risk assessments has hamstrung this agency's ability to consider as well as act against environmental injustices. The most troubling consequence of the EPA's years of inaction is that farmworker and other families trapped by poverty and racial discrimination in rural homes near sprayed fields have continued to shoulder chlorpyrifos's risks. Certainly, the health consequences that may have ensued in these cohorts need to be followed and addressed. New legislation mandating that pesticide regulation go further than either FIFRA or the FQPA to prioritize public health over agricultural practices and profits could also help.

Yet, such moves still will not fix a pattern identified in this history: how EPA risk assessment has wielded scientific standards of certainty most easily achieved in the laboratory to marginalize science and data gathered more directly from exposed places and people. Despite long-standing hopes for a more cumulative version of risk assessment, its track record with chlorpyrifos confirms Boyd's skepticism about whether "doubl[ing] down" on quantitative risk assessment will "resolve [its] shortcomings." In particular, could simply adding more calculations to the process remedy its thoroughgoing disregard for environmental inequities rooted in economic and racial injustice?[35(p223)] It thus bears asking, might there be ways of reordering risk assessment's epistemological hierarchy? Rather than revolving so centrally around the de-placed knowledge of the laboratory, might alternative or additional paths for assessing hazards and exercising EPA's regulatory power be forged, in which epidemiological and other place-based knowledge can be taken more seriously and even trigger protective actions?

Given the recent election results, more sweeping remedies await another turn in national political tides. Yet, with the Supreme Court's recent Chevron decision bound to exacerbate EPA's recent legal vulnerability, judicial battles over chlorpyrifos and other toxic chemicals are likely to intensify.[59] To counter myths about the scientific soundness of earlier EPA risk assessment we may hear in future courtrooms, advocates of public health must be ready to show how little risk assessors used to know and also how much more we know now. These arguments are not just scientific but historical—like this one. AJPH

## ABOUT THE AUTHORS

Christopher Sellers is with the History Department, Stony Brook University, Stony Brook, NY. Ellen Kohl is with the Department of Geography and Environmental Systems, University of Maryland—Baltimore County, Baltimore. Marianne Sullivan is with the Department of Public Health, William Patterson University of New Jersey, Wayne. Gretchen Gehrke is with the Environmental Data and Governance Initiative, Durham, NC. Jessica Varner is with the Weitzman School of Design, University of Pennsylvania, Philadelphia. Mark Chambers is with the History and Africana Studies Departments, Stony Brook University. Environmental Data and Governance Initiative is a research and advocacy nonprofit.

## CORRESPONDENCE

Correspondence should be sent to Christopher Sellers, History Department, N301a Social and Behavioral Sciences Building, Stony Brook University, 100 Nicholls Rd, Stony Brook, NY 11795 (e-mail: christopher.sellers@stonybrook.edu). Reprints can be ordered at https://www.ajph.org by clicking the "Reprints" link.

## PUBLICATION INFORMATION

Full Citation: Sellers C, Kohl E, Sullivan M, et al. History of risk assessments of the organophosphate pesticide chlorpyrifos at the US Environmental Protection Agency, 1980–2024. *Am J Public Health*. 2025;115(7):1074–1084.

Acceptance Date: February 12, 2025.

DOI: https://doi.org/10.2105/AJPH.2025.308073

ORCID iDs:

Christopher Sellers https://orcid.org/0000-0001-8909-4135

Ellen Kohl https://orcid.org/0000-0003-4713-6901

Marianne Sullivan https://orcid.org/0000-0002-4715-1143

Gretchen Gehrke https://orcid.org/0000-0002-1881-3291

Mark Chambers https://orcid.org/0000-0003-0772-2340

## CONTRIBUTORS

C. Sellers led the conceptualization of the project, primary research, and writing and editing of the article. E. Kohl and M. Sullivan contributed to conceptualization of the project, primary research, and writing and editing of the article, and E. Kohl to data review. G. Gehrke and J. Varner contributed to revisions of the conceptualization across drafts and to editing. M. Chambers contributed to the research and also to the drafting and editing of revisions. All authors provided critical feedback, helped shape the research, and contributed to the final article.

## ACKNOWLEDGMENTS

C. Sellers, G. Gehrke, J. Varner, and M. Chambers were supported by the National Science Foundation award 2218553. M. Sullivan and E. Kohl were supported by the National Science Foundation award 2218566.

**Note.** Any opinions, findings, and conclusions or recommendations expressed in this material are those of the authors and do not necessarily reflect the views of the National Science Foundation.

## CONFLICTS OF INTEREST

The authors have no conflicts of interest.

## REFERENCES

1. Farmworker Pesticide Project, Pesticide Action Network North America. *Poisons on the Wind: Community Air Monitoring for Chlorpyrifos in the Yakima Valley*. 2006. Available at: https://www.panna.org/wp-content/uploads/2020/07/POW12-20-06YakimaSUM-copy.pdf. Accessed May 11, 2024.
2. Rauh VA, Garfinkel R, Perera FP, et al. Impact of prenatal chlorpyrifos exposure on neurodevelopment in the first 3 years of life among inner-city children. *Pediatrics*. 2006;118(6):e1845–e1859. https://doi.org/10.1542/peds.2006-0338

3. Young JG, Eskenazi B, Gladstone EA, et al. Association between in utero organophosphate pesticide exposure and abnormal reflexes in neonates. *Neurotoxicology*. 2005;26(2):199–209. https://doi.org/10.1016/j.neuro.2004.10.004
4. Whyatt RM, Rauh V, Barr DB, et al. Prenatal insecticide exposures and birth weight and length among an urban minority cohort. *Environ Health Perspect*. 2004;112(10):1125–1132. https://doi.org/10.1289/ehp.6641
5. *Red River Valley Sugarbeet Growers Association et al. v Michael Regan, Administrator, US Environmental Protection Agency* (US Court of Appeals for the Eighth Circuit, 2023). Available at: https://ecf.ca8.uscourts.gov/opndir/23/11/221422P.pdf. Accessed April 3, 2025.
6. Graham JD, Fenner-Crisp PA. Regulation of chemicals, pesticides, and genetically engineered organisms. In: Barnes AJ, Graham JD, Konisky DM, eds. *Fifty Years at the US Environmental Protection Agency: Progress, Retrenchment, and Opportunities*. Lanham, MD: Rowman & Littlefield Publishers; 2021:309–322.
7. Van Houtzen G, Cropper M. When is a life too costly to save? The evidence from environmental regulations. *Resources for the Future*. January 1, 1994. Available at: https://www.resources.org/archives/when-is-a-life-too-costly-to-save-the-evidence-from-environmental-regulations. Accessed January 5, 2025.
8. Baker ES, Moon KJ, Branco RC. Chlorpyrifos: who paid and who profited? *Environ Justice*. 2024;17(1):79–84. https://doi.org/10.1089/env.2022.0074
9. Hites RA. The rise and fall of chlorpyrifos in the United States. *Environ Sci Technol*. 2021;55(3):1354–1358. https://doi.org/10.1021/acs.est.0c06579
10. Davis FR. Pesticides and the perils of synecdoche in the history of science and environmental history. *Hist Sci*. 2019;57(4):469–492. https://doi.org/10.1177/0073275319848964
11. Nash LL. *Inescapable Ecologies: A History of Environment, Disease, and Knowledge*. Berkeley, CA: University of California Press; 2006. https://doi.org/10.1525/9780520939998
12. Davis FR. *Banned: A History of Pesticides and the Science of Toxicology*. New Haven, CT: Yale University Press; 2014.
13. Demortain D. *The Science of Bureaucracy: Risk Decision Making and the US Environmental Protection Agency*. Cambridge, MA: MIT Press; 2019.
14. Conis E. *How to Sell a Poison: The Rise, Fall, and Toxic Return of DDT*. New York, NY: Bold Type Books; 2022.
15. Mart M. *Pesticides, A Love Story: America's Enduring Embrace of Dangerous Chemicals*. Lawrence, KS: University Press of Kansas; 2015. https://doi.org/10.1353/book42335
16. Milby TH. Prevention and management of organophosphate poisoning. *JAMA*. 1971;216(13):2131–2133. https://doi.org/10.1001/jama.1971.03180390041009
17. Namba T. Cholinesterase inhibition by organophosphorus compounds and its clinical effects. *Bull World Health Organ*. 1971;44(1-3):289–307.
18. Hodgson MJ, Block GD, Parkinson DK. Organophosphate poisoning in office workers. *J Occup Med*. 1986;28(6):434–437. https://doi.org/10.1097/00043764-198606000-00010
19. Centers for Disease Control. Organophosphate insecticide poisoning among siblings—Mississippi. *MMWR Morb Mortal Wkly Rep*. 1984;33(42):592–594.
20. Davies JE. Neurotoxic concerns of human pesticide exposures. *Am J Ind Med*. 1990;18(3):327–331. https://doi.org/10.1002/ajim.4700180314
21. Richter L, Cordner A, Brown P. Producing ignorance through regulatory structure: the case of per- and polyfluoroalkyl substances (PFAS). *Sociol Perspect*. 2021;64(4):631–656. https://doi.org/10.1177/0731121420964827
22. Office of Pesticides and Toxic Substances, Environmental Protection Agency. Pesticide fact sheet: chlorpyrifos-methyl. Washington, DC: US Environmental Protection Agency; 1985:4.
23. Henry E, Thomas V, Angeli Aguiton S, Déplaude MO, Jas N. Introduction: beyond the production of ignorance: the pervasiveness of industry influence through the tools of chemical regulation. *Sci Technol Human Values*. 2021;46(5):911–924. https://doi.org/10.1177/01622439211026749
24. Sheppard L, McGrew S, Fenske RA. Flawed analysis of an intentional human dosing study and its impact on chlorpyrifos risk assessments. *Environ Int*. 2020;143:105905. https://doi.org/10.1016/j.envint.2020.105905
25. Lerner S. The department of yes. How pesticide companies corrupted the EPA and poisoned America. *The Intercept*. June 30, 2021. Available at: https://theintercept.com/2021/06/30/epa-pesticides-exposure-opp. Accessed January 3, 2025.
26. Wargo J. *Our Children's Toxic Legacy: How Science and Law Fail to Protect Us From Pesticides*. New Haven, CT: Yale University Press; 1996.
27. Madigan DP. Setting an anti-cancer policy: risk, politics, and the Food Quality Protection Act of 1996. *Virginia Environmental Law Journal*. 1998;17(2):187–243.
28. McGarity TO. Politics by other means: law, science, and policy in EPA's implementation of the Food Quality Protection Act. *Adm Law Rev*. 2001;53(1):103–222.
29. Naidenko OV. Application of the Food Quality Protection Act children's health safety factor in the US EPA pesticide risk assessments. *Environ Health*. 2020;19(1):16. https://doi.org/10.1186/s12940-020-0571-6
30. Smegal D, Office of Pesticide Programs, Environmental Protection Agency. *Human Health Risk Assessment of Chlorpyrifos*. Washington, DC: US Environmental Protection Agency; 2000.
31. Bueschen E. An agreement between EPA and pesticide manufacturers to mitigate the risks of chlorpyrifos. *Environ Law Report*. 2001;31:10452.
32. US Environmental Protection Agency, FIFRA Scientific Advisory Panel. Meeting on Chlorpyrifos: Analysis of Biomonitoring Data; transcript. April 17, 2016. Available at: https://www.epa.gov/sites/default/files/2016-05/documents/fifra_sap_04_19_16_to_04_21_16_final_transcript.pdf. Accessed October 11, 2023.
33. Paisley-Jones C. *Chlorpyrifos (059101) National and State Summary Use and Usage Summary*. Office of Chemical Safety and Pollution Prevention, US Environmental Protection Agency. 2020. Available at: https://downloads.regulations.gov/EPA-HQ-OPP-2018-0141-0139/content.pdf. Accessed June 13, 2024.
34. Harley KG, Parra KL, Camacho J, et al. Determinants of pesticide concentrations in silicone wristbands worn by Latina adolescent girls in a California farmworker community: the COSECHA youth participatory action study. *Sci Total Environ*. 2019;652:1022–1029. https://doi.org/10.1016/j.scitotenv.2018.10.276
35. Boyd W. De-risking environmental law. *Harvard Environ Law Rev*. 2024;48(1):153–254.
36. Environmental Protection Agency. FY 2002 justification of appropriation estimates for the Committee on Appropriations, Planning, budget, and results. February 2001. Available at: https://www.epa.gov/planandbudget/fy-2021-justification-appropriation-estimates-committee-appropriations. Accessed April 3, 2025.
37. Samet JM, Muñoz A. Evolution of the cohort study. *Epidemiol Rev*. 1998;20(1):1–14. https://doi.org/10.1093/oxfordjournals.epirev.a017964
38. Doll R. Cohort studies: history of the method I. Prospective cohort studies. *Soz Praventivmed*. 2001;46(2):75–86. https://doi.org/10.1007/BF01299724
39. Engel SM, Berkowitz GS, Barr DB, et al. Prenatal organophosphate metabolite and organochlorine levels and performance on the Brazelton Neonatal Behavioral Assessment Scale in a multiethnic pregnancy cohort. *Am J Epidemiol*. 2007;165(12):1397–1404. https://doi.org/10.1093/aje/kwm029
40. Eskenazi B, Marks AR, Bradman A, et al. Organophosphate pesticide exposure and neurodevelopment in young Mexican-American children. *Environ Health Perspect*. 2007;115(5):792–798. https://doi.org/10.1289/ehp.9828
41. Slotkin TA, Tate CA, Ryde IT, Levin ED, Seidler FJ. Organophosphate insecticides target the serotonergic system in developing rat brain regions: disparate effects of diazinon and parathion at doses spanning the threshold for cholinesterase inhibition. *Environ Health Perspect*. 2006;114(10):1542–1546. https://doi.org/10.1289/ehp.9337
42. FIFRA Scientific Advisory Panel, US Environmental Protection Agency. A Set of Scientific Issues Being Considered by the Environmental Protection Agency Regarding: The Agency's Evaluation of the Toxicity Profile of Chlorpyrifos. 2008. Available at: https://www.regulations.gov/document/EPA-HQ-OPP-2008-0274-0064. Accessed April 3, 2025.
43. Office of Pesticide Programs, US Environmental Protection Agency. Office of Pesticide Programs' Framework for Incorporating Human Epidemiologic & Incident Data in Risk Assessments for Pesticides. 2016. Available at: https://www.regulations.gov/document/EPA-HQ-OPP-2008-0351-0103. Accessed April 3, 2025.
44. Chlorpyrifos: Revised Human Health Risk Assessment for Registration Review. Washington, DC: US Environmental Protection Agency; 2014.
45. US Environmental Protection Agency. Chlorpyrifos; tolerance revocations; action: proposed rule. *Fed Regist*. 2015;80(215):69080–69109.
46. Britton W, Drew D, Holman E, et al. Memorandum; Subject: Chlorpyrifos: Revised Human Health Risk Assessment for Registration Review. US Environmental Protection Agency. 2016. Available at: https://www.regulations.gov/document/EPA-HQ-OPP-2015-0653-0454. Accessed April 3, 2025.
47. Watanabe M. Comment on US EPA Federal Insecticide, Fungicide, and Rodenticide Act Scientific Advisory Panel (FIFRA SAP) April 19–21, 2016 meeting on chlorpyrifos: analysis of biomonitoring data. US Environmental Protection Agency.

2016. Available at: https://www.regulations.gov/comment/EPA-HQ-OPP-2016-0062-0100. Accessed April 3, 2025.

48. Sass J, Whyatt RM. Comment on US EPA Federal Insecticide, Fungicide, and Rodenticide Act Scientific Advisory Panel (FIFRA SAP) April 19–21, 2016 meeting on chlorpyrifos: analysis of biomonitoring data. US Environmental Protection Agency. 2016. Available at: https://www.regulations.gov/comment/EPA-HQ-OPP-2016-0062-0122. Accessed April 3, 2025.

49. Agricultural Retailers Association, Almond Hullers & Processors Association, American Farm Bureau Federation, et al. Comment on US EPA Federal Insecticide, Fungicide, and Rodenticide Act Scientific Advisory Panel (FIFRA SAP) April 19–21, 2016 meeting on chlorpyrifos: analysis of biomonitoring data. US Environmental Protection Agency. 2016. Available at: https://www.regulations.gov/comment/EPA-HQ-OPP-2016-0062-0115. Accessed April 3, 2025.

50. Collins JE. Comment on US EPA Federal Insecticide, Fungicide, and Rodenticide Act Scientific Advisory Panel (FIFRA SAP) April 19–21, 2016 meeting on chlorpyrifos: analysis of biomonitoring data. US Environmental Protection Agency. 2016. Available at: https://www.regulations.gov/comment/EPA-HQ-OPP-2016-0062-0103. Accessed April 3, 2025.

51. US Environmental Protection Agency. Order Denying Petition to Revoke All Tolerances for the Pesticide Chlorpyrifos. 2017. Available at: https://www.epa.gov/sites/default/files/2017-03/documents/chlorpyrifos3b_order_denying_panna_and_nrdc27s_petitition_to_revoke_tolerances.pdf. Accessed October 4, 2023.

52. Kaplan S, Lipton E. Trump's E.P.A. chemical safety nominee withdraws. *New York Times.* December 14, 2017. Available at: https://www.nytimes.com/2017/12/13/science/epa-chemical-safety-trump.html. Accessed August 28, 2024.

53. Goobie GC, Rice MB, Carlsten C. The Environmental Protection Agency's "Strengthening Transparency in Pivotal Science" rule: don't let history repeat itself. *Ann Am Thorac Soc.* 2021;18(10):1614–1617. https://doi.org/10.1513/AnnalsATS.202103-259VP

54. US Environmental Protection Agency. Tolerance Revocations: Chlorpyrifos. 2021. Available at: https://www.regulations.gov/document/EPA-HQ-OPP-2021-0523-0001. Accessed September 30, 2023.

55. Wołejko E, Łozowicka B, Jabłońska-Trypuć A, Pietruszyńska M, Wydro U. Chlorpyrifos occurrence and toxicological risk assessment: a review. *Int J Environ Res Public Health.* 2022;19(19):12209. https://doi.org/10.3390/ijerph191912209

56. Donley N. The USA lags behind other agricultural nations in banning harmful pesticides. *Environ Health.* 2019;18(1):44. https://doi.org/10.1186/s12940-019-0488-0

57. Woodruff TJ, Rayasam SDG, Axelrad DA, et al. A science-based agenda for health-protective chemical assessments and decisions: overview and consensus statement. *Environ Health.* 2023;21(suppl 1):132. https://doi.org/10.1186/s12940-022-00930-3

58. Michaels D. *Doubt Is Their Product: How Industry's Assault on Science Threatens Your Health.* New York, NY: Oxford University Press; 2008.

59. Davenport C, Jewett C, Rappeport A, Sanger-Katz M, Scheiber N, Weiland N. Here's what the court's Chevron ruling could mean in everyday terms. *New York Times.* June 28, 2024. Available at: https://www.nytimes.com/2024/06/28/us/politics/chevron-deference-decision-meaning.html. Accessed January 7, 2025.

# Was the Allocation of COVID-19 Vaccines Globally Fair and Equitable?

*Ezekiel J. Emanuel, MD, PhD, and Min Jung, BA*

**See also Gur-Arie, p. 993.**

Determining whether an allocation is equitable requires ethical and empirical analyses, specifically answers to 3 questions: (1) What is the ethical standard for fair allocation? (2) What is the quantitative equity metric for this standard? and (3) What do the empirical data demonstrate?

Two ethical standards for assessing the fair allocation of scarce medical resources have been delineated: the COVID-19 Vaccines Global Access initiative's population-based standard and the COVID-19 health-burden standard. The equity metric for the population-based standard is vaccine per person in each country, and for the health-burden standard it is vaccine per excess deaths per country. When using excess deaths data from the World Health Organization and vaccine data from the United Nations Children's Fund, the health-burden standard showed that middle-income countries with high excess deaths (e.g., Indonesia, Peru, Mexico, Egypt, South Africa) were treated inequitably: not provided enough vaccines given their high excess deaths.

The right standard to assess fair and equitable allocation is a health-burden assessment. According to this standard, contrary to assumptions and initial claims, low-income countries were not treated inequitably in COVID-19 vaccine allocation, and middle-income countries with high excess deaths were treated inequitably. (*Am J Public Health*. 2025;115(7):1085–1094. https://doi.org/10.2105/AJPH.2025.308077)

AJPH July 2025, Vol. 115, No. 7

After the COVID-19 pandemic began, world leaders, international organizations, nongovernmental organizations, and others preemptively called for a "fair and equitable" allocation of a future COVID-19 vaccine among countries.[1,2] They legitimately worried that a market allocation of vaccines would ensure that high-income countries acquired excessive numbers of very scarce vaccines, leaving low- and middle-income countries with few.[3] Indeed, before COVID-19 vaccines were authorized, high-income countries had reserved enough doses to immunize their own populations multiple times over.[4,5]

These concerns prompt the questions: Ultimately, was the COVID-19 vaccine allocation among countries fair and equitable? How should policymakers distribute a scarce medical intervention in the case of a future global emergency?

Answering these questions requires both ethical and empirical analyses, specifically (1) using an ethical standard for what constitutes equitable allocation of scarce medical resources, (2) using a quantitative equity metric, and (3) making an empirical assessment of whether the vaccine allocation fulfilled the equity standard (Box 1). Importantly, scarcity of medical resources necessarily means it is inevitable that initially not all people will receive the resource.[10] That some countries or people received more than others is neither prima facie nor definitive evidence that there was inequity.[4,11,12] It is simply the definition of scarcity.

## TWO EQUITABLE VACCINE ALLOCATION STANDARDS

Two different frameworks for allocating scarce medical resources among countries have been delineated. The COVID-19 Vaccine Global Access (COVAX) adopted the World Health Organization's (WHO's) population-based standard, which it described on September 9, 2020 (Box 1).[13,14] The population-based standard recommends that the supply of vaccines be allocated to countries so that initially 3% of the population is covered and

**BOX 1— Two Conceptions of Fair and Equitable Allocation of Scarce Medical Resources**

| Author and Date | Best Standard for Fair and Equitable Allocation | Metric Used to Determine Equity | Unfair and Inequitable Vaccine Distribution During the COVID-19 Pandemic |
|---|---|---|---|
| COVAX (sponsored by WHO, GAVI, and CEPI),[3,6] September 9, 2020 | Population based | Vaccines per person in a country | High-income countries received significantly more vaccines per population than did low-income countries |
| Independent Group (fair priority model),[7–9] September 3, 2020 | Health burden based | Three conceivable equity metrics:<br>1. Vaccines per future excess deaths based on models of likely surges and "hot spots" (prospective)<br>2. Vaccine per standard expected years of life lost averted<br>3. Vaccines per excess deaths (retrospective) | • The countries that received too few vaccines were largely middle-income countries with high excess deaths, e.g., Peru, Mexico, Indonesia<br>• Countries with negative or few excess deaths (< 15 000) received too many vaccines<br>• The US and UK did not receive too many vaccines<br>• Generally, low-income and sub-Saharan countries, except South Africa and Nigeria, did not receive too few vaccines |

*Note*. CEPI = Coalition for Epidemic Preparedness Innovations; COVAX = COVID-19 Vaccines Global Access; GAVI = Gavi, the Vaccine Alliance; WHO = World Health Organization.

then up to 20% of the population is vaccinated.[3,6] Subsequently, COVAX proposed that COVID-19 vaccines should be allocated based on the number of COVID-19 cases.[3]

On September 3, 2020, an independent group delineated the Fair Priority Model (FPM), which specifies that equitable allocation among countries be based on COVID-19 health burden: scarce medical resources should be allocated based on where they will save the most lives or standard expected life-years (Box 1).[7,8] (E. J. E. was one of the authors of the FPM.)

## EQUITY METRICS

According to COVAX's population-based standard, the appropriate equity metric is vaccines per person in a country until 20% of each country's population is vaccinated.[3,6] According to the FPM's health-burden standard, the ideal equity metric should reflect how many deaths or life-years lost in a country each additional vaccine can prevent.[7–9] The FPM had 3 potential equity metrics on fair distribution of resources. One potential metric was prospective, assessing the likely impact of the COVID-19 pandemic in countries in the subsequent months.[7] A second potential metric was based on trying to "minimize standardized life-years lost to excess deaths (SEYLL)."[7–9,15,16] A third potential equity metric was retrospective, allocating vaccines among countries based on excess deaths.[7,8] We evaluate the third equity metric as a more equitable metric than COVAX's population-based standard.

## EMPIRICAL EVALUATION OF EQUITY METRICS

We conducted an empirical assessment of the COVAX population-based standard and the fair priority model to determine which approach is more equitable in the context of vaccine allocations during a global pandemic.

### Population-Based Standard

According to the population-based standard, the COVID-19 vaccine allocation among countries was inequitable (Figure 1).[17,18] The United Nations declared the vaccine allocation "morally unconscionable":

> Of the 832 million vaccine doses administered, 82 per cent have gone to high- or upper-middle-income countries, while only 0.2 per cent have been sent to their low-income counterparts. In high-income countries alone, 1 in 4 people have been vaccinated, a ratio that drops precipitously to 1 in 500 in poorer countries.[19]

By mid-2021, the WHO noted that 2% of the population in 50 African nations received 1 dose whereas in the United Kingdom, more than 70% of the adult population had.[20]

### Health-Burden Standard

*Methods.* We evaluated the FPM through vaccines per excess deaths. During an emergency, excess deaths serve as a more appropriate metric than direct COVID-19 deaths for 3 reasons. First, excess deaths are easier and more reliably measured since determining a cause of death—and thus confirming viral infection among decedents—is not needed. More importantly, "indirect"

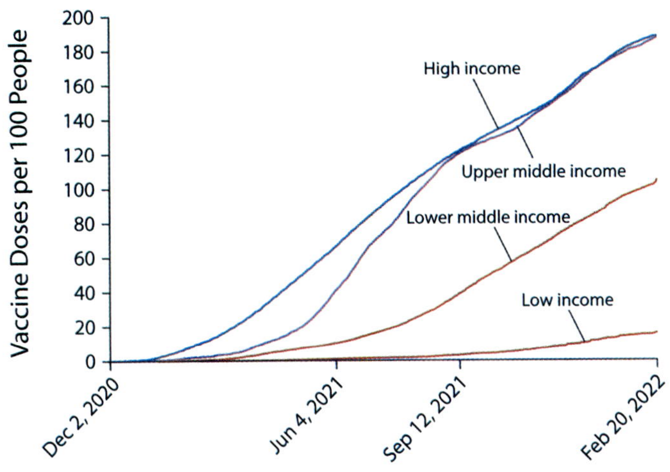


**FIGURE 1— Worldwide Allocation of COVID-19 Vaccines Based on Population Standard**

*Source.* Hunter et al.[17]

deaths from other diseases that result from overwhelmed health systems and other factors should be considered. Finally, as excess deaths is already extensively used in global health policy, the strengths and limitations of this metric for global health policy decision-making are well established.[21,22]

Our analysis used excess deaths data at the end of 2020 and vaccine distribution data at several points in 2021. We chose December 2020, as vaccines were just becoming available but were of insufficient supply, making prioritization necessary. By the end of 2021, prioritization of vaccines was unnecessary, as there was more supply of vaccines than demand. The WHO, *The Economist*,[23] and the Institute for Health Metrics and Evaluation[24] reported excess death data. We used the updated WHO excess death data for 179 countries, excluding China, India, Russia, small nations, and other countries not reporting or providing only partial data, such as Tanzania (Table C, available as a supplement to the online version of this article at http://www.ajph.org).[25] To calculate excess deaths, the WHO used all-cause mortality data that are available for only 100 countries. We used an extensive modeling method to estimate the excess deaths for the remaining countries. Although excess death estimates for these countries may be less robust than those for countries with all-cause mortality data, the WHO has confidence that their data are in the probable range of excess deaths (by March 2022, 140 countries were consulted and had direct input into the model).[26]

Analyses of excess deaths from other data sources (e.g., the initial WHO report and *The Economist*) did not alter our conclusions (Table C). We did not use the Institute for Health Metrics and Evaluation because it did not provide data on deaths in calendar year 2020 (Table D, available as a supplement to the online version of this article at http://www.ajph.org). The WHO published their first COVID-19–related modeled estimates of global excess deaths in May 2021.[25] The WHO updated its excess death estimates in May 2023 (Table B, available as a supplement to the online version of this article at http://www.ajph.org).

We determined the amount of vaccines available in each country using the United Nations Children's Fund's COVID-19 Market Dashboard.[27] This dashboard includes vaccine data from COVAX, bilateral and multilateral agreements, and donations.

The metric of vaccine per excess death is controversial. First, some argue death data do not reflect COVID-19's impact in low-income countries.[28] Many countries have limited vital statistics infrastructure. In Zambia, for instance, COVID-19 was rarely listed as the cause of death, yet 32% of the deceased tested positive for COVID-19 antibodies, although this does not mean the people died of COVID-19. In addition, a survey by the United Nations Economic Commission for Africa showed that "official registration systems captured only one in three deaths."[29] Conversely, India criticized WHO estimates of COVID-19 deaths as excessively inflated.

Importantly, using the number of excess deaths simplifies and increases the reliability of comparisons. By not requiring confirmation of COVID-19 infection as the cause of death, it addresses major differences in countries' capacity to report disease-specific cause of deaths, and thus does not penalize low-income countries that cannot do viral testing on all decedents to confirm infectious causes. By using the number of excess deaths, problems related to deceased Zambians not classified as dying from COVID-19 and India's complaint about WHO's inflated COVID-19 deaths are minimized. Further, there are ways of corroborating excess deaths during the COVID-19 pandemic even in countries with low vital statistic infrastructure, such as high rates of visits to health facilities, hospitalizations, and funerals. Increasingly, even satellite photographs can show new grave and cremation sites.[30]

Overall, despite much scrutiny and perplexity, clinics, hospitals, and funeral homes in sub-Saharan countries did not report substantial increases in deaths.[29] Thus, although data on COVID-19–specific deaths in low-income countries might be relatively unreliable and reflect poor data infrastructure, the low excess deaths among low-income countries is unlikely to be an artifact of unreliable data. Further, international health organizations have some experience in addressing undercounting of deaths because of infrastructure and consistently use and report on excess deaths.[31] Indeed both WHO and *The Economist* report on excess deaths during the COVID-19 pandemic in low-income countries, indicating they have confidence in these data.[26]

A second empirical complication is that excess deaths vary widely among countries in the same income stratum (Table A, available as a supplement to the online version of this article at http://www.ajph.org; Figure 2). For instance, in December 2020, the United States was the country with the most cumulative excess deaths, 467 313, whereas Japan had −21 921 excess deaths. Overall deaths actually declined compared with pre–COVID-19 pandemic levels (Table A). Similarly, Zambia had 2018 excess deaths, whereas Rwanda had −1670 excess deaths (Table A).[25]

***Findings.*** Empirical assessment shows that middle-income countries had the majority of excess deaths (Tables A and B). As the *British Medical Journal* summarized the revised WHO data: "Middle income countries accounted for 81% of the excess deaths, whereas high-income countries accounted for 15% and low-income countries 4%."[33(p1)] Among countries ranked by excess deaths, the top 25 account for more than 80% of all excess deaths in the world and include 8 high-income, 8 upper-middle-income, and 9 lower-middle-income countries (Table B). (*The Economist* included 1 low-income country [Sudan] in its top 25.) Similarly, among the top 25 countries with excess deaths per 100 000 population from March 2020 to December 2020, none was a low-income country, 2 (8%) were low-middle-income countries, 12 (48%) were upper-middle, and 11 (44%) were high-income countries (Table A).[25,32] Indeed, the low-income country with the most deaths per 100 000 population was Afghanistan (29th). There were only 2 sub-Saharan countries among the top 25 countries ranked by excess deaths: South Africa and Nigeria.

Analyzing excess deaths and vaccine allocation engendered 4 conclusions (Table A). First, United Nations Children's Fund's data on vaccine distribution from June 2021 showed that largely middle-income countries with high excess deaths, such as Indonesia, Peru, Mexico, and Egypt, did not receive sufficient vaccines (Table A; Figure 2).[25,27] In early 2021, when COVID-19 vaccines were in extremely short supply, the top 25 countries in terms of excess deaths received too few vaccines. Importantly, every country in the top 25 in excess deaths that received fewer than 200 vaccines per excess death was middle income.[25,27,32]

Another way to understand the burden on middle-income countries is that Mexico was 3rd in excess deaths at the end of 2020 but 139th in vaccines per excess deaths in June 2021, and Peru was 9th in excess deaths but 155th in vaccines per excess deaths (Table A). On average, the top 10 countries in excess deaths slipped about 120 ranks in vaccines per excess death.[25,27,32] By December 2021, the situation was similar (Table E). That middle-income countries received too few vaccines probably relates to not having resources to outbid high-income countries and, unlike low-income countries, not receiving sizable donations.

Second, 2 groups of countries received a greater share of vaccines relative to their COVID-19 health burden: the 25 countries with negative excess deaths in December 2020, including Vietnam, the Philippines, Kenya, and Rwanda, and the 105 countries with fewer than 10 000 cumulative excess deaths; this list includes 32 high-income countries, 26 upper-middle-income countries, 29 lower-middle-income countries, and 18 low-income countries (Table B).[25,27,32] Because of the low COVID-19 health burden, the FPM suggests that these countries should have received minimal allocation of scarce vaccines in early to mid-2021, when vaccines were most scarce.

Third, the data suggest that countries that manufactured vaccines were not receiving too many given their high excess deaths. In December 2020, the United States had the most excess deaths and received 817.3 vaccines per excess death by June 2021. Similarly, the United Kingdom, with the 10th most excess deaths, received 925.3 vaccines per excess death. Other countries received more vaccines per excess death, including the United Arab Emirates, Israel, Denmark, Ireland, Cambodia, and Zimbabwe (Table A).[25,27,32]

Finally, most low-income and sub-Saharan countries, except South Africa and Nigeria, were not treated inequitably by vaccine allocation (Table A; Figure 3). Cumulatively, by December 2020, the group of 29 low-income countries had 120 503 excess deaths (3.7% of total excess deaths) and had

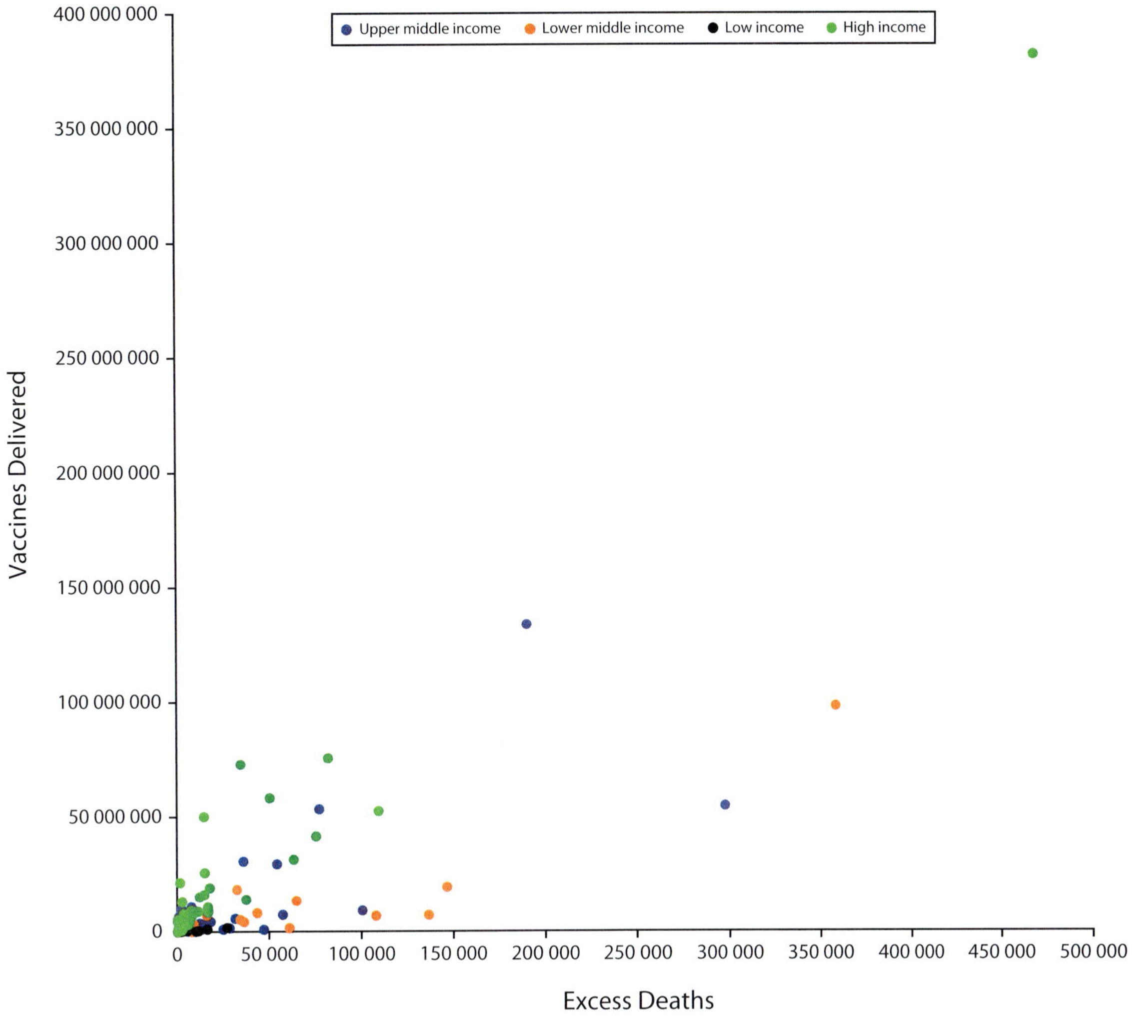


**FIGURE 2—** **Worldwide Allocation of Vaccines From 2021 and Excess Deaths From December 2020**

*Source.* World Health Organization,[25] United Nations Children's Fund,[27] and World Bank and lending groups.[32]

received 119.4 vaccines per excess death by June 2021.[25,27,32] Similarly, between March 2020 and December 2021, the group of all sub-Saharan countries, excluding South Africa and Nigeria, had 495 171 excess deaths (3.3% of total excess deaths) and received 603.0 vaccines per excess deaths.[25,27,32] Indeed, the WHO's revision of COVID-19's impact actually decreased the number of excess deaths in low-income and sub-Saharan countries. For instance, Zambia's excess deaths were initially reported by the WHO as 5294 but lowered by more than 50% to 2018. Similarly, Rwanda's −320 excess deaths were lowered further to −1670.

The question of inequity in vaccine distribution may be best captured by the case of Ghana, a low-middle-income, sub-Saharan country and the first country in the world to receive COVAX vaccines (February 2021). By December 2020, Ghana cumulatively had 3255 excess deaths—just 0.09% of the world's excess deaths (ranked 81st). (Initially, the WHO reported 6461 excess deaths.) By June 2021, Ghana had received 421.5 vaccines per excess death (rank 113; Table A). Ghana had neither a substantial number of excess deaths nor a very low level of vaccines per excess death, especially compared with Mexico, Peru, Ecuador, Iran, Egypt, Nigeria, and South Africa (Table A).[25,27,33]

Although low-income and sub-Saharan countries did not receive many vaccines by June 2021, these countries were fortunate in not suffering many excess deaths related to COVID-19 to justify prioritizing them for scarce vaccines. Why low-income and sub-Saharan countries had low excess deaths while having high infection rates remains unresolved.

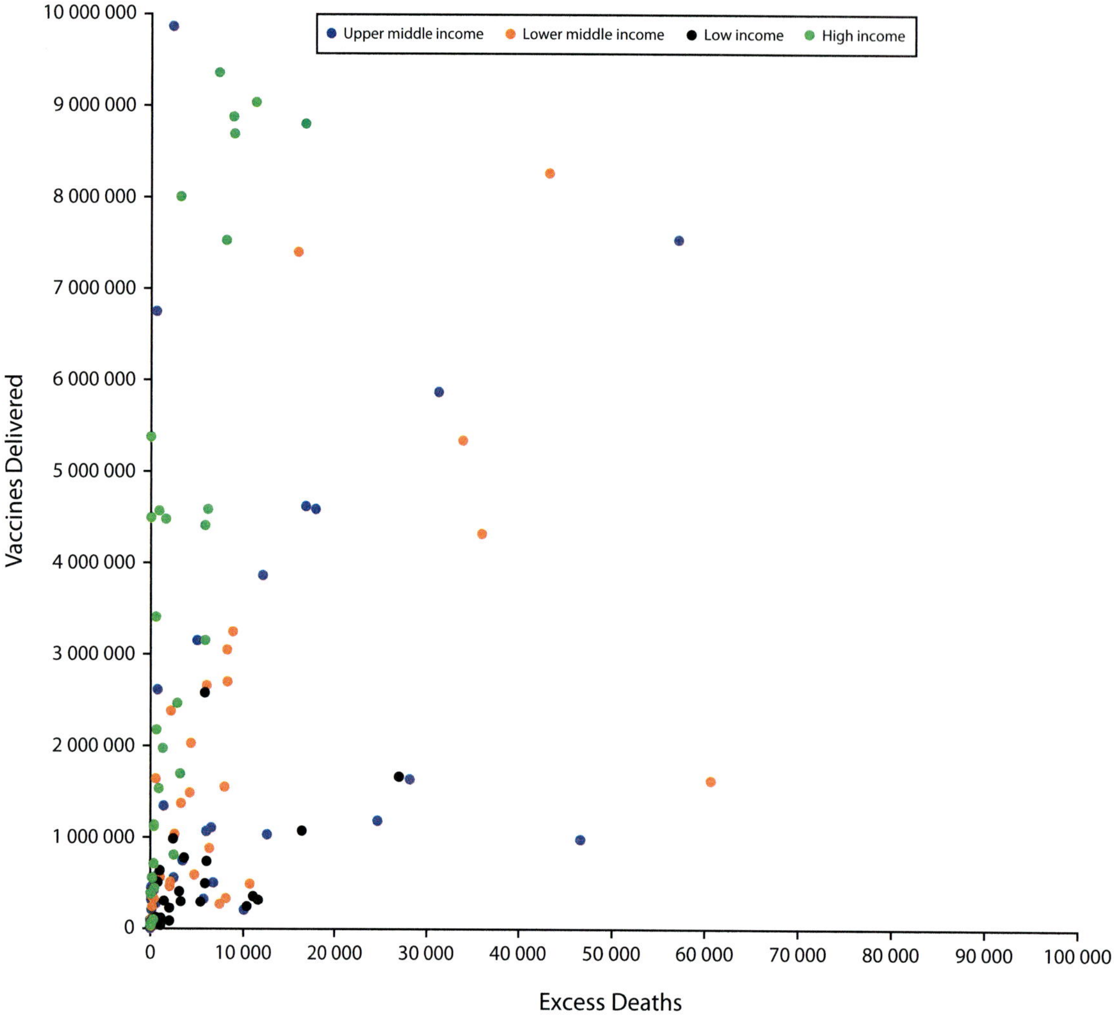


**FIGURE 3— Worldwide Allocation of Vaccines per Excess Deaths From December 2020 and Vaccines From June 2021 Expanded for < 100 000 Excess Deaths and < 10 000 000 Vaccines Delivered**

*Source.* World Health Organization,[25] United Nations Children's Fund,[27] and World Bank and lending groups.[32]

Potential explanations include a younger age distribution of the population; less obesity, diabetes, and other comorbidities; immunity from previous infections; or some other factor.[34] Regardless, these countries were largely spared excess deaths from COVID-19.

## THE ETHICALLY RIGHT STANDARD

The COVAX population-based standard indicates that low-income countries were unfairly treated, whereas the FPM health-burden standard indicates that middle-income countries were unfairly treated in the COVID-19 vaccine allocation. For myriad reasons—particularly the legacy of colonialism and exploitation—there is wider acceptance of the population-based standard's conclusion that low-income and sub-Saharan countries were inequitably treated.[1–3,17–20,35]

Is the population-based standard the right ethical standard for allocating scarce medical resources among countries? COVAX's population-based standard has never been defended by an appeal to ethical principles.[13,14] Its defense has been pragmatic.[3,6] The WHO claimed it guarantees each country some vaccines, thereby incentivizing participation in a global allocation mechanism such as COVAX.[3]

This raises 2 problems. Why participation in COVAX should be the ethical goal of vaccine distribution is never justified. It hardly seems a valid standard in a pandemic when millions of people are dying. Furthermore, pragmatic considerations are not ethical

AJPH July 2025, Vol. 115, No. 7

considerations and do not suffice to justify claims about the justice and equity of vaccine allocation. Nonetheless, the vaccines per population metric has advantages. Population data cannot be easily manipulated. Such objectivity decreases conflict among countries and promotes acceptance of the actual allocation.

However, in a global pandemic, does higher objectivity mean a more ethical or equitable distribution of vaccines? In the aim to make the allocation process "more objective," a population-based metric ignores any differences in severity of the pandemic in a country. However, by focusing on an objective allocation, the standard produces scenarios in which countries with a high health burden do not receive enough, whereas countries with a low health burden receive more than they need. Thus, a population-based metric is a pragmatic compromise that fails to target inequity.

Conversely, the health-burden metric is widely recognized as an ethical approach to allocating scarce medical resources among countries. The Pan-American Healthcare Organization,[36] the draft WHO Treaty on Pandemic Preparedness, and the WHO in allocating other scarce resources, such as the RTS,S malaria vaccine,[7] all support allocating scarce resource "based on public health risks and needs."

Unlike the population-based standard, the health-burden standard appeals to widely shared ethical values, specifically minimizing harms and optimizing benefits, mitigating disparities, and treating all individuals with equal moral concern.[7–9] The health-burden standard fulfills a moral concern: that all people count equally regardless of the country they live in.[7] Consequently, the standard affirms that vaccines should go to countries likely to experience the most excess deaths, regardless of their income. "A fair distribution of COVID-19 vaccines should respond to the pandemic's differential severity in different countries."[7(p1311)]

It is true that determining health burden is more complicated than measuring population. The infrastructure to record deaths varies widely among countries, and future health emergencies may present different characteristics in terms of vaccine and data availability. However, the merit of the health-burden standard is that it can be updated and refined over time. As determination of excess deaths among countries evolves with better data—as they did during the COVID-19 pandemic—the allocation of vaccines or other interventions can be adjusted to ensure that resources are linked to health burden.[25]

## OBJECTIONS CONSIDERED

Several objections can be raised to the COVID-19 health-burden standard.

First, distributing vaccines based on excess deaths may punish countries with inadequate resources for recording deaths, surveillance, and viral registration. Despite gaps in death-reporting capabilities, extensive modeling and direct country input allow researchers to accurately estimate excess deaths in each country.[26] Furthermore, the excess deaths metric requires far less infrastructure and surveillance capabilities than does determining COVID-19–related deaths or viral registration, making it a valid option as countries continue to develop their public health infrastructure.

Death reporting is a crucial public health tool that deserves equal—or greater—priority than vaccine distribution. Inadequate resources for recording deaths likely indicates a bigger gap in public health system abilities, such as limited absorption capacity and ability to adequately store and effectively distribute vaccines. For instance, by the end of 2021, more than a million doses were estimated to be wasted in Nigeria owing to a "lack of appropriate storage facilities, poor electricity supply, [and] insecurity challenges."[37(p229)] Objecting to the health-burden standard because some countries lack death-reporting capabilities and will be at a disadvantage because they underreport deaths is not decisive. Those same countries are likely to lack infrastructure to receive, store, and effectively distribute vaccines, leading to the waste of a life-saving resource. The health-burden standard could prompt countries to improve their death-reporting capability because receiving vaccines would be an incentive to countries such as Nigeria to improve their vaccine distribution infrastructure. If concerns about the health-burden standard's feasibility are related to public health infrastructure that countries should have, there should be an effort to address those gaps to use the framework that would save more lives.

Today, the excess death metric is the most reliable and valid metric and is already used regularly in global health and allocation of resources. Policymakers understand its limitations, make analytic adjustments for accuracy, and can accommodate the limitations in implementing policies. Finally, the health-burden standard becomes stronger as each country continues to improve its public health infrastructure, whereas the population-based standard does not.

Second, what if at the start of the COVID-19 pandemic or some other global health emergency, interventions like a vaccine were readily available and there were no data on excess deaths? How would the FPM's health-burden standard suggest that vaccines be distributed without excess death data? In response, excess deaths are not the only measure of health burden that can be used. For instance, early in the COVID-19 pandemic, some countries were overwhelmed with high numbers of COVID-19 cases and hospitalizations. Wuhan, China, as the first area severely affected by COVID-19, would have been prioritized for vaccines under the health-burden standard. In late February 2020, Lombardy, Italy, had a large number of cases and hospitalizations, which would have made it the next priority for resources. As other "hot spots" developed, vaccines would have been shipped until reliable estimates of excess deaths could be obtained.

Third, vaccine allocation should rely on prospective models rather than the retrospective number of excess deaths.[7] Future allocation decisions will likely occur within 12 months of an emergency, when the data are insufficient for accurate modeling. During the COVID-19 pandemic, predictive models systematically underestimated the total number of US deaths from June 2020 to March 2021—just the time needed for vaccine allocation decisions.[38] Furthermore, the 25 countries with the majority of excess deaths by December 2020 also experienced very high excess deaths between January 2021 and December 2021 (Table C). This suggests that the number of excess deaths is a very good indicator of prospective burden.

Fourth, in their retroactive modeling of vaccine allocation based on COVAX's population-based standard, Moore et al. claim it could have saved 1.3 million lives. The authors state that adopting the health-burden standard might have saved fewer people.[39] However, these researchers did not model COVAX's population-based standard, but the allocation based on countries' population age structure, with more going to countries with older populations. Consistent with the health-burden standard, the model of Moore et al. predicted that targeting middle-income rather than low-income countries—because of their larger and older populations and higher COVID-19 excess deaths—would have saved more total lives.[39] Furthermore, Moore et al. argue that vaccine distribution should be based on need, not wealth, consistent with the health-burden standard.[39]

Fifth, the health-burden standard could disincentivize countries to impose mitigation measures in hopes of gaining vaccine priority. During the COVID-19 pandemic, some countries did not impose mitigation measures, not to obtain more vaccines but under the belief that this approach would create herd immunity. Furthermore, high-income countries are unlikely to adopt this strategy because they can purchase vaccines. For other countries, this approach would be self-contradictory and self-defeating. A country seeking vaccines to reduce deaths would not fail to impose mitigation measures with the hope—with no certainty—of getting more vaccines because this approach would ultimately generate more harm. Nothing in the world ensures against having reckless leaders who are willing to sacrifice their own populations currently for a slightly higher chance of getting vaccines in the future. But there were no such leaders during the COVID-19 pandemic.

Finally, that low-income and sub-Saharan countries were not treated inequitably in vaccine allocation was accidental; this was neither intentional nor because of adherence to ethical principles. Additionally, even if they did not experience inequity in actual vaccine allocation, low-income countries experienced procedural inequity. The allocation method excluded many low-income countries' perspectives, failing to consider their interests in the decision-making process.

Both the intention and the outcome matter in the ethical evaluation of COVID-19 vaccine allocation. However, in public health practice, if death is the result, outcomes should be the preeminent consideration.[7,8] Importantly, in preparing for the next health emergency, in which disease burden may not be concentrated in high- and upper-middle-income countries, agreeing on the ethical allocation standard and an accepted mechanism to implement it is critical.[40] These standards must not entrench the same procedural neglect of low-income countries and their interests.

## POLICY IMPLICATIONS

Our findings about the fairness of COVID-19 vaccine allocation lead to 2 conclusions. First, global leaders should not automatically assume and use faulty ethical standards and data to proclaim that low-income countries are necessarily treated unfairly. Ethical evaluations should be objective, using agreed on ethical standard and metrics. In future emergencies, these will be the health-burden standard and scarce interventions per excess deaths or similar outcome.[9] Second, announcing the health-burden standard should incentivize countries to upgrade their data collection infrastructure to collect more accurate mortality data.

Future studies could build on our work by incorporating more factors related to resource allocation and health outcomes. For instance, assessing the marginal cost of the COVID-19 emergency response and incorporating a broad array of resources, such as vaccines and therapeutics, would enable a more comprehensive evaluation of the fairness of the health-burden standard.

## CONCLUSIONS

During the COVID-19 pandemic, there was genuine worry that low-income and sub-Saharan countries would be treated unfairly when effective vaccines were produced.[1–3] Many have cited the low vaccines per population among low-income countries as evidence of inequity.[17,19] However, the number of vaccines per population is not a valid ethical standard in an emergency.[8,9] Invoking vaccines per person to condemn vaccine allocation as unethical is mistaken.

Equity is a matter of ethics not pragmatics. Using a health-burden standard, middle-income countries with high excess deaths, such as Peru, Mexico, Indonesia, Egypt, and South Africa, were treated inequitably during the COVID-19 pandemic. Their proportion of vaccines was not commensurate with their high COVID-19 health burden. Low-income and sub-Saharan countries—except South Africa and Nigeria—had low excess deaths, and their initial low vaccine allocation was therefore not inequitable. That low-income countries cannot be assumed to be treated inequitably is a very important conclusion to guide future emergencies. This conclusion may not be the popular or politically favored one, but it is the ethical one. AJPH


### ABOUT THE AUTHORS

Ezekiel J. Emanuel is with the Department of Medical Ethics and Health Policy, University of Pennsylvania, Philadelphia. At the time of writing, Min Jung was with the University of Pennsylvania, Philadelphia.

### CORRESPONDENCE

Correspondence should be sent to Ezekiel J. Emanuel, MD, PhD, 423 Guardian Dr, Philadelphia, PA 19104 (e-mail: zemanuel@upenn.edu). Reprints can be ordered at https://www.ajph.org by clicking the "Reprints" link.



### PUBLICATION INFORMATION

Full Citation: Emanuel EJ, Jung M. Was the allocation of COVID-19 vaccines globally fair and equitable? *Am J Public Health*. 2025;115(7): 1085–1094.

Acceptance Date: February 12, 2025.

https://doi.org/10.2105/AJPH.2025.308077


### CONTRIBUTORS

The authors contributed equally to this essay.


### ACKNOWLEDGMENTS

We thank the fair priority model researchers, especially Daniel Halliday, Joseph Heath, Lisa Herzog, R. J. Leland, Florencia Luna, Govind Persad, Henry Richardson, Owen Schaeffer, and Kit Wellman as well as Michael Parker, Maxwell Smith, Amaya Diana, Matt Guido, and Patricia Hong for all their help through criticisms and comments and assistance in preparing the essay. We also thank the 3 reviewers for their criticisms, which strengthened this essay.

### CONFLICTS OF INTEREST

E. J. Emanuel reports payment or honoraria for lectures, presentations, government testimony, speakers bureaus, writing, or educational events from President's Biden's Transition COVID-19 Committee; the World Health Organization (WHO) COVID-19 Ethics and Governance Working Group; the WHO Expert Group Ethics and Governance Outbreaks and Emergencies; the US House of Representatives Committee on Science, Space, and Technology (Subcommittee on Investigations and Oversight); the Health Action Alliance; Yale University; the University of California, San Francisco; the Consortium on Law and Values University of Minnesota; the Hawaii Medical Service Association; the Faith Health Alliance Project; the American Academy of Political and Social Science; the 16th World Congress of Bioethics; the Blue Cross/Blue Shield Alliance for Health Research Annual Meeting; Arnold D. Kates Lecture Bowdoin College; the National Academies of Sciences, Engineering, and Medicine Forum on Microbial Threats; the University of Oklahoma (as recipient of the Patricia Price Browne Prize in Biomedical Ethics); the College of Medicine (Oklahoma City, OK); the Suntory Foundation (Tokyo, Japan); National Taiwan University, School of Public Health (Taipei, Taiwan); the National Institutes of Health Ethics Grand Rounds Use of COVID-19 Vaccines; the Penn India Engagement Forum New Delhi, Delhi, India.

M. Jung has no conflicts of interest to declare.


### HUMAN PARTICIPANT PROTECTION

No protocol approval was necessary because no human participants were involved in this study.

### REFERENCES


1. Katz IT, Weintraub R, Bekker LG, Brandt AM. From vaccine nationalism to vaccine equity—finding a path forward. *N Engl J Med*. 2021; 384(14):1281–1283. https://doi.org/10.1056/NEJMp2103614
2. Emanuel EJ, Persad G, Upshur R, et al. Fair allocation of scarce medical resources in the time of COVID-19. *N Engl J Med*. 2020;382(21):2049–2055. https://doi.org/10.1056/NEJMsb2005114
3. World Health Organization. WHO concept for fair access and equitable allocation of COVID-19 health products. 2020. Available at: https://www.who.int/publications/m/item/fair-allocation-mechanism-for-covid-19-vaccines-through-the-covax-facility. Accessed April 17, 2025.
4. Goldhill O. We have enough COVID-19 vaccines for most of the world. But rich countries are stockpiling more than they need for boosters. December 13, 2021. Available at: https://www.statnews.com/2021/12/13/we-have-enough-covid-vaccines-for-most-of-world-but-rich-countries-stockpiling-more-than-they-need. Accessed April 17, 2025.
5. Schaefer GO, Leland RJ, Emanuel EJ. Making vaccines available to other countries before offering domestic booster vaccinations. *JAMA*. 2021;326(10):903. https://doi.org/10.1001/jama.2021.13226
6. World Health Organization. Access and allocation: how will there be fair and equitable allocation of limited supplies? January 12, 2021. Available at: https://www.who.int/news-room/feature-stories/detail/access-and-allocation-how-will-there-be-fair-and-equitable-allocation-of-limited-supplies. Accessed June 21, 2023.
7. Emanuel EJ, Persad G, Kern A, et al. An ethical framework for global vaccine allocation. *Science*. 2020;369(6509):1309–1312. https://doi.org/10.1126/science.abe2803
8. Herzog LM, Norheim OF, Emanuel EJ, McCoy MS. COVAX must go beyond proportional allocation of COVID-19 vaccines to ensure fair and equitable access. *BMJ*. 2021;372:m4853. https://doi.org/10.1136/bmj.m4853
9. Emanuel EJ, Luna F, Schaefer GO, Tan KC, Wolff J. Enhancing the WHO's proposed framework for distributing COVID-19 vaccines among countries. *Am J Public Health*. 2021;111(3):371–373. https://doi.org/10.2105/AJPH.2020.306098
10. Persad G, Wertheimer A, Emanuel EJ. Principles for allocation of scarce medical interventions. *Lancet*. 2009;373(9661):423–431. https://doi.org/10.1016/S0140-6736(09)60137-9
11. Feinmann J. How the world is (not) handling surplus doses and expiring vaccines. *BMJ*. 2021;374: n2062. [Erratum in: *BMJ*. 2021;374:n2127.

https://doi.org/10.1136/bmj.n2127]. https://doi.org/10.1136/bmj.n2062

12. Taylor A. Amid low demand, global coronavirus vaccination set to slow in 2023 amid low demand. *Washington Post*. January 4, 2023. Available at: https://www.washingtonpost.com/world/2023/01/04/covid-vaccine-demand-covax-2023. Accessed June 19, 2023.
13. Boost for global response to COVID-19 as economies worldwide formally sign up to COVAX facility. Available at: https://www.who.int/news/item/21-09-2020-boost-for-global-response-to-covid-19-as-economies-worldwide-formally-sign-up-to-covax-facility. Accessed November 2, 2024.
14. Fair allocation mechanism for COVID-19 vaccines through the COVAX facility. Available at: September 9, 2020. https://www.who.int/publications/m/item/fair-allocation-mechanism-for-covid-19-vaccines-through-the-covax-facility. Accessed November 2, 2024.
15. Sharp D, Millum J. Prioritarianism for global health investments: identifying the worst off. *J Appl Philos*. 2018;35(1):112–132. https://doi.org/10.1111/japp.12142
16. Marshall RJ. Standard expected years of life lost as a measure of mortality: norms and reference to New Zealand data. *Aust N Z J Public Health*. 2004;28(5):452–457. https://doi.org/10.1111/j.1467-842X.2004.tb00027.x
17. Hunter DJ, Abdool Karim SS, Baden LR et al. Addressing vaccine inequity—COVID-19 vaccines as a global public good. *N Engl J Med*. 2022;386(12):1176–1179. https://doi.org/10.1056/NEJMe2202547
18. Rouw A, Wexler A, Kates J, Michaud J. Global COVID-19 vaccine access: a snapshot of inequality. March 17, 2021. Available at: https://www.kff.org/policy-watch/global-covid-19-vaccine-access-snapshot-of-inequality. Accessed June 19, 2023.
19. United Nations. Unequal vaccine distribution self-defeating, World Health Organization chief tells Economic and Social Council's special ministerial meeting. Available at: https://press.un.org/en/2021/ecosoc7039.doc.htm. Accessed April 17, 2025.
20. Burki T. Global COVID-19 vaccine inequity. *Lancet Infect Dis*. 2021;21(7):922–923. https://doi.org/10.1016/S1473-3099(21)00344-3
21. Islam N. "Excess deaths" is the best metric for tracking the pandemic. *BMJ*. 2022;376:o285. https://doi.org/10.1136/bmj.o285
22. Leon DA, Shkolnikov VM, Smeeth L, Magnus P, Pechholdová M, Jarvis CI. COVID-19: a need for real-time monitoring of weekly excess deaths. *Lancet*. 2020;395(10234):e81. https://doi.org/10.1016/S0140-6736(20)30933-8
23. Economist. The pandemic's true death toll. October 25, 2022. Available at: https://www.economist.com/graphic-detail/coronavirus-excess-deaths-estimates. Accessed June 28, 2023.
24. Wang H, Paulson KR, Pease SA, et al. Estimating excess mortality due to the COVID-19 pandemic: a systematic analysis of COVID-19-related mortality, 2020–21. *Lancet*. 2022;399(10334):1513–1536. https://doi.org/10.1016/S0140-6736(21)02796-3
25. World Health Organization. Global excess deaths associated with COVID-19 (modelled estimates) May 21, 2023. Available at: https://www.who.int/data/sets/global-excess-deaths-associated-with-covid-19-modelled-estimates. Accessed June 28, 2023.
26. Msemburi W, Karlinsky A, Knutson V, Aleshin-Guendel S, Chatterji S, Wakefield J. The WHO estimates of excess mortality associated with the COVID-19 pandemic. *Nature*. 2023;613(7942):130–137. https://doi.org/10.1038/s41586-022-05522-2
27. United Nations Children's Fund. COVID-19 market dashboard. Available at: https://www.unicef.org/supply/covid-19-market-dashboard. Accessed April 17, 2025.
28. Ioannidis JPA, Zonta F, Levitt M. Flaws and uncertainties in pandemic global excess death calculations. *Eur J Clin Investig*. 2023;53(8):e14008. https://doi.org/10.1111/eci.14008
29. Nolen S. Trying to solve a COVID-19 mystery: Africa's low death rates. *New York Times*. March 23, 2022. Available at: https://www.nytimes.com/2022/03/23/health/covid-africa-deaths.html. Accessed June 19, 2023.
30. Besson ESK, Norris A, Ghouth ASB, et al. Excess mortality during the COVID-19 pandemic: a geospatial and statistical analysis in Aden governorate, Yemen. *BMJ Glob Health*. 2021;6(3):e004564. https://doi.org/10.1136/bmjgh-2020-004564
31. Karanikolos M, McKee M. How comparable is COVID-19 mortality across countries? Available at: https://iris.who.int/bitstream/handle/10665/336295/Eurohealth-26-2-45-50-eng.pdf. Accessed April 17, 2025.
32. World Bank. Country and lending groups. Available at: https://datahelpdesk.worldbank.org/knowledgebase/articles/906519-world-bank-country-and-lending-groups. Accessed June 19, 2023.
33. Taylor L. COVID-19: True global death toll from pandemic is almost 15 million, says WHO. *BMJ*. 2022;377:o1144. https://doi.org/10.1136/bmj.o1144
34. Cabore JW, Karamagi HC, Kipruto HK, et al. COVID-19 in the 47 countries of the WHO African region: a modelling analysis of past trends and future patterns. *Lancet Glob Health*. 2022;10(8):e1099–e1114. https://doi.org/10.1016/S2214-109X(22)00233-9
35. Bollyky TJ, Bown CP. The tragedy of vaccine nationalism. December 10, 2021. Available at: https://www.foreignaffairs.com/articles/united-states/2020-07-27/vaccine-nationalism-pandemic. Accessed August 2, 2022.
36. Pan American Health Organization. Update on monkeypox in the region of the Americas and access to vaccines. August 5, 2022. Available at: https://www.paho.org/sites/default/files/cdss2-2-e-monkeypox_0.pdf. Accessed April 17, 2025.
37. Musa MK, Abdulsalam A, Haruna UA, et al. COVID-19 vaccine wastage in Africa: a case of Nigeria. *Int J Health Plann Manage*. 2024;39(2):229–236. https://doi.org/10.1002/hpm.3749
38. Coroneo L, Iacone F, Paccagnini A, Santos Monteiro P. Testing the predictive accuracy of COVID-19 forecasts. *Int J Forecast*. 2023;39(2):606–622. https://doi.org/10.1016/j.ijforecast.2022.01.005
39. Moore S, Hill EM, Dyson L, Tildesley MJ, Keeling MJ. Retrospectively modeling the effects of increased global vaccine sharing on the COVID-19 pandemic. *Nat Med*. 2022;28(11):2416–2423. https://doi.org/10.1038/s41591-022-02064-y
40. Emanuel EJ, Persad G. The shared ethical framework to allocate scarce medical resources: a lesson from COVID-19. *Lancet*. 2023;401(10391):1892–1902. https://doi.org/10.1016/S0140-6736(23)00812-7

# Self-Reported Versus County-Based Rurality of People Who Gave Birth in 6 US States, 2020

Katy Backes Kozhimannil, PhD, MPA, Emily C. Sheffield, MPH, Julia D. Interrante, PhD, MPH, Chen Liu, MHS, and Jamie R. Daw, PhD

**Objectives.** To measure concordance between postpartum people's self-reported residence in rural, urban, or suburban areas and county-based measurement of rurality.

**Methods.** We used survey data (collected January 2021–March 2022) from a representative sample of postpartum people with a live birth in 2020 in 6 US states (n = 3225), comparing respondents' self-report to county designations based on Rural–Urban Continuum Codes (RUCCs).

**Results.** Nearly 80% of postpartum people had concordant self-reported and RUCC-based residency. That is, 70% lived in counties that matched their self-report as urban (19%) or suburban (51%), and 9% lived in counties that matched their self-report as rural. However, almost 20% were rural discordant (lived in urban RUCC counties and self-reported as rural); these residents were more likely to lack a high-school degree and to have Medicaid-paid births compared with concordant respondents living in the same RUCC counties.

**Conclusions.** County-based measures of rurality may incorrectly categorize substantial portions of rural residents, and those potentially misclassified are of lower socioeconomic status.

**Public Health Implications.** Maternal health programs and policies using county-based definitions of rurality should account for rural residents living in areas designated as urban. (*Am J Public Health*. 2025;115(7):1095–1105. https://doi.org/10.2105/AJPH.2025.308058)

AJPH July 2025, Vol. 115, No. 7

Rural US residents face greater risks for maternal and infant morbidity and mortality than residents of urban areas,[1–4] and rural hospital closures and workforce shortages limit access to care for pregnant people living in rural areas.[5,6] Hospital-based obstetric care access is declining in rural communities.[7] From 2010 to 2022, 238 rural hospitals stopped providing obstetric care,[8] leaving many rural patients to travel long distances to care. Ensuring access to maternal health services and supports for rural residents is an urgent priority for health care delivery systems and state and federal policymakers.[9–11]

Various definitions of rurality are used by researchers and federal and state governments to describe populations, to determine access to and eligibility for programs, and to develop targeted policies to address rural health inequities.[12,13] This measurement variation affects estimations of rural–urban disparities and the distribution of resources intended for rural or urban places and people.[13,14]

There are strengths and drawbacks to each definition of rurality, including the potential for misclassification. Rural–Urban Continuum Codes (RUCCs), a county-based measure, are commonly used because counties align with administrative units and are consistently measured.[15] However, a drawback to county-based measures like RUCCs is that US counties vary widely in size and population density.[12,14] Individuals living in remote areas of a county may logically consider themselves to be rural residents but may potentially be classified as urban residents if their county contains an urban center and is defined as "metropolitan" according to county-based schemes. This has implications for statistics reported for both rural and urban residents.

Rural health experts have noted the salience of self-report as a meaningful measure to better capture individuals' lived experiences of rurality compared with administrative classifications such as RUCCs.[12,15] Despite potential benefits of using self-report, there are currently no national standards for collecting or using self-reported rurality in programs or research.[15] Thus, self-report has been underutilized, including in research on rural maternity care. Given the drawbacks to commonly used administrative definitions, there is growing interest in collecting data on self-reported rurality (e.g., the American Housing Survey[16]) and developing validated measures of self-reported rurality.[17]

Attention to addressing maternal health challenges has increased, but rural maternity care access continues to decline.[7,18,19] It is not clear whether programs and policies targeting resources to rural communities are reaching those who self-identify as rural residents because they may live in sparsely populated communities, outside of towns, or far from health care facilities. To our knowledge, no previous studies have compared self-reported rurality to a county-based definition among people who give birth in the United States. The goal of this analysis was to measure the concordance between postpartum people's self-reported residence in a rural, urban, or suburban area and RUCC county-based definitions and to describe the characteristics of people with self-reports that are discordant from this common definition.

# METHODS

We used survey data from the Postpartum Assessment of Health Survey (PAHS), a representative sample of postpartum individuals in 6 states (KS, MI, NJ, PA, UT, VA) and New York City.[20] The PAHS is a 12- to 14-month follow-up survey to the Centers for Disease Control and Prevention (CDC) Pregnancy Risk Assessment Monitoring System (PRAMS), the largest representative survey on pregnancy risk factors and outcomes in the United States. The PRAMS sampling frame is a stratified random sample drawn monthly from state and city birth certificate files.[21] Individuals in the 2020 PRAMS sampling frame had a live birth between January and December 2020 and completed the PRAMS survey 2- to 6-months postpartum. PRAMS respondents could opt out of being recontacted at 1-year postpartum for the PAHS survey. PAHS recruitment and data collection then occurred 12 to 14 months after their live birth from January 2021 to March 2022. Of those contacted for PAHS (n = 6021; 71.1% of 2020 PRAMS respondents), 4598 completed the survey (76.4% response rate).

## Outcomes

This analysis compared 2 measures of rurality, both collected in PAHS at 12- to 14-months postpartum: the 2023 RUCC, a county-based measure that accounts for the size of a population center within a county as well as adjacency to a metropolitan area,[22] and self-reported perceived rurality. We converted zip codes self-reported on PAHS to counties using the US Department of Housing and Urban Development Zip Code Crosswalk Files[23] and classified respondents as metropolitan (RUCC codes 1–3) or nonmetropolitan (RUCC codes 4–9).

Self-reported rurality measured respondents' own perceptions of the rurality of their communities based on responses to the question: "How would you describe the community where you currently live?" Response options were "rural," "suburban," "urban," and "I don't know."

We assessed concordance between self-reported rurality and county classification. We defined 6 mutually exclusive groups: rural concordant (self-reported rural people living in nonmetropolitan counties), rural discordant (self-reported rural people living in metropolitan counties), urban concordant (self-reported urban people living in metropolitan counties), urban discordant (self-reported urban people living in nonmetropolitan counties), suburban concordant (self-reported suburban people living in metropolitan counties), and suburban discordant (self-reported suburban people living in nonmetropolitan counties). For parsimony in some comparisons, we combined urban and suburban concordant and discordant into metropolitan concordant and discordant.

## Sociodemographic Characteristics

We included individual-level sociodemographic variables associated with rurality, based on self-reported data from the PAHS survey: age (18–24, 25–29, 30–34, or ≥ 35 years), race/ethnicity (non-Hispanic White; non-Hispanic Black; Hispanic/Latinx; Asian/Native Hawaiian or Pacific Islander [NHPI]/Southwest Asian, Middle Eastern, or North African [SWMENA];

Native American/Alaska Native; multiple races), marital status (married/domestic partner, not married/no domestic partner), education (< high school, high school, > high school), primary language (English, Spanish, other), and primary payer at childbirth (commercial, Medicaid/public, uninsured). For PAHS demographic variables with missing values, information was imputed from the PRAMS-linked birth certificate. We also merged county-level data from publicly available sources to describe the communities where respondents lived. These included dichotomous indicators of majority Black, Indigenous, or People of Color (BIPOC) populations; population density; and county area from the Area Health Resources File. We also included dichotomous indicators of whether the county of residence was above, at, or below the US mean for the following measures: infant mortality rate, life expectancy, percentage of people who were uninsured, and median household income from the County Health Rankings.

## Analysis

We estimated rates of and concordance between self-reported geography and RUCC-designated metropolitan and nonmetropolitan counties. We further examined the individual- and county-level sociodemographic characteristics of respondents by self-reported geography, county designation, and concordance between self-report and county designation. Next, we identified individual- and county-level predictors of rural discordance (self-reported rural people living in metropolitan counties). To do so, among people with a metropolitan county classification, we used survey-weighted logistic regression to estimate adjusted differences in the predicted probability of rural self-report (i.e., rural discordance) by individual- and county-level characteristics. Adjusted models included age, race/ethnicity, marital status, education, primary language, health insurance at birth, and county-level characteristics (life expectancy, uninsured rate, and median household income relative to the US mean, low population density, and large county area). We estimated adjusted differences in the predicted probability of rural discordance by individual-level and county-level characteristics using the Stata MARGINS command, with adjustment of standard errors for county-level clustering. This analysis focused on the characteristics of people living in metropolitan areas who described their community as rural; these individuals may be the most likely to be harmed by misclassification in county-based measures (e.g., by not having access to rural-specific programs despite living in a self-described rural area).

We conducted 4 supplemental analyses. First, we compared sociodemographic characteristics of respondents with missing geography to those with complete self-reported geography. Second, we estimated concordance rates between self-reported geography and another common federal measure for assessing rurality, the National Center for Health Statistics (NCHS) 6-category scheme for counties; categories 1 to 4 (large central metro, large fringe metro, medium metro, and small metro) are considered metropolitan (urban or suburban), and categories 5 and 6 (micropolitan and noncore) are considered nonmetropolitan (rural).[24] Third, we compared rural discordant with rural concordant individuals. Finally, we stratified rates of and concordance between self-report and RUCC designations by state.

We used PAHS survey weights to generate estimates that are representative of live births in 2020 in the 6 jurisdictions included in our study. PAHS survey weights were built on the CDC PRAMS analytic weights to account for the PRAMS stratified survey design, PRAMS nonresponse, and PAHS nonresponse. PAHS weights were also calibrated to known population totals by maternal age, race, ethnicity, education, marital status, sampling strata, and infant birth weight based on live birth records for 2020 in each jurisdiction.[20] We performed analyses by using Stata version 18 (StataCorp LP, College Station, TX).

## RESULTS

Among 4598 PAHS respondents, we excluded New York City respondents (n = 645) because all resided in a metropolitan area, as well as respondents missing zip code (n = 177) or self-reported geography (n = 551), resulting in a study sample size of 3225.

Table 1 presents the prevalence of self-reported geography categories and RUCC county designations. Most postpartum respondents (72%; n = 2377) self-reported as suburban or urban (53.6% and 18.7%, respectively), and 28% self-reported as rural (n = 848). Based on county, 88% of respondents were classified as metropolitan (suburban or urban) residents (n = 2796), and 12% were classified as nonmetropolitan (rural) residents (n = 429). Approximately 9% of respondents were rural concordant (self-reporting as rural with a nonmetropolitan county), 19% were rural discordant (self-reporting as rural with a metropolitan county), and 70% were metropolitan concordant (self-reporting as urban or suburban with a metropolitan county). Metropolitan

**TABLE 1— Sample Geography Based on Self-Report and Rural-Urban Continuum Codes (RUCCs): United States, Postpartum Assessment of Health Survey, January 2021–March 2022**

| | No. | Weighted % (95% CI) |
|---|---|---|
| **Self-reported geography** | | |
| Rural | 848 | 27.8 (25.0, 30.7) |
| Suburban | 1739 | 53.6 (50.6, 56.5) |
| Urban | 638 | 18.7 (16.9, 20.6) |
| **RUCC designation** | | |
| Nonmetropolitan (rural) | 429 | 11.8 (9.9, 14.0) |
| Metropolitan (urban or suburban) | 2796 | 88.2 (86.0, 90.1) |
| **Concordance of self-report and RUCC designation** | | |
| Rural concordant | 345 | 9.2 (7.7, 11.1) |
| Rural discordant | 503 | 18.5 (16.3, 21.0) |
| Metropolitan concordant | 2293 | 69.7 (66.7, 72.5) |
| Suburban concordant | 1669 | 51.2 (48.3, 54.1) |
| Urban concordant | 624 | 18.5 (16.7, 20.4) |
| Metropolitan discordant | 84 | 2.6 (1.6, 4.0) |
| Suburban discordant | 70 | 2.4 (1.4, 3.8) |
| Urban discordant | 14 | 0.2 (0.1, 0.4) |

*Note.* CI = confidence interval. The sample size was n = 3225. Rural concordant is rural self-report and nonmetropolitan RUCC. Rural discordant is rural self-report and metropolitan RUCC. Metropolitan concordant is urban or suburban self-report and metropolitan RUCC. Metropolitan discordant is urban or suburban self-report and nonmetropolitan RUCC. Respondents with missing geography (either self-report [n = 586; 14.8% missing] or zip code [n = 177; 4.5% missing]) are excluded from the main analyses and their characteristics are presented in Tables C and D (available as supplements to the online version of this article at https://ajph.org).

discordance was rare: only 2.4% of the sample were suburban discordant, and 0.2% were urban discordant (i.e., self-reporting as suburban or urban with a nonmetropolitan county). Discordance was much more common among self-reported rural residents; approximately 60% of self-reported rural people were potentially misclassified as metropolitan (503 of 848). In contrast, only 2% of self-reported suburban people (70 of 1739) and 4% of self-reported urban people (14 of 638) were potentially misclassified as nonmetropolitan.

Table 2 presents individual- and county-level characteristics of postpartum respondents stratified by self-reported geography. Compared with self-reported suburban respondents, self-reported rural respondents were more likely to be younger (18–24 years; 27% rural vs 12% suburban), non-Hispanic White (72% rural vs 68% suburban), unmarried or not in a domestic partnership (22% rural vs 12% suburban), have a lower education level (< high school; 12% rural vs 2% suburban), speak Spanish as a primary language (8% rural vs 3% suburban), and be insured by Medicaid or other public insurance (38% rural vs 21% suburban) or be uninsured (4% rural vs 1% suburban) at the time of childbirth. County-level characteristics also varied by self-reported geography. Self-reported rural respondents were more likely to live in counties with lower life expectancy (22% rural vs 11% suburban), higher uninsured populations (49% rural vs 26% suburban), lower median household incomes (73% rural vs 41% suburban), and lower population density (36% rural vs 5% suburban) compared with self-reported suburban respondents.

Table 3 presents the individual- and county-level characteristics of postpartum respondents stratified by the concordance between self-reported geography and county designation. Compared with metropolitan concordant residents, rural discordant residents were more likely to be younger (18–24 years; 13% vs 24%, respectively), non-Hispanic White (59% vs 66%, respectively), have a lower education level (< high school; 4% vs 13%, respectively), and be insured by Medicaid or other public insurance at the time of childbirth (29% vs 40%, respectively). County-level characteristics also varied between rural discordant and metropolitan concordant respondents. Compared with metropolitan concordant respondents, rural discordant residents were more likely to live in counties with higher infant mortality rates (40% vs 53%, respectively), lower median household incomes (43% vs 62%, respectively), and lower population density (3% vs 14%, respectively); furthermore, they were less likely to live in counties with majority BIPOC populations (28% vs 15%, respectively).

Figure 1 presents the differences in adjusted predicted probabilities of rural discordance by individual- and county-level characteristics among respondents living in metropolitan counties. Among metropolitan residents, respondents who were younger (18–24 vs 30–34 years; marginal difference = 13.2%) and those who had a lower education level (< high school vs > high school; marginal difference = 21.6%) were more

**TABLE 2—** Sample Characteristics by Self-Reported Geography: United States, Postpartum Assessment of Health Survey, January 2021–March 2022

| | Self-Reported Rural (n = 848; 27.8%), Weighted % (95% CI) | Self-Reported Suburban (n = 1739; 53.6%), Weighted % (95% CI) | Self-Reported Urban (n = 638; 18.7%), Weighted % (95% CI) |
|---|---|---|---|
| **Individual-level characteristics** | | | |
| Age, y | | | |
| 18–24 | 26.7 (21.9, 32.1)* | 11.7 (9.6, 14.3) | 17.3 (13.5, 22.1)* |
| 25–29 | 27.6 (23.5, 32.3) | 25.5 (22.6, 28.6) | 30.6 (25.5, 36.3) |
| 30–34 | 26.5 (22.7, 30.7)* | 39.6 (36.5, 42.9) | 30.7 (25.2, 36.7)* |
| ≥ 35 | 19.2 (16.2, 22.6)* | 23.1 (20.7, 25.8) | 21.4 (17.3, 26.1) |
| Race/ethnicity | | | |
| Non-Hispanic White | 71.6 (67.0, 75.8) | 68.1 (65.1, 70.9) | 33.6 (29.0, 38.7)* |
| Non-Hispanic Black | 11.0 (8.1, 14.9) | 9.4 (7.7, 11.4) | 27.7 (23.2, 32.7)* |
| Hispanic/Latinx | 13.0 (10.2, 16.6) | 9.2 (7.6, 11.2) | 28.4 (24.0, 33.3)* |
| Asian/NHPI/SWMENA | 2.7 (1.4, 4.9)* | 11.5 (9.7, 13.4) | 8.4 (5.7, 12.3) |
| Native American/Alaska Native | 1.3 (0.6, 2.6) | 0.9 (0.3, 2.8) | 0.2 (0.0, 0.8) |
| Multiple races | 0.4 (0.1, 1.1) | 0.9 (0.4, 2.0) | 1.7 (0.8, 3.6) |
| Marital status | | | |
| Not married/no domestic partner | 22.3 (17.5, 28.0)* | 11.6 (9.3, 14.2) | 32.9 (27.4, 38.9)* |
| Married/domestic partner | 77.7 (72.0, 82.5)* | 88.4 (85.8, 90.7) | 67.1 (61.1, 72.6)* |
| Education | | | |
| < High school | 12.3 (8.2, 18.1)* | 2.2 (1.4, 3.5) | 7.9 (5.0, 12.5)* |
| High school | 24.1 (20.0, 28.6)* | 13.8 (10.8, 17.4) | 27.0 (21.0, 34.1)* |
| > High school | 63.6 (58.0, 68.8)* | 84.0 (80.4, 87.1) | 65.0 (58.7, 70.9)* |
| Primary language | | | |
| English | 88.7 (83.9, 92.2) | 91.2 (88.6, 93.3) | 76.7 (72.1, 80.7)* |
| Spanish | 8.1 (5.5, 11.8)* | 2.9 (2.0, 4.1) | 15.7 (12.5, 19.5)* |
| Other | 2.1 (1.1, 3.9)* | 5.6 (3.9, 8.0) | 7.1 (4.8, 10.6) |
| Health insurance at birth | | | |
| Commercial/military/other | 57.2 (51.2, 63.1)* | 77.9 (74.7, 80.9) | 43.4 (38.1, 48.9)* |
| Medicaid/public | 38.3 (32.6, 44.3)* | 21.0 (18.0, 24.3) | 52.0 (46.5, 57.5)* |
| Uninsured | 4.4 (2.6, 7.3)* | 1.1 (0.6, 1.8) | 4.6 (2.9, 7.1)* |
| **County-level characteristics** | | | |
| Infant mortality rate > US mean | 39.7 (33.9, 45.8) | 34.3 (30.8, 38.0) | 51.2 (45.4, 57.1)* |
| Life expectancy < US mean | 21.5 (16.7, 27.2)* | 11.4 (8.7, 14.7) | 27.2 (22.2, 32.7)* |
| % uninsured > US mean | 49.3 (44.1, 54.5)* | 26.4 (24.0, 29.0) | 44.6 (38.7, 50.6)* |
| Median household income < US mean | 73.4 (68.9, 77.5)* | 40.5 (36.9, 44.3) | 55.8 (50.7, 60.8)* |
| Majority BIPOC | 10.7 (7.1, 14.2)* | 19.1 (16.5, 21.7) | 49.8 (44.2, 55.4)* |
| Low population density (< 100 people/sq mi) | 36.4 (31.6, 41.4)* | 5.4 (4.1, 7.0) | 2.6 (1.3, 5.0)* |
| Large area (> US mean ~1000 sq mi) | 18.3 (1.4, 22.9)* | 10.7 (9.1, 12.5) | 5.0 (3.4, 7.3)* |

*Note.* BIPOC = Black, Indigenous or People of Color; CI = confidence interval; NHPI = Native Hawaiian or Pacific Islander; SWMENA = Southwest Asian, Middle Eastern or North African. The sample size was n = 3225. Respondents with missing geography (either self-report [n = 586; 14.8% missing] or zip code [n = 177; 4.5% missing]) are excluded from the main analyses and their characteristics are presented in Tables C and D (available as supplements to the online version of this article at https://ajph.org).

*Difference compared with suburban reference group is statistically significant, $P < .05$.

**TABLE 3—** **Sample Characteristics by Concordance Between Self-Reported Geography and RUCC Designation: United States, Postpartum Assessment of Health Survey, January 2021–March 2022**

| | Rural Concordant (n = 345; 9.2%), Weighted % (95% CI) | Rural Discordant (n = 503; 18.5%), Weighted % (95% CI) | Metropolitan Concordant (n = 2293; 69.7%), Weighted % (95% CI) |
|---|---|---|---|
| **Individual-level characteristics** | | | |
| Age, y | | | |
| 18–24 | 31.5 (22.9, 41.6)* | 24.3 (18.7, 30.8)* | 12.6 (10.6, 15.0) |
| 25–29 | 26.0 (18.9, 34.6) | 28.5 (23.1, 34.5) | 27.3 (24.7, 30.1) |
| 30–34 | 27.4 (19.6, 36.9) | 26.0 (21.4, 31.2)* | 37.3 (34.5, 40.2) |
| ≥ 35 | 15.1 (10.1, 22.0) | 21.2 (17.3, 25.7) | 22.8 (20.9, 24.8) |
| Race/ethnicity | | | |
| Non-Hispanic White | 83.0 (73.8, 89.4)* | 66.0 (59.1, 72.2) | 59.4 (57.0, 61.7) |
| Non-Hispanic Black | 8.8 (3.8, 19.1) | 12.1 (8.5, 17.1) | 14.3 (12.6, 16.1) |
| Hispanic/Latinx | 5.4 (3.3, 8.6)* | 16.8 (12.6, 22.1) | 14.6 (12.9, 16.4) |
| Asian/NHPI/SWMENA | 1.0 (0.2, 4.8)* | 3.5 (1.9, 6.5) | 10.5 (9.2, 12.0) |
| Native American/Alaska Native | 1.7 (0.6, 4.6)* | 1.1 (0.4, 3.1) | 0.2 (0.1, 0.5) |
| Multiple races | 0.2 (0.0, 1.0) | 0.4 (0.1, 1.6) | 1.1 (0.6, 1.9) |
| Marital status | | | |
| Not married/no partner | 21.7 (14.5, 31.1) | 22.7 (16.7, 30.0) | 17.2 (15.0, 19.7) |
| Married/domestic partner | 78.3 (68.9, 85.5) | 77.3 (70.0, 83.3) | 82.8 (80.3, 85.0) |
| Education | | | |
| < High school | 11.1 (5.3, 21.8)* | 12.9 (8.0, 20.3)* | 3.6 (2.6, 5.1) |
| High school | 24.4 (16.7, 34.2) | 23.9 (18.5, 30.3) | 17.0 (14.4, 20.0) |
| > High school | 64.5 (53.8, 73.9)* | 63.2 (55.7, 70.0)* | 79.3 (76.6, 81.9) |
| Primary language | | | |
| English | 96.5 (92.2, 98.4)* | 86.4 (81.0, 90.5) | 87.4 (85.4, 89.2) |
| Spanish | 1.9 (0.8, 4.6)* | 11.2 (7.4, 16.5) | 6.4 (5.3, 7.6) |
| Other | 1.6 (0.4, 6.4) | 2.4 (1.1, 4.9) | 6.2 (4.8, 8.0) |
| Health insurance at birth | | | |
| Commercial/military/other | 59.3 (49.0, 68.8) | 56.3 (48.8, 63.6)* | 69.3 (66.5, 72.0) |
| Medicaid/public | 35.5 (26.3, 45.8) | 39.7 (32.3, 47.6)* | 28.7 (26.1, 31.6) |
| Uninsured | 5.2 (1.9, 13.8) | 3.9 (2.0, 7.7) | 2.0 (1.4, 2.8) |
| **County-level characteristics** | | | |
| Infant mortality rate > US mean | 64.1 (44.3, 80.0)* | 53.4 (45.4, 61.2)* | 39.7 (36.7, 42.9) |
| Life expectancy < US mean | 22.2 (15.1, 31.5) | 21.1 (15.4, 28.3) | 15.3 (12.9, 18.0) |
| % uninsured > US mean | 74.4 (62.5, 83.5)* | 36.8 (31.1, 42.9) | 29.7 (27.4, 32.2) |
| Median household income < US mean | 96.3 (93.8, 97.8)* | 62.1 (56.2, 67.7)* | 42.9 (40.0, 46.0) |
| Majority BIPOC | 2.0 (1.1, 3.5)* | 15.0 (10.5, 21.0)* | 27.9 (25.3, 30.7) |
| Low population density (< 100 people/sq mile) | 80.6 (72.0, 87.0)* | 14.4 (10.8, 19.0)* | 2.8 (2.0, 3.8) |
| Large area (> US mean ~1000 sq mi) | 37.9 (28.5, 48.3)* | 8.5 (6.0, 12.0) | 8.7 (7.5, 10.0) |

*Note.* BIPOC = Black, Indigenous, or People of Color; CI = confidence interval; NHPI = Native Hawaiian or Pacific Islander; RUCC = Rural-Urban Continuum Code; SWMENA = Southwest Asian, Middle Eastern, or North African. The sample size was n = 3225. Rural concordant is rural self-report and nonmetropolitan RUCC. Rural discordant is rural self-report and metropolitan RUCC. Metropolitan concordant is urban or suburban self-report and metropolitan RUCC. Respondents with missing geography (either self-report [n = 586; 14.8% missing] or zip code [n = 177; 4.5% missing]) are excluded from the main analyses and their characteristics are presented in Tables C and D (available as supplements to the online version of this article at https://ajph.org). Metropolitan discordant respondents (n = 84; < 3%) were excluded from this table.

*Difference compared with metropolitan concordant reference group is statistically significant, $P < .05$.

| Comparative Dimensions | Marginal Predicted Probability Difference (95% CI) |
|---|---|
| **Individual-level characteristics** | |
| **Age, y (Ref = 30–34)** | |
| 18–24 | 13.2 (3.2, 23.3) |
| 25–29 | 4.5 (−1.2, 10.3) |
| ≥35 | 4.7 (−0.7, 10.2) |
| **Race/ethnicity (Ref = non-Hispanic White)** | |
| Non-Hispanic Black | −8.8 (−16.2, −1.4) |
| Hispanic/Latinx | −8.2 (−15.7, −0.8) |
| Asian/NHPI/SWMENA | −12.4 (−22.2, −2.5) |
| Native American/Alaska Native | 23.8 (−22.7, 70.3) |
| Multiple races | −14.9 (−37.8, 8.0) |
| **Marital status (Ref = married/domestic partner)** | |
| Not married/No domestic partner | −0.1 (−6.1, 6.4) |
| **Education (Ref = >high school)** | |
| <high School | 21.6 (5.7, 37.6) |
| High school | 3.5 (−4.2, 11.2) |
| **Primary language (Ref = English)** | |
| Spanish | 10.1 (−3.5, 23.8) |
| Other | −3.4 (−18.6, 11.7) |
| **Health insurance at birth (Ref = commerical/military/other)** | |
| Medicaid/public | 1.8 (−5.2, 8.8) |
| Uninsured | 4.2 (−12.3, 20.7) |
| **County-level characteristics** | |
| Life expectancy < US mean | −0.9 (−8.1, 6.4) |
| % uninsured > US mean | −0.9 (−6.1, 4.3) |
| Median household income < US mean | 9.0 (2.7, 15.2) |
| Low population density (< 100 people per sq mile) | 32.7 (20.5, 44.8) |
| Large area (> US mean of 1000 sq miles) | −7.4 (-13.9, −1.0) |

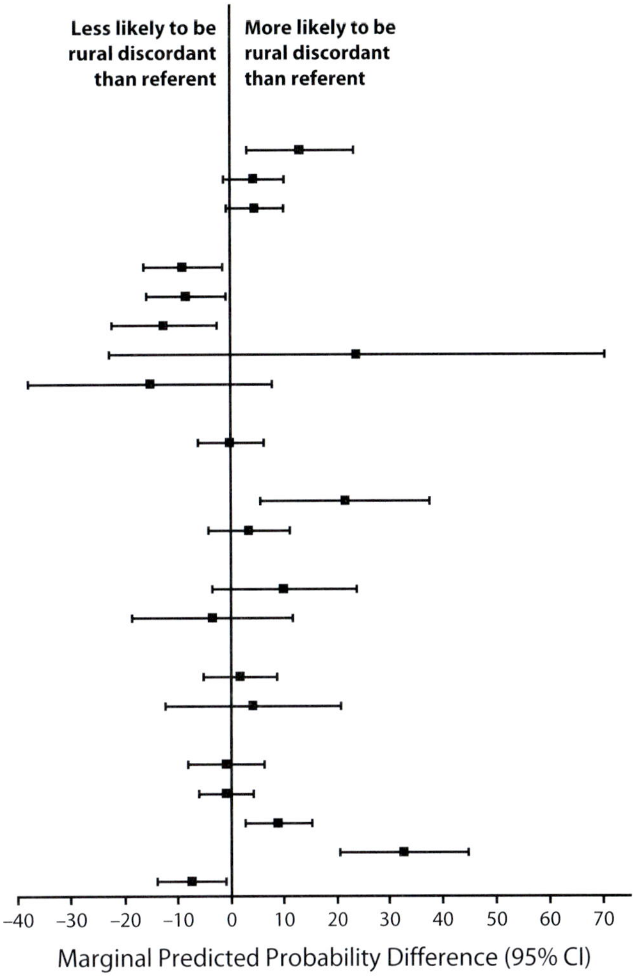


**FIGURE 1— Differences in Adjusted Predicted Probabilities of Rural Discordance Among Respondents Living in RUCC-Designated Metropolitan Counties: United States, Postpartum Assessment of Health Survey, January 2021–March 2022**

*Note.* CI = confidence interval; NHPI = Native Hawaiian or Pacific Islander; RUCC = Rural–Urban Continuum Code; SWMENA = Southwest Asian, Middle Eastern, or North African. Estimates for this figure can be found in Table A (available as a supplement to the online version of this article at https://www.ajph.org). The sample size was n = 2796.

likely to be rural discordant. Metropolitan residents who identified as non-Hispanic Black (marginal difference = −8.8%), Hispanic/Latinx (marginal difference = −8.2%), or Asian/NHPI/SWMENA (marginal difference = −12.4%) were less likely to be rural discordant compared with metropolitan residents who identified as non-Hispanic White. In addition, metropolitan respondents living in counties with median household incomes lower than the US mean (marginal difference = 9.0%) and with low population density (marginal difference = 32.7%) were more likely to be rural discordant, and those living in large counties of greater than 1000 square miles (marginal difference = −7.4%) were less likely to be rural discordant. Estimates for Figure 1 can be found in Table A (available as a supplement to the online version of this article at https://ajph.org).

Results from the sensitivity analysis using the NCHS measure instead of the RUCC measure to assess concordance or discordance between self-reported and county-based measures of rurality were consistent (Table B, available as a supplement to the online version of this article at https://ajph.org). A substantial portion of respondents were missing self-reported geography. Table C (available as a supplement to the online version of this article at https://ajph.org) shows the distribution of respondents with missing and complete self-reported geography, stratified by RUCC designation. Individuals with missing responses on self-reported geography were more likely to be aged younger than 25 years, non-Hispanic Black, Hispanic/Latinx, unmarried or not in a domestic partnership, have a high-school or less than high-school education, have Medicaid or other public insurance at the time of childbirth, and speak Spanish as a primary language (Table D, available as a supplement to the online version of this article at https://ajph.org). Table E (available as a supplement to the online version of this article at https://ajph.org) shows the individual- and county-level characteristics of postpartum respondents stratified by their RUCC county designation. Figure A (available as a supplement to the online version of this article at https://ajph.org) compares characteristics for rural concordant and rural discordant individuals. Rural discordance was highest in Pennsylvania (22.0%) and lowest in Utah (9.2%; Table F, available as a supplement to the online version of this article at https://ajph.org).

## DISCUSSION

According to commonly used RUCC county-based designations, 88% of postpartum people in this study lived in metropolitan counties (comprising both urban and suburban areas), and 12% lived in nonmetropolitan (rural) counties. When asked to describe the community where they currently live, 19% said urban, 54% said suburban, and 28% said rural.

Most respondents identified their community in a way that was concordant with RUCC definitions. Most postpartum people lived in metropolitan counties and self-identified as either urban (19%) or suburban (51%). In addition, 9% of postpartum people in this sample were residents of nonmetropolitan counties that identified as rural residents. Many people who described themselves as living in a rural community were located in a county that would be defined as metropolitan by many researchers, programs, and policies. This group of people with a self-identity that was discordant from a county-based definition was sizeable: almost 1 in 5 postpartum people lived in metropolitan counties but identified themselves as rural residents. In addition, in this sample, the discordance between self-report and county designations served to misclassify rural people almost exclusively—less than 3% of postpartum people who lived in nonmetropolitan counties identified themselves as urban (0.2%) or suburban (2.4%) residents. These findings among postpartum people are consistent with studies showing sizeable populations of self-identified rural residents living in metropolitan-designated counties among the general population.[17,25,26]

While there is not a gold standard for determining rurality, self-report is an important way of ascertaining the type of community where a person lives.[12] However, differences in health outcomes and health care access are not frequently assessed using self-report and, thus, are not well-documented. In public health and health care, it is not always possible to ask individuals to describe where they live, and reliance on other measures is the only practical solution. It is therefore essential to understand the challenges of using RUCC and other common measures. This analysis provides evidence that access and outcomes may differ because self-reported rural postpartum people were more likely than others living in metropolitan counties to have characteristics associated with lower socioeconomic status and greater maternal health risks. In addition, rural discordant individuals generally live in different types of metropolitan counties compared with those who are metropolitan concordant. Specifically, the counties themselves are lower income and have lower population density, suggesting that they may be metropolitan counties that contain remote areas where some residents live. Previous research shows that lower-income and less-populated communities have more limited access to hospital-based maternity care.[5]

## Public Health Implications

Attention to rural maternal health inequities in public health and health policy is warranted,[7,19,27] and policy attention has been increasing.[9,10,18] This analysis found that a substantial portion of postpartum people—nearly 20%—would be classified as residents of metropolitan counties, despite self-identifying as rural residents. Some rural residents (up to 60% of those who self-identify as rural) may not be counted as rural in research, affecting estimates of health burdens in both metropolitan and nonmetropolitan counties. In addition, they may lack access to programs that are intended for rural residents if living in a metropolitan county excludes them from those services. Reaching rural residents—whether they live in metropolitan or nonmetropolitan counties—may require more resources per capita.

Because of the different definitions used by rural-specific programs, determining eligibility for individuals, organizations, groups, or communities that consider themselves rural is not straightforward; as such, the Rural Health Information Hub hosts an online tool called "Am I Rural?," which can be used to understand a community's category and eligibility for rural programs under a range of definitions.[28] For example, this tool can generate reports that outline how a location is defined by common definitions of rurality (e.g., RUCCs, Urban Influence Codes, Frontier and Remote Area Codes), as well as whether the area is classified as rural with regard to eligibility for rural-specific programs, such as the Centers for Medicare and Medicaid Services' Rural Health Clinics Program.[28]

Importantly, this analysis found that rural discordant respondents have specific characteristics that are associated with limited access to maternity care and with maternal morbidity and mortality.[3,29–32] Rural discordant residents were statistically more likely to be younger (18–24 years) and have a lower level of education. While not statistically significant, it is important for equity purposes to note that those who were rural discordant in this study were also more likely to identify as Native American/Alaska Native, speak Spanish as a primary language, or be uninsured at the time of childbirth. Postpartum residents with these characteristics who are living in metropolitan counties may not be the highest risk populations in terms of maternity care access compared with the most remote rural residents; however, many rural discordant individuals have individual characteristics associated with poor maternal health outcomes. Research methods and public health efforts should account for the likelihood that a substantial portion of postpartum individuals living in what they describe as "rural" communities are residing in metropolitan counties. Indeed, postpartum people living in metropolitan counties differ in important ways. In addition to self-reported rural individuals living in these counties, there are notable differences between suburban- and urban-identifying metropolitan residents that may require greater attention in maternal health–related research and policy.

## Limitations

This analysis provides new information on the potential for misclassification of rural postpartum people using a common definition of rurality, with implications for measurement in both metropolitan and nonmetropolitan counties. There are some important limitations. First, while findings are representative of births in the 6 states represented in this analysis, they may not be generalizable to other states. While rates of concordance were similar across states in our sample, there was some variation (Table F). Second, missingness in the self-report variable was substantial (14.8%), and was much higher for non–English-speaking respondents and for respondents who identified as Hispanic/Latinx; this suggests that the question wording may not have translated well, despite similar wording having been used by the US Census and the US Department of Housing and Urban Development (e.g., in the 2017 Neighborhood Description Study).[16] Future research should use self-report variables that can be interpreted across cultures and languages.

Third, sample sizes limited analytic capacity, particularly among Asian/NHPI/SWMENA, Native American/Alaska Native, or multiracial people and respondents whose primary language was not English. Fourth, although we used RUCC designations for comparison against self-report and found nearly identical results when using NCHS measures, we did not assess all commonly used measures of rurality. However, our findings are similar to those of previous studies showing substantial proportions of rural discordance when comparing self-reported rurality with both county-based and zip code–based measures among the general population.[25,26,33,34] Fifth, this analysis did not account for the distribution of clinicians or health care facilities. Finally, there is no gold standard for measuring rurality in research, which creates difficulty in assessing rurality and using it as a criterion in program and policy eligibility determinations and research[35]; still, recognizing measured geographic inequities is imperative to target resources toward those experiencing barriers to access and adverse maternal and infant health outcomes.

## Conclusions

County-based measures of rurality may incorrectly categorize a substantial portion of postpartum people who are rural residents living in metropolitan counties. Using self-identified rurality in research may improve understanding of differences in health and health care access for people living in metropolitan and nonmetropolitan counties, and maternal health programs and policies using common county-based definitions of metropolitan areas should account for the presence of rural residents in these communities. AJPH

### ABOUT THE AUTHORS

Katy Backes Kozhimannil, Emily C. Sheffield, and Julia D. Interrante are with the University of Minnesota Rural Health Research Center, Division of Health Policy and Management, University of Minnesota School of Public Health, Minneapolis. Chen Liu was with the Department of Health Policy and Management, Columbia University

Mailman School of Public Health, New York, NY, at the time of this study. Jamie R. Daw is with the Department of Health Policy and Management, Columbia University Mailman School of Public Health.

## CORRESPONDENCE

Correspondence should be sent to Katy Backes Kozhimannil, PhD, MPA, 2221 University Ave SE #350, Minneapolis, MN 55414 (e-mail: kbk@umn.edu). Reprints can be ordered at https://www.ajph.org by clicking the "Reprints" link.

## PUBLICATION INFORMATION

Full Citation: Kozhimannil KB, Sheffield EC, Interrante JD, Liu C, Daw JR. Self-reported versus county-based rurality of people who gave birth in 6 US states, 2020. *Am J Public Health*. 2025;115(7): 1095–1105.

Acceptance Date: February 3, 2025.

DOI: https://doi.org/10.2105/AJPH.2025.308058

ORCID iDs:

Katy Backes Kozhimannil https://orcid.org/0000-0002-5734-9049

Emily C. Sheffield https://orcid.org/0009-0008-7355-3219

Julia D. Interrante https://orcid.org/0000-0001-8579-6623

Chen Liu https://orcid.org/0000-0001-8889-0105

## CONTRIBUTORS

K. B. Kozhimannil, E. C. Sheffield, J. D. Interrante, C. Liu, and J. R. Daw made substantial contributions to the conceptualization or design of the work or the acquisition, analysis, or interpretation of data for the work; drafted the work or revised it critically for important intellectual content; and gave final approval of the version to be published.

## ACKNOWLEDGMENTS

This research was supported in part by Columbia World Projects and by the National Institutes of Health's National Institute of Minority Health and Health Disparities (grant 5R01MD017460).

**Note.** The content is solely the responsibility of the authors and does not necessarily represent the official views of the National Institutes of Health.

## CONFLICTS OF INTEREST

The authors have no relevant conflicts of interest to disclose.

## HUMAN PARTICIPANT PROTECTION

This study was approved by the Columbia University institutional review board.

## REFERENCES

1. Ehrenthal DB, Kuo HHD, Kirby RS. Infant mortality in rural and nonrural counties in the United States. *Pediatrics*. 2020;146(5):e20200464. https://doi.org/10.1542/peds.2020-0464
2. Kozhimannil KB, Leonard SA, Handley SC, et al. Obstetric volume and severe maternal morbidity among low-risk and higher-risk patients giving birth at rural and urban US hospitals. *JAMA Health Forum*. 2023;4(6):e232110. https://doi.org/10.1001/jamahealthforum.2023.2110
3. Kozhimannil KB, Interrante JD, Henning-Smith C, Admon LK. Rural-urban differences in severe maternal morbidity and mortality in the US, 2007–15. *Health Aff (Millwood)*. 2019;38(12): 2077–2085. https://doi.org/10.1377/hlthaff.2019.00805
4. Womack LS, Rossen LM, Hirai AH. Urban–rural infant mortality disparities by race and ethnicity and cause of death. *Am J Prev Med*. 2020;58(2): 254–260. https://doi.org/10.1016/j.amepre.2019.09.010
5. Hung P, Henning-Smith CE, Casey MM, Kozhimannil KB. Access to obstetric services in rural counties still declining, with 9 percent losing services, 2004–14. *Health Aff (Millwood)*. 2017;36(9): 1663–1671. https://doi.org/10.1377/hlthaff.2017.0338
6. Kozhimannil KB, Interrante JD, Admon LK, Basile Ibrahim BL. Rural hospital administrators' beliefs about safety, financial viability, and community need for offering obstetric care. *JAMA Health Forum*. 2022;3(3):e220204. https://doi.org/10.1001/jamahealthforum.2022.0204
7. Kozhimannil KB, Interrante JD, Fritz AH, Sheffield EC. Loss of Hospital-Based Obstetric Services in Rural Counties in the United States, 2010–2022. University of Minnesota Rural Health Research Center. July 2024. Available at: https://rhrc.umn.edu/wp-content/uploads/2024/07/UMN-Infographic-OB-Closures_7.3_final.pdf. Accessed November 16, 2024.
8. Kozhimannil KB, Interrante JD, Carroll C, et al. Obstetric care access at rural and urban hospitals in the United States. *JAMA*. 2025;333(2):166–169. https://doi.org/10.1001/jama.2024.23010
9. The White House. *White House Blueprint for Addressing the Maternal Health Crisis*. June 2022. Available at: https://bidenwhitehouse.archives.gov/wp-content/uploads/2022/06/Maternal-Health-Blueprint.pdf. Accessed March 17, 2025.
10. Centers for Medicare and Medicaid Services. *Advancing Rural Maternal Health Equity*. May 2022. Available at: https://www.cms.gov/files/document/maternal-health-may-2022.pdf. Accessed December 17, 2024.
11. Office of the Surgeon General. *The Surgeon General's Call to Action to Improve Maternal Health*. US Department of Health and Human Services. 2020. Available at: https://www.hhs.gov/sites/default/files/call-to-action-maternal-health.pdf. Accessed September 3, 2024.
12. Bennett KJ, Borders TF, Holmes GM, Kozhimannil KB, Ziller E. What is rural? Challenges and implications of definitions that inadequately encompass rural people and places. *Health Aff (Millwood)*. 2019;38(12): 1985–1992. https://doi.org/10.1377/hlthaff.2019.00910
13. Danek R, Blackburn J, Greene M, Mazurenko O, Menachemi N. Measuring rurality in health services research: a scoping review. *BMC Health Serv Res*. 2022;22(1):1340. https://doi.org/10.1186/s12913-022-08678-9
14. Long JC, Delamater PL, Holmes GM. Which definition of rurality should I use? The relative performance of 8 federal rural definitions in identifying rural–urban disparities. *Med Care*. 2021;59(suppl 5):S413–S419. https://doi.org/10.1097/MLR.0000000000001612
15. Kozhimannil KB, Sheffield EC, Adole MJ, et al. *Resources for Measuring Rurality in Research on Maternity Care*. University of Minnesota Rural Health Research Center. January 2025. Available at: https://rhrc.umn.edu/wp-content/uploads/2025/01/PracticalImplications_measuring-rurality_final-1.pdf. Accessed January 13, 2025.
16. Office of Policy Development and Research. The 2017 AHS Neighborhood Description Study. US Department of Housing and Urban Development. Available at: https://www.huduser.gov/portal/AHS-neighborhood-description-study-2017.html. Accessed August 2, 2024.
17. Oser CB, Strickland J, Batty EJ, Pullen E, Staton M. The Rural Identity Scale (RIS): development and validation. *J Rural Health*. 2022;38(1):303–310. https://doi.org/10.1111/jrh.12563
18. US Government Accountability Office. Maternal health: availability of hospital-based obstetric care in rural areas. October 19, 2022. Available at: https://www.gao.gov/products/gao-23-105515. Accessed December 17, 2024.
19. Kozhimannil KB. Declining access to US maternity care is a systemic injustice. *BMJ*. 2023;382:2038. https://doi.org/10.1136/bmj.p2038
20. Columbia World Projects. *PAHS 2020 Technical Documentation*. Columbia University. March 1, 2023. Available at: https://www.publichealth.columbia.edu/file/15116/download?token=h3OrI__u. Accessed July 19, 2024.
21. Shulman HB, D'Angelo DV, Harrison L, Smith RA, Warner L. The Pregnancy Risk Assessment Monitoring System (PRAMS): overview of design and methodology. *Am J Public Health*. 2018;108(10): 1305–1313. https://doi.org/10.2105/AJPH.2018.304563
22. Economic Research Service, US Department of Agriculture. Rural-Urban Continuum Codes. Data Products. January 2024. Available at: https://www.ers.usda.gov/data-products/rural-urban-continuum-codes. Accessed August 20, 2024.
23. Office of Policy Development and Research. HUD USPS ZIP Code Crosswalk Files. US Department of Housing and Urban Development. Available at: https://www.huduser.gov/portal/datasets/usps_crosswalk.html. Accessed December 15, 2024.
24. National Center for Health Statistics. NCHS Urban-Rural Classification Scheme for Counties. Centers for Disease Control and Prevention. 2017. Available at: https://www.cdc.gov/nchs/data_access/urban_rural.htm. Accessed August 20, 2024.
25. Igielnik R, Grieco E, Castillo A. Evaluating what makes a US community urban, suburban or rural. Pew Research Center. November 22, 2019. Available at: https://www.pewresearch.org/decoded/2019/11/22/evaluating-what-makes-a-us-community-urban-suburban-or-rural. Accessed August 20, 2024.
26. Castle ME, Tak CR. Self-reported vs RUCA rural-urban classification among North Carolina pharmacists. *Pharm Pract (Granada)*. 2021;19(3):2406. https://doi.org/10.18549/PharmPract.2021.3.2406
27. Kozhimannil KB, Interrante JD, Tuttle MS, Henning-Smith C, Admon L. Characteristics of US rural hospitals by obstetric service availability, 2017. *Am J Public Health*. 2020;110(9):1315–1317. https://doi.org/10.2105/AJPH.2020.305695

28. Rural Health Information Hub. Am I Rural? - Tool. Available at: https://www.ruralhealthinfo.org/am-i-rural. Accessed June 3, 2024.
29. Interrante JD, Tuttle MS, Admon LK, Kozhimannil KB. Severe maternal morbidity and mortality risk at the intersection of rurality, race and ethnicity, and Medicaid. *Womens Health Issues*. 2022;32(6):540–549. https://doi.org/10.1016/j.whi.2022.05.003
30. Interrante JD, Pando C, Fritz AH, Kozhimannil KB. Perinatal care among Hispanic birthing people: differences by primary language and state policy environment. *Health Serv Res*. 2024:59(5):14339. https://doi.org/10.1111/1475-6773.14339
31. Kozhimannil KB, Interrante JD, Tofte AN, Admon LK. Severe maternal morbidity and mortality among Indigenous women in the United States. *Obstet Gynecol*. 2020;135(2):294–300. https://doi.org/10.1097/AOG.0000000000003647
32. Thorsen ML, Harris S, Palacios JF, McGarvey RG, Thorsen A. American Indians travel great distances for obstetrical care: examining rural and racial disparities. *Soc Sci Med*. 2023;325:115897. https://doi.org/10.1016/j.socscimed.2023.115897
33. Krutsinger DC, Yadav KN, Hart JL. Self-identified rurality in a nationally representative population in the US. *Rural Remote Health*. 2024;24(1):8483. https://doi.org/10.22605/RRH8483
34. Onega T, Weiss JE, Alford-Teaster J, Goodrich M, Eliassen MS, Kim SJ. Concordance of rural-urban self-identity and ZIP code-derived Rural-Urban Commuting Area (RUCA) designation. *J Rural Health*. 2020;36(2):274–280. https://doi.org/10.1111/jrh.12364
35. Health Resources and Services Administration. Defining rural population. January 2024. Available at: https://www.hrsa.gov/rural-health/about-us/what-is-rural. Accessed November 14, 2024.

# State-Level Estimates of Nonfatal Firearm Injury Hospitalizations, 2000–2021

Rosanna Smart, PhD, James Murphy, PhD, Terry L. Schell, PhD, Andrew R. Morral, PhD, and Nancy Nicosia, PhD

See also Braga, p. 990.

**Objectives.** To create a comprehensive, publicly available data set of state-level nonfatal firearm injury inpatient hospitalizations (NFIIHs) in the United States from 2000 to 2021.

**Methods.** We used Bayesian modeling to impute missing NFIIH rates for 334 state–year observations and correct for incomplete injury mechanism coding in 766 observations.

**Results.** NFIIH rates increased nationally, with the largest rise between 2019 and 2020, up by one third to reach 1.31 (95% credibility interval [CrI] = 1.27, 1.35) per 10 000 population. State prevalences ranged from 0.18 (95% CrI = 0.14, 0.22) in Hawaii to 2.18 (2.04, 2.33) in Louisiana. South Central states (Mississippi, Arkansas, Missouri) had the largest increases. Twelve states—predominantly in the Northeast and West—experienced decreases. NFIIH rates correlated more strongly with firearm homicide rates (correlation = 0.86) than other intents (correlations < 0.28). Nationwide, there were 2.4 NFIIHs for every firearm homicide, but this ratio varied more than fourfold across states.

**Conclusions.** NFIIH rates varied substantially across and within states. Despite strong correlation, many states diverged from the national NFIIH to firearm homicide ratio.

**Public Health Implications.** Firearm deaths systematically underrepresent serious firearm injuries in some states. This new data set can inform how policies affect serious firearm injuries and injury lethality.
(*Am J Public Health*. 2025;115(7):1106–1114. https://doi.org/10.2105/AJPH.2025.308069)

AJPH July 2025, Vol. 115, No. 7

Firearm violence is an urgent public health problem in the United States. In 2022, 48 204 people were shot and killed by a firearm, a 21% increase from 3 years before.[1] However, these deaths are a fraction of the total burden of firearm violence. Estimates suggest that nonfatal firearm crimes outnumber firearm deaths by a factor of 10 and that the number of nonfatal firearm injuries treated in hospitals and emergency departments (EDs) is double that of firearm deaths.[2,3] Growing research demonstrates that survivors of nonfatal shootings experience serious negative consequences to their physical, psychological, social, and economic well-being[4–6] and that these adverse effects extend to survivors' friends, family, and broader communities.[7–9] These nonfatal firearm injuries thus impose substantial costs on communities where such violence is concentrated[10] and on the health care systems tasked with treating them.[3,11]

Despite their importance, nonfatal firearm injuries have received limited attention in the policy evaluation literature, largely because of inadequacies in the existing data infrastructure. Unlike data on firearm mortality, there is no comprehensive national source of reliable, complete, and comparable state-level data on nonfatal firearm injuries.[12,13] Although several data sources capture subsets of nonfatal firearm injury incidents nationwide (e.g., hospitalizations, ED visits), each has serious limitations, including inadequate sample size (e.g., number of included hospitals or states) to support state-level estimates or cross-state comparisons.[14] Other sources collect complete data on ED visits or hospitalizations from participating facilities or jurisdictions, but year-to-year variability in the sample of participants renders comparisons over time and across jurisdictions unreliable. Even with near-census data (i.e., with minimal missing data across states and years) on hospitalizations, identifying firearm injuries through hospital data sets remains challenging because of incomplete or inaccurate coding, errors that vary over time and across states.[15,16] Consequently, most studies evaluating the effects of state policies on nonfatal firearm injuries have been limited to cross-sectional analyses or have been longitudinal studies involving incomplete, nonrepresentative, or unbalanced state panels.[17–19]

Improved data on nonfatal firearm injury could enhance our understanding of how the burden of serious firearm injuries varies by location and over time as well as the effectiveness of strategies aimed at reducing firearm-related harms or treating firearm injuries. We aimed to address this gap by creating a state-level panel database of NFIIH from 2000 through 2021. We have improved on previous work by combining the most comprehensive available inpatient data on firearm injury, correcting for biases owing to incomplete coding of injuries, and imputing data for state–years with missing hospital data using a model with excellent predictive accuracy. We generated a publicly available, complete state-level panel data set of nonfatal firearm injury inpatient hospitalizations (NFIIHs) from 2000 to 2021, and we used these data to describe how NFIIH rates have varied over time, across states, and relative to firearm mortality trends.

## METHODS

We built on earlier imputation efforts,[20] extending and improving the analyses in several ways. Our new analyses extend the data series through 2021, separate fatal and nonfatal injuries, and simplify the imputation model without loss of predictive accuracy. Analytic code and the final data set are available on Open Science Framework (http://bit.ly/42EWxNO).

### Data Sources and Population

*Hospitalizations.* Most data on firearm injury hospitalizations came from HCUPnet, a query system that uses data from the Healthcare Cost and Utilization Project (HCUP) State Inpatient Databases to produce aggregate statistics on inpatient hospitalizations for participating states over time. The current system provides state-level estimates starting in 2000 and based on Clinical Classification Software Refined codes. We classified firearm injuries from 2016 onward using the Clinical Classification Software Refined code specific to firearm injuries. For data before 2016, we relied on a previous iteration of the HCUPnet system that allowed classification of firearm injury hospitalizations based on *ICD-9-CM* (*International Classification of Diseases, Ninth Revision, Clinical Modification.* Hyattsville, MD: National Center for Health Statistics; 1980) codes. The data pulled from this earlier HCUPnet system, which we used to develop the imputation model in Smart et al.,[20] were more consistent with the new Clinical Classification Software Refined definitions than were the Clinical Classification Software data currently available through the HCUPnet system for that period. Further details on these data decisions and the harmonization process between the old and the new HCUPnet data can be found in Appendix A and Figure A (available as a supplement to the online version of this article at http://www.ajph.org).

Fourteen states had no hospitalization data available through HCUPnet; for 6 of these, we identified alternative sources, most commonly state departments of health. Additionally, for 4 states with data available through HCUPnet, we supplemented with information from state hospitalization data systems to resolve possible errors in the HCUPnet data (Table A, available as a supplement to the online version of this article at http://www.ajph.org). Of the final set of 795 state–year observations obtained, 29 state–years had extreme outliers that suggested possible problems with the administrative data. We set those to missing (Appendix B; Table B [available as a supplement to the online version of this article at http://www.ajph.org]), yielding 334 of 1100 possible state–year observations that needed to be fully imputed.

*Deaths.* Annual state-level mortality data came from Centers for Disease Control and Prevention Wide-Ranging Online Data for Epidemiologic Research (CDC WONDER). We used the query fields for injury intent, mechanism, and place of death to identify all firearm deaths, firearm deaths by particular intent types (homicide, suicide, unintentional, legal intervention), and firearm deaths occurring in medical facilities or in inpatient facilities specifically. We used per capita rates of nonsuicide firearm deaths and of firearm deaths in medical facilities as predictors in the imputation model, and we used data on firearm deaths by intent to assess the correlation between our final imputed measure of NFIIHs and firearm deaths by specific intent types. To construct measures of NFIIHs, we also identified firearm injury deaths occurring in inpatient facilities based on the information on place of death available in CDC WONDER; we subtracted these from the hospitalization counts, which included both fatal and nonfatal injuries, to construct a count of NFIIHs.

We scaled firearm injury deaths and NFIIHs as population rates per 10 000 person–years using population data published through CDC WONDER (Appendix A).

*Additional measures.* In the imputation model, we also used the following state-level measures: household firearm ownership rates, percentage of the population without health insurance, poverty rate, per capita income, percentage of the population that is non-Hispanic White, percentage of the population living in urban areas, violent crime rate, percentage of the population that is female, and proportion of inpatient hospitalizations owing to externally caused injuries that lacked a specific code indicating the injury mechanism. This last measure, sourced from published reports,[21,22] was particularly important, as it reflected the proportion of inpatient injuries for which firearm involvement could not be determined and affected all state–year observations (regardless of outcome missingness). Table C (available as a supplement to the online version of this article at http://www.ajph.org) provides details on data sources for these additional measures.

## Statistical Analysis

We simultaneously imputed the missing hospitalization data and corrected for incomplete injury mechanism in a single, hierarchical Bayesian regression model. The model generated multiple imputed data sets, each corresponding to a sample from the Markov chain Monte Carlo process. The final model was the product of a lengthy model development process and included 13 standard predictors and several interactions. The model employed a complex error structure designed to account for key characteristics of the data, including the correlation of values in each state over time, larger variance in NFIIH rates for state–years with smaller populations, and larger variance for state–years with larger error in the estimated nonsuicide firearm homicide rate (the most important predictor in the model).

For states with nonmissing hospitalization data, we included a term for the proportion of hospital discharges missing an injury code. We included this measure of the incomplete coding of injuries as a predictor in the model in a manner that constrained the relationship between completeness and observed hospitalizations, and we allowed this relationship to vary across a state. This allowed us to estimate completeness-corrected firearm hospitalization rates for state–years that recorded hospital discharges but had missing injury codes for some discharges. Appendix B provides details on the imputation model and the previous distributions for model parameters.

We present results that treat the underlying data as a census of hospital discharges: without variability owing to sampling but with variability owing to uncertainty in the imputed missing or incomplete data for some state–years. The 95% credibility intervals (CrIs) presented correspond to the 2.5th and 97.5th quantiles of the posterior distribution of imputed values.

# RESULTS

The final model fully imputed 334 state–year observations with missing hospitalization data and applied completeness correction to the remaining 766 state–year observations. Our model had excellent fit with the observed NFIIH data, with a model $R^2$ of 0.90. The strongest state-level predictor of NFIIHs was the rate of nonsuicide firearm deaths. Full parameter estimates are provided in Table D (available as a supplement to the online version of this article at http://www.ajph.org). Posterior predictive checks also indicated that the model was well calibrated (e.g., 97% of the actual observations fell within the central 95% of their respective posterior predictive distributions).

Figure 1 highlights that interstate variation in NFIIH rates far exceeded temporal variation. Over the study period, the annual national rate per 10 000 population ranged from a low of 0.84 (95% CrI = 0.82, 0.86) in 2014 to a high of 1.37 (95% CrI = 1.33, 1.41) in 2021, with an SD across years of 0.13. By comparison, averaging over the full period from 2000 to 2021, state rates of NFIIHs varied by more than an order of magnitude: from 0.18 (95% CrI = 0.14, 0.22) in Hawaii to 2.18 (95% CrI = 2.04, 2.33) in Louisiana, with an SD across states of 0.35 (Table E, available as a supplement to the online version of this article at http://www.ajph.org).

Nationally, the time trends in NFIIH per 10 000 population showed an increase from 2000 (1.01; 95% CrI = 0.97, 1.05) through the mid-2000s, followed by a decline that reached a minimum in 2014 (0.84; 95% CrI = 0.82, 0.86; Figure 1). NFIIH rates then increased, with the largest year-over-year rise occurring between 2019 and 2020, when rates increased by one third

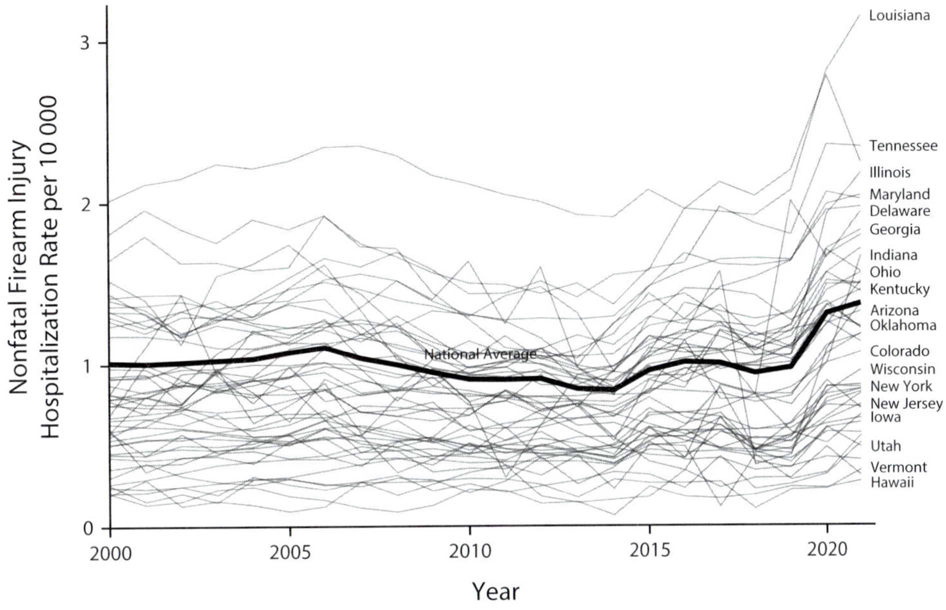


**FIGURE 1— National and State Trends in the Nonfatal Firearm Injury Inpatient Hospitalization Rate: United States, 2000–2021**

*Note.* For legibility, the following states are not labeled: Missouri (2021 rate: 2.24 per 10 000), South Carolina (2.02), Alabama (1.97), Mississippi (1.79), Pennsylvania (1.71), North Carolina (1.56), New Mexico (1.51), Florida (1.49), Texas (1.49), Arkansas (1.44), Michigan (1.38), Nevada (1.37), West Virginia (1.22), Alaska (1.21), California (1.18), Virginia (1.18), Kansas (1.13), Minnesota (0.87), South Dakota (0.84), Connecticut (0.84), Oregon (0.82), Washington (0.81), Nebraska (0.73), North Dakota (0.72), Montana (0.68), Rhode Island (0.64), Idaho (0.57), Wyoming (0.55), Maine (0.51), Massachusetts (0.41), and New Hampshire (0.31). The bold line represents the national rate.

(from 0.98 [95% Cr = 0.94, 1.01] in 2019 to 1.31 [95% CrI = 1.27, 1.35] in 2020). Aggregated to the national level, our NFIIH estimates are highly similar to, and much more precisely estimated than, the weighted estimates produced from the Nationwide Inpatient Sample. Agreement in estimated counts is particularly notable after 2011, when the Nationwide Inpatient Sample was redesigned to improve its ability to make national estimates (Table F, available as a supplement to the online version of this article at http://www.ajph.org).

National trends obscure substantial variability across states in both the levels of NFIIHs and the time trends. Figure 2 compares differences across states in average hospitalization rates for the 2000 to 2004 period versus the 2017 to 2021 period (see Figure B for the full time series of each state [available as a supplement to the online version of this article at http://www.ajph.org]). Most states experienced increases in NFIIH rates over the period, with particularly pronounced increases in the South Central states of Mississippi, Arkansas, and Missouri, where rates increased by more than 0.50 per 10 000, reflecting an increase of more than 60%.

Twelve states—predominantly in the Northeast and West—had lower rates of NFIIHs in the 2017 to 2021 period than in the 2000 to 2004 period. Some of the largest decreases were in the West. NFIIH rates in California, Nevada, and Arizona decreased by approximately 0.34 per 10 000, corresponding to a reduction of approximately 25% relative to their earlier rates. NFIIH rates in Wyoming fell from 0.53 (95% CrI = 0.26, 0.80) to 0.34 (95% CrI = 0.20, 0.49), an approximately 35% reduction. Substantial declines also occurred in New Jersey (21% reduction) and New York (28% reduction). For some of these states (e.g., California and New York), these large declines in NFIIH rates occurred despite spikes in NFIIHs starting in 2020 (Figure C, available as a supplement to the online version of this article at http://www.ajph.org).

These trends contribute to the distinct regional patterning in NFIIH rates observed in 2021 (Figure 3), with generally higher rates in the Southeast and East Central regions and lower rates in the Mountain West, the Pacific, and New England. Differences in NFIIH rates across states contribute to a misalignment in the extent to which firearm death rates reflect serious firearm injuries, defined here as the sum of NFIIHs and firearm deaths in the state.

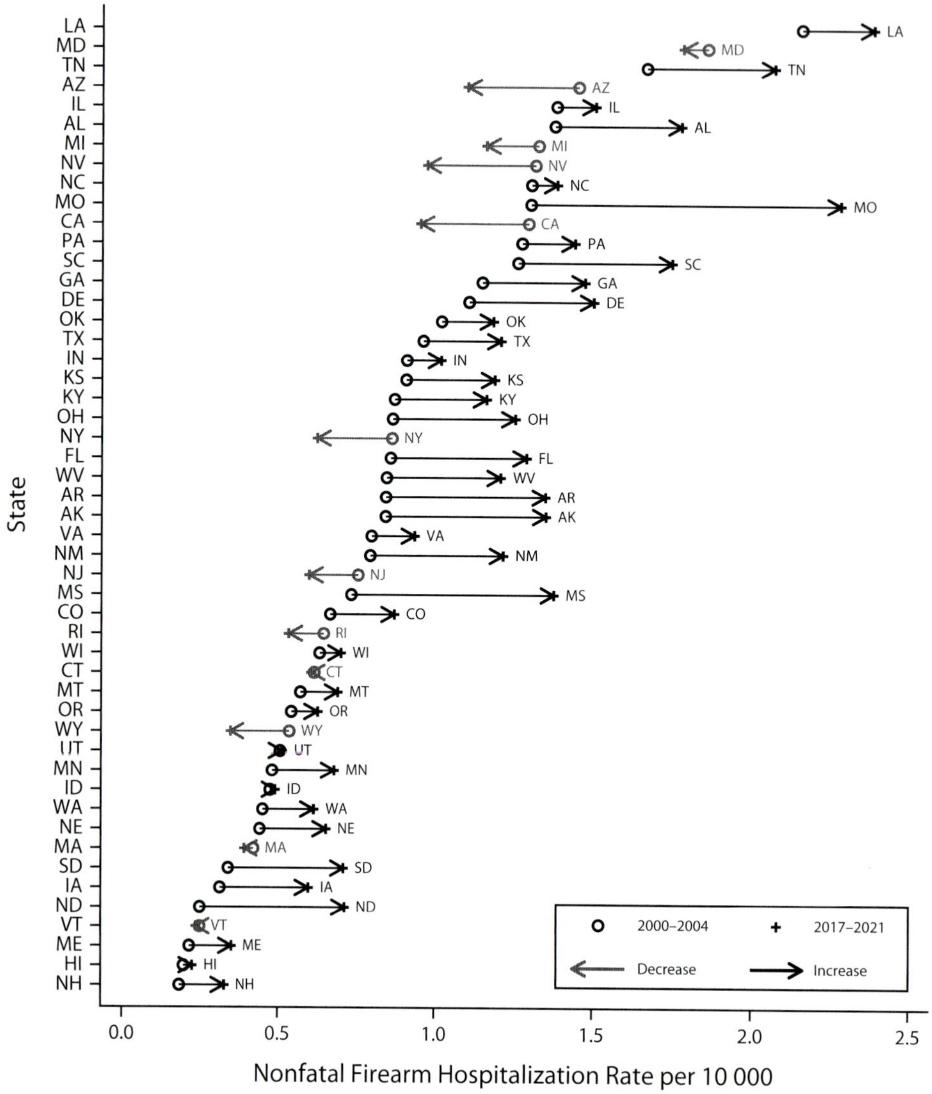


**FIGURE 2— Nonfatal Firearm Injury Inpatient Hospitalization Rate Over Time, by State: United States, 2000–2021**

*Note.* States are ordered from the highest (top) to the lowest (bottom) rate in 2000–2004. Arrows indicate the directionality of changes in average nonfatal firearm injury inpatient hospitalization rates in 2000–2004 and 2017–2021.

In some states, particularly those in the Mountain West, more than 65% of serious firearm injuries are fatal (Figure 3). This contrasts sharply with several other states—such as California, Illinois, and those in the mid-Atlantic region—where firearm deaths account for less than half of all serious firearm injuries.

These patterns reflect systematic differences in how NFIIHs and firearm deaths vary across states and over time. Indeed, the correlation of state–year NFIIH rates with firearm mortality rates varies by type of death. The correlation between NFIIH rates and total firearm mortality rates was 0.54 (95% CrI = 0.50, 0.58), far lower than the correlation with firearm homicide rates ($\rho = 0.86$; 95% CrI = 0.81, 0.89). Correlations with firearm-related accidental ($\rho = 0.27$; 95% CrI = 0.22, 0.32), undetermined ($\rho = 0.22$; 95% CrI = 0.17, 0.27), and suicide ($\rho = 0.11$; 95% CrI = 0.07, 0.15) death rates were much lower.

The higher correlation of NFIIHs with firearm deaths from homicides than from other intents is reflected in national patterns: nationally, the number of NFIIHs annually is similar to total firearm mortality, but the pattern in the NFIIH trend more closely mirrors the firearm homicide trend, albeit at a

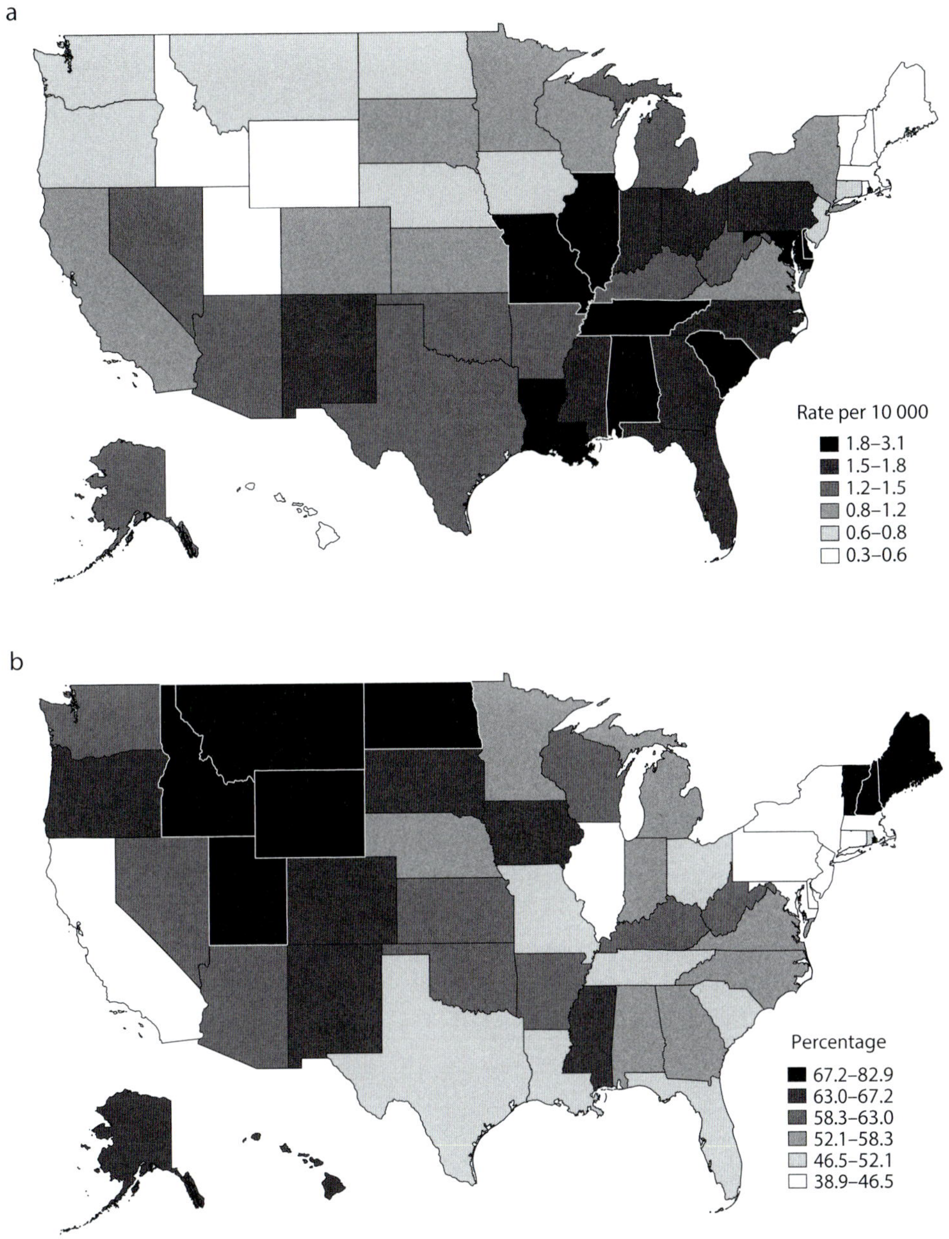


**FIGURE 3— US State Variation in (a) Nonfatal Firearm Injury Inpatient Hospitalization Rates per 10 000 Population and (b) Percentage of Serious Firearm Injuries That Were Fatal: 2021**

*Note.* Serious injuries are defined here as the sum of fatal firearm injuries and nonfatal firearm injuries resulting in inpatient hospitalization.

higher level (2.2–2.7 NFIIHs per firearm homicide death in a given year; Figures D and E, available as a supplement to the online version of this article at http://www.ajph.org). Although it might be reasonable to expect that firearm homicides could thus serve as a sufficient statistic for assessing variation in NFIIH, there is substantial variability in this relationship when evaluating it at the state level. Averaging over the study period (Figure 3), the ratio of NFIIHs to firearm homicides varied from 1.05 (95% CrI = 0.68, 1.44) in Mississippi to 4.55 (95% CrI = 3.01, 6.11) in South Dakota (median = 2.6; interquartile range = 2.3–3.0). Generally, Southern states tend to have fewer firearm injury hospitalizations per homicide than Northern states, although there is considerable variation in this ratio within regions and within states over time, although the general pattern has been a declining trend in this ratio (Figure 4;

AJPH July 2025, Vol. 115, No. 7

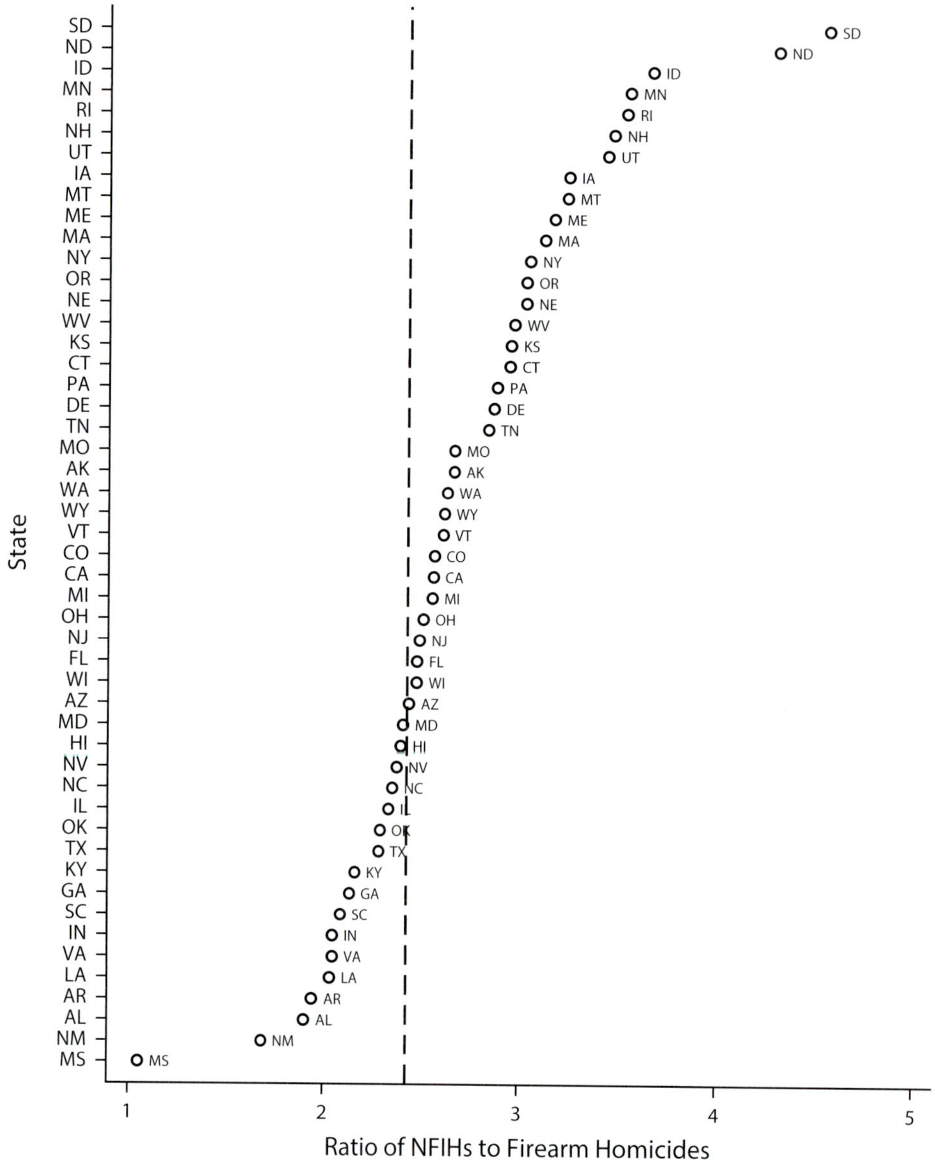


**FIGURE 4— Ratio of Nonfatal Firearm Injury Inpatient Hospitalizations (NFIIHs) to Firearm Homicides, by State and Averaged: United States, 2000–2021**

*Note.* Vertical dashed line represents the national average.

Figure E, available as a supplement to the online version of this article at http://www.ajph.org).

## DISCUSSION

Firearm injuries impose tremendous costs on health care systems, with national costs of inpatient hospitalizations estimated at nearly 1 billion dollars annually.[23–25] Although national estimates provide insight into scope, addressing these harms requires an understanding of how they are distributed by location and over time. We constructed the first, to our knowledge, comprehensive state-level data set of NFIIHs for 2000 through 2021. The 10-fold variation in NFIIH rates across states reveals that the burden is disproportionately borne by states in the Southeast and the Midwest. But even some of these highly affected states have experienced much larger increases over time than other states in their regions. The substantial geographic variation in NFIIHs suggests that relying solely on national data to assess firearm injury hospitalization trends obscures the uneven burden of health care costs owing to firearm violence across different regions, which may also limit our ability to identify effective state and local policy interventions.

A potential assumption for epidemiological research and policy evaluations is that mortality captures the main variation in consequences resulting from firearms because other firearm consequences (e.g., nonfatal injuries) are likely to closely mirror trends in mortality. Our analyses suggest that this assumption is not wholly accurate. To the extent that patterns for nonfatal injuries diverge, efforts to direct resources or to interpret results from policy evaluations based on total firearm mortality may systematically miss policy effects on the more prevalent nonfatal injuries. The spatial and temporal variation in NFIIHs has far greater commonality with firearm homicides than with firearm suicides; this may reflect the fact that firearm suicide attempts are very likely to be fatal,[26] and thus people who engage in self-harm may be more likely than victims of interpersonal violence to die before hospital admission. Consequently, a state such as Wyoming, which had the highest firearm suicide rate in the country but a relatively low firearm homicide rate in 2021, also has the highest percentage of serious firearm injuries that are fatal. Although firearm homicides appear to mirror nonfatal injuries more closely overall, there are nontrivial differences between these trends across states and over time that could affect estimates of policy effects.

## Limitations

Although our study is the most comprehensive effort to date toward generating a complete time series of state-level data on NFIIHs, our results are subject to limitations. First, we did not capture nonfatal firearm injuries that did not result in hospital admission (i.e., those treated only in EDs or other nonhospital medical settings) or for which treatment was not sought. Thus, our analyses more directly inform how policies affect firearm injuries resulting in inpatient hospitalization (including incidents of individuals admitted through an ED), which are likely to capture the most serious nonfatal incidents. Second, our estimates are limited by inaccuracies in hospital coding of firearm injuries. Research has shown a high rate of external cause code reporting in the HCUP databases.[27] Firearm injuries in particular have been found to be coded with high validity,[28] and our models include a direct adjustment for incomplete injury mechanism coding. However, we do not have information on coding completeness specific to firearm injuries or for every state and year. Furthermore, owing to greater issues of coding disagreement regarding firearm injury intent (i.e., classifying assault vs accident vs undetermined),[15,29] combined with limitations in the level of detail on diagnostic codes that would support querying injuries by intent type using the HCUPnet system (Appendix A), we cannot disaggregate our estimates of firearm injury hospitalizations by intent.

Finally, we are presenting our results as a multiply imputed data set to facilitate additional research on firearm injury. This data set addresses many of the limitations caused by partially or completely missing hospital injury records, but we emphasize that the data have substantial imputation and must be interpreted and analyzed carefully. In particular, future analyses using these data will have accurate confidence intervals or *P* values only if they use multiple imputation analytic methods.

## Public Health Implications

Efforts to understand the burden of firearms on communities and to evaluate the efficacy of policy interventions should incorporate nonfatal hospitalizations to provide a more complete portrayal. The state-level data produced in this study, which are publicly available on Open Science Framework, can facilitate research that incorporates these nonfatal injuries when examining epidemiologic trends and the costs associated with firearm violence, previous efforts toward which have focused primarily on national trends.[13,30] Furthermore, the substantial geographic disparities in NFIIHs identified by this study highlight the need to evaluate how state policies or other state-level factors—such as economic mobility, health care infrastructure, and firearm availability—drive these differences. Evaluating the outcome of NFIIHs along with firearm deaths can improve our understanding of how interventions influence the prevalence and lethality of firearm injuries. AJPH

**ABOUT THE AUTHORS**

Rosanna Smart, James Murphy, and Terry L. Schell are with the RAND Corporation, Santa Monica, CA. Andrew R. Morral is with the RAND Corporation, Arlington, VA. Nancy Nicosia is with the RAND Corporation, Boston, MA.

**CORRESPONDENCE**

Correspondence should be sent to Rosanna Smart, 1776 Main St, Santa Monica, CA 90401 (e-mail: rsmart@rand.org). Reprints can be ordered at https://www.ajph.org by clicking the "Reprints" link.

**PUBLICATION INFORMATION**

Full Citation: Smart R, Murphy J, Schell TL, Morral AR, Nicosia N. State-level estimates of nonfatal firearm injury hospitalizations, 2000–2021. *Am J Public Health*. 2025;115(7):1106–1114.

Acceptance Date: February 6, 2025.

DOI: https://doi.org/10.2105/AJPH.2025.308069

ORCID iDs:

Rosanna Smart https://orcid.org/0000-0002-1568-2097

Terry L. Schell https://orcid.org/0000-0001-8484-5462

Andrew R. Morral https://orcid.org/0000-0001-9091-3724

## CONTRIBUTORS

R. Smart wrote the original draft of the article. J. Murphy performed the formal analyses. All authors supervised the study; contributed to writing, review, and editing; administered the project; designed the study, performed data acquisition, analysis, and interpretation; and gave final approval of the version to be published.

## ACKNOWLEDGMENTS

This work was supported by the National Institutes of Health (NIH; grant R61AA029064) and Arnold Ventures.

The findings of this study were presented at the 2024 National Research Conference for the Prevention of Firearm Related Harms, Seattle, Washington; December 10, 2024.

We thank Sam Peterson for contributions to an earlier version of the imputation model, and we thank Rose Kerber and Jason Mastbaum for research assistance. Finally, we are grateful for the provision of data to include in this study obtained from officials from the Delaware Department of Health and Social Services, Indiana State Department of Health, Louisiana Department of Health, New Hampshire Department of Health and Human Services, and New Mexico Department of Health; and from staff at Virginia Health Information.

**Note.** The contents of this article are solely the responsibility of the authors and do not necessarily represent the official views of the NIH or Arnold Ventures.

## CONFLICTS OF INTEREST

The authors have no actual or potential conflicts of interest to declare.

## HUMAN PARTICIPANT PROTECTION

This study was approved by the RAND Corporation's institutional review board (expedited category 5: data collected for nonresearch purposes).

## REFERENCES

1. Centers for Disease Control and Prevention. National Vital Statistics System, mortality 2018–2022. 2024. Available at: http://wonder.cdc.gov/mcd-icd10-expanded.html. Accessed June 10, 2024.
2. Kena G, Truman JL. Trends and patterns in firearm violence, 1993–2018. Available at: https://bjs.ojp.gov/content/pub/pdf/tpfv9318.pdf. Accessed April 13, 2025.
3. Miller GF, Barnett SBL, Florence CS, Harrison KM, Dahlberg LL, Mercy JA. Costs of Fatal and nonfatal firearm injuries in the US, 2019 and 2020. *Am J Prev Med.* 2024;66(2):195–204. https://doi.org/10.1016/j.amepre.2023.09.026
4. Song Z, Zubizarreta JR, Giuriato M, Paulos E, Koh KA. Changes in health care spending, use, and clinical outcomes after nonfatal firearm injuries among survivors and family members: a cohort study. *Ann Intern Med.* 2022;175(6):795–803. https://doi.org/10.7326/M21-2812
5. Czaja MP, Kraus CK, Phyo S, et al. Injury characteristics, outcomes, and health care services use associated with nonfatal injuries sustained in mass shootings in the US, 2012–2019. *JAMA Netw Open.* 2022;5(5):e2213737. https://doi.org/10.1001/jamanetworkopen.2022.13737
6. Cabral M, Kim B, Rossin-Slater M, Schnell M, Schwandt H. *Trauma at School: The Impacts of Shootings on Students' Human Capital and Economic Outcomes*; 2024. NBER working paper 28311. https://doi.org/10.3386/w28311
7. Paruk J, Semenza D. Gun violence exposure and quality of life in nine US states. *J Urban Health.* 2024;101(5):942–950. https://doi.org/10.1007/s11524-024-00891-7
8. Semenza DC, Stansfield R, Silver IA, Savage B. Reciprocal neighborhood dynamics in gun violence exposure, community health, and concentrated disadvantage in one hundred US cities. *J Urban Health.* 2023;100(6):1128–1139. https://doi.org/10.1007/s11524-023-00796-x
9. Magee LA, Aalsma MC, Fortenberry JD, Gharbi S, Wiehe SE. Mental health outcomes from direct and indirect exposure to firearm violence: a cohort study of nonfatal shooting survivors and family members. *J Crim Justice.* 2022;83:101961. https://doi.org/10.1016/j.jcrimjus.2022.101961
10. Cook PJ, Ludwig J. *Gun Violence: The Real Costs.* New York, NY: Oxford University Press; 2000.
11. Davoudi A, Woodworth L. The burden of firearm injuries on the hospital system, 2000–2020. *Inj Epidemiol.* 2023;10(1):12. https://doi.org/10.1186/s40621-023-00420-1
12. Barber C, Cook PJ, Parker ST. The emerging infrastructure of US firearms injury data. *Prev Med.* 2022;165(pt A):107129. https://doi.org/10.1016/j.ypmed.2022.107129
13. Kaufman EJ, Delgado MK. The epidemiology of firearm injuries in the US: the need for comprehensive, real-time, actionable data. *JAMA.* 2022;328(12):1177–1178. https://doi.org/10.1001/jama.2022.16894
14. Cook PJ, Rivera-Aguirre AE, Cerdá M, Wintemute G. Constant lethality of gunshot injuries from firearm assault: United States, 2003–2012. *Am J Public Health.* 2017;107(8):1324–1328. https://doi.org/10.2105/AJPH.2017.303837
15. Barber C, Goralnick E, Miller M. The problem with ICD-coded firearm injuries. *JAMA Intern Med.* 2021;181(8):1132–1133. https://doi.org/10.1001/jamainternmed.2021.0382
16. Stewart CC, Simon G, Ahmedani BK, et al. Variation in completeness of coding external cause of injuries under *ICD-10-CM*. *Inj Prev.* 2024; Epub ahead of print. https://doi.org/10.1136/ip-2023-045164
17. DeSimone J, Markowitz S, Xu J. Child access prevention laws and nonfatal gun injuries. *South Econ J.* 2013;80(1):5–25. https://doi.org/10.4284/0038-4038-2011.333
18. McClellan C, Tekin E. Stand your ground laws, homicides, and injuries. *J Hum Resour.* 2017;52(3):621–653. https://doi.org/10.3368/jhr.52.3.0613-5723R2
19. Simonetti JA, Rowhani-Rahbar A, Mills B, Young B, Rivara FP. State firearm legislation and nonfatal firearm injuries. *Am J Public Health.* 2015;105(8):1703–1709. https://doi.org/10.2105/AJPH.2015.302617
20. Smart R, Peterson S, Schell TL, Kerber R, Morral AR. *Inpatient Hospitalizations for Firearm Injury.* Santa Monica, CA: RAND Corporation; 2021.
21. Barrett M, Steiner C, Sheng M, Bailey M. Healthcare Cost and Utilization Project (HCUP) external cause of injury code (E Code) evaluation report (updated with 2013 HCUP data). July 26, 2016. Available at: https://hcup-us.ahrq.gov/reports/methods/2016-03.pdf. Accessed April 13, 2025.
22. Healthcare Cost and Utilization Project. Injuries and external causes: reporting of causes on the HCUP State Inpatient Databases, 2016–2019. September 29, 2021. Available at: https://hcup-us.ahrq.gov/reports/ataglance/HCUPanalysisInjuryReporting.pdf. Accessed April 13, 2025.
23. Barry LE, Crealey GE, Nguyen NT, Weiser TG, Spitzer SA, O'Neill C. Hospital costs and fatality rates of traumatic assaults by mechanism in the US, 2016–2018. *JAMA Netw Open.* 2022;5(6):e2218496. https://doi.org/10.1001/jamanetworkopen.2022.18496
24. Spitzer SA, Vail D, Tennakoon L, Rajasingh C, Spain DA, Weiser TG. Readmission risk and costs of firearm injuries in the United States, 2010–2015. *PLoS One.* 2019;14(1):e0209896. https://doi.org/10.1371/journal.pone.0209896
25. Spitzer SA, Staudenmayer KL, Tennakoon L, Spain DA, Weiser TG. Costs and financial burden of initial hospitalizations for firearm injuries in the United States, 2006–2014. *Am J Public Health.* 2017;107(5):770–774. https://doi.org/10.2105/AJPH.2017.303684
26. Wang J, Sumner SA, Simon TR, et al. Trends in the incidence and lethality of suicidal acts in the United States, 2006 to 2015. *JAMA Psychiatry.* 2020;77(7):684–693. https://doi.org/10.1001/jamapsychiatry.2020.0596
27. Coben JH, Steiner CA, Barrett M, Merrill C, Adamson D. Completeness of cause of injury coding in healthcare administrative databases in the United States, 2001. *Inj Prev.* 2006;12(3):199–201. https://doi.org/10.1136/ip.2005.010512
28. LeMier M, Cummings P, West TA. Accuracy of external cause of injury codes reported in Washington State hospital discharge records. *Inj Prev.* 2001;7(4):334–338. https://doi.org/10.1136/ip.7.4.334
29. Miller M, Azrael D, Yenduri R, et al. Assessment of the accuracy of firearm injury intent coding at 3 US hospitals. *JAMA Netw Open.* 2022;5(12):e2246429. https://doi.org/10.1001/jamanetworkopen.2022.46429
30. Kaufman EJ, Wiebe DJ, Xiong RA, Morrison CN, Seamon MJ, Delgado MK. Epidemiologic trends in fatal and nonfatal firearm injuries in the US, 2009–2017. *JAMA Intern Med.* 2021;181(2):237–244. https://doi.org/10.1001/jamainternmed.2020.6696

# Sequencing-Based Detection of Measles in Wastewater: Texas, January 2025

Sara Javornik Cregeen, PhD, Michael J. Tisza, PhD, Blake Hanson, PhD, Marissa Cook, BS, Anil Surathu, MSc, Rebecca Schneider, MSc, Jingjing Wu, PhD, Kirstin Short, MPH, Kaavya Domakonda, BS, Loren Hopkins, PhD, Matthew C. Ross, PhD, Joseph F. Petrosino, PhD, Jennifer Deegan, MPAff, Lauren B. Stadler, PhD, Eric Boerwinkle, PhD, and Anthony Maresso, PhD

Measles is a potentially deadly viral infection spread via respiratory droplets from infected individuals. Outbreaks occur when vaccine coverage drops below the threshold of herd, or community, immunity. Using a sequencing-based approach, we report the prospective (January 7, 2025) detection of measles in nucleic acid extracts from 2 wastewater treatment plants in Houston, Texas, with a population of more than 218 000 residents. The sequencing data from 2 samples contained 53 unique reads mapping to 11 different regions of the measles virus genome with a 99.4% match to genotype B3. Importantly, no detections were observed from 821 previous samples from the same city spanning nearly 3 years of monitoring. The findings were confirmed using droplet digital polymerase chain reaction. A concomitant investigation identified 2 unvaccinated measles-positive travelers living within the same sewershed as the wastewater detection event. This work suggests that sequencing-based wastewater analysis is valuable as a comprehensive early detection warning system that facilitates more targeted epidemiological investigation. (*Am J Public Health*. 2025;115(7):1115–1119. https://doi.org/10.2105/AJPH.2025.308146)

AJPH July 2025, Vol. 115, No. 7

Measles is a highly contagious RNA virus. Symptoms include fever, runny nose, and rash, similar to other respiratory or skin infections,[1] but, in some cases, measles can be fatal, especially in children and those who are immunocompromised.[2] Before there was an effective vaccine in 1968, the number of new measles cases per year was highly variable but averaged more than 300 cases per 100 000 population. In comparison, the number of new cases per year between 2000 and 2009 was less than 0.05 per 100 000.[3] It is now well established that local outbreaks can occur when vaccine coverage falls below 95%.[4] In recent years, lower vaccine uptake has contributed to overall higher incidence rates.[5] Its extraordinary transmission rate, lower vaccination rates, and an aging population warrant effective surveillance of this concerning virus.

There have been reports of wastewater-based epidemiology for measles. The measles D8 genotype was detected by polymerase chain reaction (PCR) in the Netherlands.[6] Estimates based on urine shed rates suggest routine measles detection can be effective with wastewater-based epidemiology.[7] However, there is concern that wastewater-based epidemiology detections may be attributable to strains used in the vaccine, particularly measles genotype A, leading to false-positive findings.[8] Targeted assays that differentiate vaccine from nonvaccine strains have been developed.[9] Multiplexed assays of PCR have also been developed that detect measles in combination with respiratory viruses (e.g., severe acute respiratory coronavirus 2 [SARS-CoV-2] and influenza A and B).[10] As far as we understand, there is no sequencing-based method for measles detection as part of a routine wastewater monitoring program. In this brief report, we summarize the prospective detection of measles in Houston, Texas, using a novel sequencing-based approach as a part of a statewide wastewater surveillance initiative. The a priori detection of viruses without knowledge of cases or PCR surveillance may facilitate more targeted epidemiological investigation.

## METHODS

Detailed methods for sample collection and extraction are in the references[11,12] and the Appendix (available as a supplement to the online version of this article at https://ajph.org). Briefly, the positive samples were prospectively taken January 7, 2025, from 2 different wastewater treatment plants (WWTPs 1 and 2) that include more than 218 000 people. Samples were centrifuged at 3500 to 4100 × relative centrifugal force (g) for 10 minutes, and the supernatant was filtered using an electronegative filter. Filters were washed, bead-beated, and centrifuged at 17 000 revolutions per minute, and nucleic acid was extracted using a Qiagen RNA Mini Kit (Qiagen, Germantown, MD) and sequenced.

Probe capture, sequencing, and data analysis were performed after processing over 72 hours.[11] Briefly, RNA extracts were converted to cDNA, and the cDNA was used for library construction. The libraries were pooled and hybridized using the Twist Comprehensive Viral Research Panel (Twist Biosciences, San Francisco, CA). The postcapture pool was amplified for 12 cycles and sequenced on an Illumina NovaSeq 6000 SP flowcell (Illumina, San Diego, CA). Input reads were aligned to the Virus Pathogen Database (version 2.0.2) with Minimap2. For reverse transcriptase droplet digital PCR (RT-ddPCR), quantification of measles RNA was performed using one-step RT-ddPCR (Bio-Rad, Hercules, CA) targeting the M gene (Figure 1, purple bar).[9]

## RESULTS

With a sequencing-based approach, measles virus was detected in 2 wastewater treatment plants' samples taken January 7, 2025, from the city of Houston. The first sample contained 51 unambiguous, deduplicated reads aligning with the measles genome. The second sample contained 2 unambiguous, deduplicated reads (Figure 1). The 51 reads mapped to 11 different genomic regions of the measles L gene, which codes for the polymerase (Figure 1). The 2 additional reads mapped to 1 region of the H gene, which codes for the hemagglutinin protein. Importantly, no evidence of measles was detected in 821 previous wastewater samples between May 2022 and January 2025, suggesting this detection was unique. The reads were 99.44% identical to measles genotype B3 (accession KX838946.2), a nonvaccine strain and circulating lineage that emerged globally in 1976. Two independent laboratories computationally verified the sequence data. The read sequences are presented in Appendix Table A.

To orthogonally validate the measles detections, a second team analyzed the wastewater using a different method—RT-ddPCR.[9] Pooled samples tested positive for wild-type measles with 4 to 8 positive droplets across replicates, which corresponds to a concentration of 2596 ± 1178 genome copies per liter of wastewater (Figure 2). Notably, a synthetic measles amplicon (short stretch of measles nucleic acid) added to another reaction also yielded positive droplets (positive control) while another reaction without this nucleic acid added showed no signal (negative control).

Concomitantly, the City of Houston Health Department (HHD) investigated 2 clinical cases of suspected measles. On Friday, January 17, 2025, HHD confirmed and reported 2 cases of measles in unvaccinated adults (ages 18–49) associated with recent international travel. One individual was hospitalized and recovered. HHD conducted an investigation, performed contact tracing, reported locations visited, and

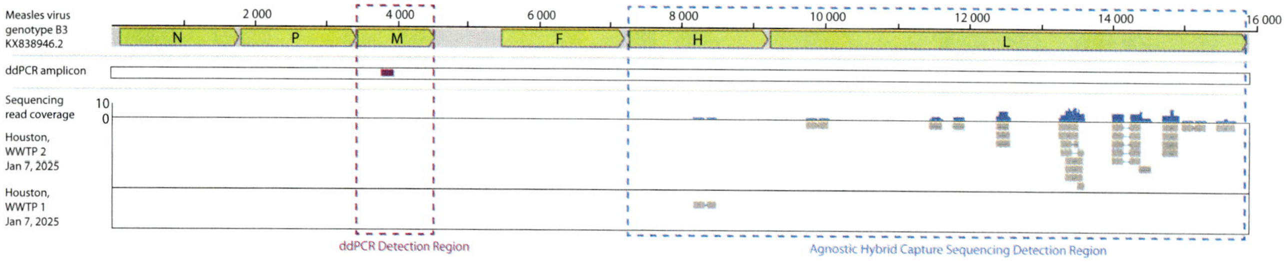


**FIGURE 1— Agnostic Hybrid Sequencing Measles Detection in Wastewater: Houston, TX, January 2025**

*Note.* WWTP = wastewater treatment plant. The measles genome showing the reads from probe-capture sequencing (gray) stacked across the L (11 separate regions) and H genes (1 region). A coverage map is displayed in blue, which shows the regions of the measles genome for which we have sequencing data ("agnostic hybrid capture sequencing detection region"). For reverse transcriptase droplet digital polymerase chain reaction (RT-ddPCR), the genomic region where the primers will anneal is shown in pink, which targets the M gene ("ddPCR detection region").

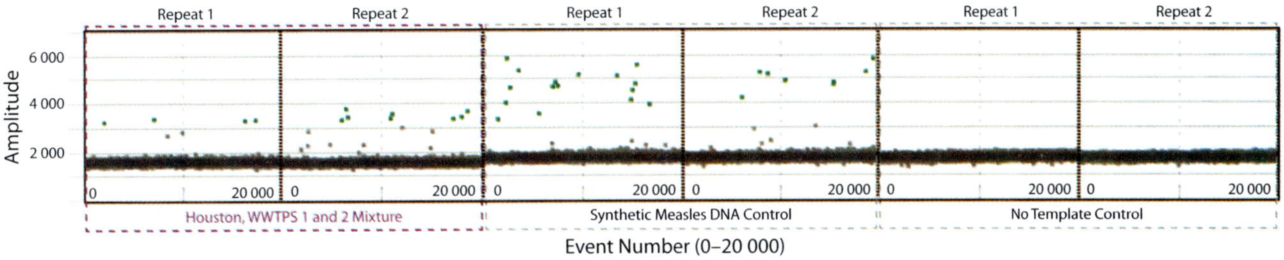


**FIGURE 2— RT-ddPCR Measles Detection in Wastewater: Houston, TX, January 2025**

*Note.* RT-ddPCR = reverse transcriptase droplet digital polymerase chain reaction; WWTP = wastewater treatment plant. RT-ddPCR results of the 2 replicate wastewater samples that were an equal volume mixture of the 2 Houston sites. The positive control is a synthetic measles nucleic acid RNA amplicon from the M gene of the D8 measles wild-type strain. The negative control is a reaction that has no wastewater sample and no RNA amplicon template. Y-axis = amplitude (strength of detection event); x-axis = event number from 0 to 20 000 in the partition well.

issued a health alert for medical providers and a media advisory for the public. Importantly, the individuals resided in the catchment area where the wastewater detections occurred, providing reasonable evidence that the detections were from 1 or both of these cases and highlighting the sensitivity of this sequencing approach. An approximate timeline is presented in Figure 3.

## DISCUSSION

We report the detection of wild-type measles using a sequencing-based approach in samples taken before epidemiological reporting. These 2 findings are novel. The results were confirmed by PCR. A concomitant investigation found measles virus in 2 travelers residing in the same wastewater catchment area. If the signal originated (likely) from the 2 travelers in a catchment area containing more than 218 000 residents, these results suggest that measles may be shed at much higher rates than previously estimated or that the agnostic hybrid-capture method is quite sensitive, or both. Similar approaches have been developed into a high-throughput sequencing–based pipeline for the agnostic detection of human viruses.[13]

Even though the current application focuses on a single virus, measles, implementation of the agnostic approach in a real public health setting is important for 2 reasons. First, because the data are part of a regular pathogen surveillance program, the pivot from the current focus of the program to measles was very quick because the raw data were readily available. Besides the independent validation, no new laboratory work was required. Second, because the method is sequence-based, we were able to determine that the 2 traveler cases in Houston were likely independent from the co-occurring outbreak in West Texas and New Mexico. The measles genotype from the Houston wastewater was B3, whereas the Centers for Disease Control and Prevention released that the cases in West Texas and New Mexico were genotype D8. In addition, a benefit of agnostic sequencing is the ability to detect emerging viruses of significant concern—for instance, the recent identification of avian H5N1 influenza.[12] Other benefits include routine tracking of viruses of seasonal importance (e.g., influenza, COVID-19), viruses not normally on the clinical



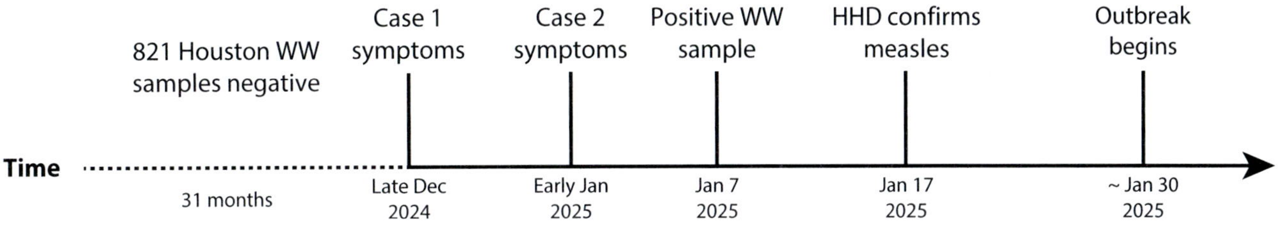


**FIGURE 3— Approximate Timeline for the Clinical Manifestation and Wastewater Detection of Measles: Houston, TX, January 2025**

*Note.* HHD = Houston Health Department; WW = wastewater.

radar (e.g., measles), and the ability to monitor the evolution of concerning viral variants.[13] Although the measles-positive wastewater sample was collected before the epidemiological investigation was complete, one enhancement to this program would be if the samples were analyzed in near-real time, which would allow reporting of the finding 2 to 3 days earlier than what is currently practiced.

The RT-ddPCR method used herein targets the M gene and yielded a positive result, but no reads from the M gene were detected using the sequencing approach. Because the probes in hybrid capture are tiled across the genome, it suggests our approach may provide comprehensive capture of nucleic acid that survived wastewater transit or processing or both, thereby providing signal from genomic regions not targeted by PCR. It may also be valuable for public health laboratories to consider designing primers for PCR against regions detected by hybrid capture sequencing as reported here, especially in cases where the PCR result is negative, but sequencing is positive. In general, on a per-sample basis, PCR is less expensive than the sequencing approach used herein. However, when one considers that PCR is often used to detect a single virus at a time, whereas probe capture and sequencing can report on tens to hundreds of viruses in the same sample, on a per-target basis, the approach used here is potentially much more economical. Routine wastewater PCR monitoring of measles is likely not justified owing to the low probability of outbreaks in highly vaccinated areas. However, as a part of a comprehensive sequencing program (as reported here), it adds no cost to the analysis and, thus, should be considered as an early warning system for the emergence of outbreaks.

One limitation of our study is that we were unable to sequence the measles strain from the infected travelers because of low sample quantity. This may have allowed for an unambiguous match to the clinical cases. However, because no other cases have been reported and the detections occurred in the same area where the travelers resided (the first in nearly 3 years of sampling), it is reasonable to assume the signal is from the infected cases. Collectively, this report demonstrates the sensitivity and specificity of agnostic sequencing as a next-generation technology to expand wastewater-based viral detection and epidemiology. Such an approach might have broader implications for public health, particularly as a sentinel surveillance system to detect viruses before widespread outbreaks occur. AJPH


## ABOUT THE AUTHORS

Sara Javornik Cregeen, Michael J. Tisza, Marissa Cook, Anil Surathu, Matthew C. Ross, Joseph F. Petrosino, and Anthony Maresso are with The Alkek Center for Metagenomics and Microbiome Research and the Department of Molecular Virology and Microbiology at Baylor College of Medicine, Houston, TX. Blake Hanson, Jennifer Deegan, and Eric Boerwinkle are with the School of Public Health at University of Texas Health Science Center at Houston. Rebecca Schneider, Kirstin Short, Kaavya Domakonda, and Loren Hopkins are with the Houston Health Department. Jingjing Wu and Lauren B. Stadler are with the Department of Civil and Environmental Engineering at Rice University, Houston.

## CORRESPONDENCE

Correspondence should be sent to Anthony Maresso, Department of Molecular Virology and Microbiology, Baylor College of Medicine, 1 Baylor Plaza, Houston, TX 77030 (e-mail: maresso@bcm.edu) or Eric Boerwinkle, School of Public Health, University of Texas Health Science Center at Houston, Houston, TX 77030 (e-mail: eric.boerwinkle@uth.tmc.edu). Reprints can be ordered at https://ajph.org by clicking the "Reprints" link.



## PUBLICATION INFORMATION

Full Citation: Javornik Cregeen S, Tisza MJ, Hanson B, et al. Sequencing-based detection of measles in wastewater: Texas, January 2025. *Am J Public Health*. 2025;115(7):1115–1119.

Acceptance Date: March 30, 2025.

DOI: https://doi.org/10.2105/AJPH.2025.308146



ORCID iDs:

Sara Javornik Cregeen https://orcid.org/0009-0000-2698-6478

Michael J. Tisza https://orcid.org/0000-0003-1168-1617

Blake Hanson https://orcid.org/0000-0003-2949-7818

Marissa Cook https://orcid.org/0009-0005-0096-0858

Anil Surathu https://orcid.org/0000-0002-4780-3746

Rebecca Schneider https://orcid.org/0000-0001-8435-7426

Jingjing Wu https://orcid.org/0000-0003-0531-1353

Kirstin Short https://orcid.org/0000-0002-8597-4773

Matthew C. Ross https://orcid.org/0000-0002-7621-8829

Jennifer Deegan https://orcid.org/0009-0004-9988-966X

Lauren B. Stadler https://orcid.org/0000-0001-7469-1981

Anthony Maresso https://orcid.org/0000-0002-4452-3490


## CONTRIBUTORS

S. Javornik Cregeen and M. J. Tisza contributed equally. S. Javornik Cregeen, M. J. Tisza, L. B. Stadler, and A. Maresso carried out the main data analysis and drafted the initial article. R. Schneider, J. Wu, K. Short, K. Domakonda, L. Hopkins, and L. B. Stadler performed the digital droplet polymerase chain reaction data generation and processing, looked into the epidemiological findings, and reviewed the article. S. Javornik Cregeen, M. C. Ross, B. Hanson, M. Cook, A. Surathu, and A. Maresso performed the sequencing data generation and processing and reviewed the article. J. F. Petrosino, L. B. Stadler, E. Boerwinkle, and A. Maresso obtained funding and reviewed and revised the article. All authors contributed to the article and approved the final article as submitted.


## ACKNOWLEDGMENTS

This study was supported by funds from SB 1780, 87th Legislature, 2021 Reg Sess (Texas, 2021; to Boerwinkle, Maresso, and Petrosino), Baylor College of Medicine Joseph Melnick seed funds (to Maresso), Alkek Foundation seed funds (to Petrosino), and Centers for Disease Control and Prevention grant NU50CK000557 (to the Houston Health Department).

The authors would also like to acknowledge the Houston Wastewater Epidemiology team and Houston Water for their support in providing samples.

## CONFLICTS OF INTEREST

The authors declare no conflict of interest.

## HUMAN PARTICIPANT PROTECTION

This was not human participants' research. All samples and information are deidentified.

## REFERENCES


1. De Vries RD, Mesman AW, Geijtenbeek TB, Duprex WP, de Swart RL. The pathogenesis of measles. *Curr Opin Virol.* 2012;2(3):248–255. doi:10.1016/j.coviro.2012.03.005
2. Misin A, Antonello RM, Di Bella S, et al. Measles: An overview of a re-emerging disease in children and immunocompromised patients. *Microorganisms.* 2020;8(2):276. doi:10.3390/microorganisms8020276
3. John Elflein. Rate of new measles cases in the US from 1919 to 2024 (per 100,000 population). Statista. March 6, 2025. Available at: https://www.statista.com/statistics/186409/cases-of-measles-in-the-us-since-1950. Accessed April 28, 2025.
4. Moss WJ, Strebel P. Biological feasibility of measles eradication. *J Infect Dis.* 2011;2041(suppl 1):S47–S53. doi:10.1093/infdis/jir065
5. Gambrell A, Sundaram M, Bednarczyk RA. Estimating the number of US children susceptible to measles resulting from COVID-19-related vaccination coverage declines. *Vaccine.* 2022; 40(32):4574–4579. doi:10.1016/j.vaccine.2022.06.033
6. Benschop KSM, van der Avoort HG, Jusic E, Vennema H, van Binnendijk R, Duizer E. Polio and measles down the drain: environmental enterovirus surveillance in the Netherlands, 2005 to 2015. *Appl Environ Microbiol.* 2017;83(13):e00558-17. doi:10.1128/AEM.00558-17
7. Chen W, Bibby K. Temporal, spatial, and methodological considerations in evaluating the viability of measles wastewater surveillance. *Sci Total Environ.* 2025;959:178141. doi:10.1016/j.scitotenv.2024.178141
8. Tomalty E, Mercier É, Pisharody L, et al. Detection of measles virus genotype A in a non-endemic wastewater setting: insights from measles wastewater and environmental monitoring in Canada's capital region. *Environ Sci Technol Lett.* 2025;12(2):124–129. doi:10.1021/acs.estlett.4c00945
9. Wu J, Wang MX, Kalvapalle P, et al. Multiplexed detection, partitioning, and persistence of wild-type and vaccine strains of measles, mumps, and rubella viruses in wastewater. *Environ Sci Technol.* 2024;58(50):21930–21941. doi:10.1021/acs.est.4c05344
10. Hayes EK, Gouthro MT, LeBlanc JJ, Gagnon GA. Simultaneous detection of SARS-CoV-2, influenza A, respiratory syncytial virus, and measles in wastewater by multiplex RT-qPCR. *Sci Total Environ.* 2023;889:164261. doi:10.1016/j.scitotenv.2023.164261
11. Tisza M, Javornik Cregeen S, Avadhanula V, et al. Wastewater sequencing reveals community and variant dynamics of the collective human virome. *Nat Commun.* 2023;14(1):6878. doi:10.1038/s41467-023-42064-1
12. Tisza MJ, Hanson BM, Clark JR, et al. Sequencing-based detection of avian influenza A(H5N1) virus in wastewater in ten cities. *N Engl J Med.* 2024; 391(12):1157–1159. doi:10.1056/NEJMc2405937
13. Clark JR, Terwilliger A, Avadhanula V, et al. Wastewater pandemic preparedness: Toward an end-to-end pathogen monitoring program. *Front Public Health.* 2023;11:1137881. doi:10.3389/fpubh.2023.1137881

# World Trade Center (WTC) Exposures and Cardiometabolic Risk Among WTC Health Program General Responders

Helena Krasnov, PhD, Krupa Ambalal Patel, Pablo Knobel, PhD, Hsiao-Hsien Leon Hsu, ScD, Susan L. Teitelbaum, PhD, MPH, Mary Ann McLaughlin, MD, MPH, Allan C. Just, PhD, and Maayan Yitshak Sade, PhD

**Objectives.** To assess the association between World Trade Center (WTC) exposures, cardiometabolic diseases (CMDs), and trajectories of glucose and systolic blood pressure (SBP) among WTC Health Program general responders (WTHPGR).

**Methods.** We included monitoring visits (2003–2021) of WTHPGR who participated in the operations in New York City after the September 11, 2001, attack (n = 47 795). The WTC Health Program assessed WTC exposures using questionnaires and measured trajectories during monitoring study visits; CMDs were self-reported. We assessed associations with CMDs (hazard ratios and their corresponding 95% confidence intervals [CIs]) using survival analyses. We assessed associations with trajectories (odds ratios and their corresponding 95% CIs) using logistic regressions.

**Results.** Interquartile range (IQR) increases in the number of days on-site in the 9 months following the attack were associated with increased diabetes (1.057; 95% CI = 1.025, 1.089) and hypertension (1.035; 95% CI = 1.014, 1.057) risks. IQR increases in hours on-site during September 2001 were associated with worsening glucose (1.040; 95% CI = 1.017, 1.064) and SBP (1.006; 95% CI = 1.001, 1.010) trajectories.

**Conclusions.** WTC exposures are associated with higher CMD risk and worsening cardiometabolic trajectories among WTHPGR.

**Public Health implications.** Linking WTC exposures to emerging diseases is vital because of its impact on health care costs and treatment access among WTHPGR. (*Am J Public Health*. 2025;115(7):1120–1128. https://doi.org/10.2105/AJPH.2025.308079)

AJPH July 2025, Vol. 115, No. 7

The September 11, 2001 (9/11), attacks on the World Trade Center (WTC) resulted in nearly 3000 fatalities in their immediate aftermath. Additionally, the health of responders who engaged in the search, rescue, recovery, service restoration, and cleanup operations in New York City has been negatively affected in the years since. More than 100 000 responders were exposed to smoke, fumes, dust, and debris in the air because of these attacks,[1] and to date, these exposures have not been fully described.[2] Adequate respiratory protective equipment was not consistently available, so these exposures contributed to health consequences arising years later.[3] Alongside the chemical and environmental exposures, responders have experienced psychosocial stress resulting from working long hours and completing challenging tasks in hectic environments, as well as fear for their safety, illness, or injury.[4]

The WTC Health Program provides medical monitoring, treatment, and assistance to eligible responders. In the past 2 decades, 48 389 responders were assessed, forming the General Responder Cohort. The cohort repository includes physical examinations, laboratory tests, and exposure and health questionnaires. Several studies associated WTC exposures with adverse health outcomes, focusing mostly on respiratory diseases,[5,6] cancer,[7] and mental health.[8–10] Only a few studies have investigated the associations between WTC exposures and cardiometabolic diseases. A 2013 study reported a higher risk of diabetes following 9/11 dust cloud exposure and posttraumatic stress.[11] Another study found a higher risk of cardiovascular disease among responders who arrived at the WTC on 9/11 than among those who arrived on or after September 12, 2001.[10]

Additionally, a recent investigation found higher cholesterol and glucose levels among responders categorized into a higher WTC exposure index category, which represents longer time on-site and more intense dust exposure.[12] Other studies, however, reported lower than expected cardiovascular disease,[13,14] metabolic syndrome,[15] and diabetes rates[16] compared with the general population. Furthermore, there is limited literature associating WTC exposures with cardiometabolic biomarkers.[12]

Given these mixed results, further studies are needed to understand the impact of 9/11 on long-term cardiometabolic diseases risk. Therefore, we assessed the associations of various WTC exposures with diabetes, hypertension, and coronary artery disease risk. In addition to these self-reported diseases, we investigated objective cardiometabolic biomarkers and evaluated the associations with long-term trajectories of blood glucose and systolic blood pressure (SBP).

## METHODS

The study population included 47 795 WTC Health Program general responders from 2003 to 2021.

### Study Population and Outcome

The cohort consisted of responders who participated in rescue, recovery, and cleanup efforts following the 9/11 attack on the WTC and were monitored over more than 20 years. The WTC Health Program administered an exposure assessment questionnaire at the initial monitoring visit. The WTC Health Program administered a medical questionnaire during all annual monitoring visits, which included self-reported information on the diagnosis date of various chronic conditions. The WTC Health Program asked the responders about numerous conditions and whether a physician had ever told them they had the condition. The data additionally contain sociodemographic variables, habits (e.g., smoking, alcohol consumption), laboratory results (e.g., blood glucose, lipids), and physical examinations (e.g., body mass index and blood pressure). Details regarding study eligibility criteria are described elsewhere.[17]

*Subcohorts for cardiometabolic diseases survival analyses.* We constructed subcohorts to analyze long-term associations with hypertension, diabetes, and coronary artery disease. In each subcohort, we followed responders annually until disease occurrence, death, or last documented visit (whichever came first). The observation period started in 2003, and we excluded responders diagnosed with the studied outcome within 2 years of the WTC attack (1.85%) to account for the potential induction period. We assigned hypertension, diabetes, and coronary artery diseases to responders based on self-reports. We also assigned diabetes to responders with at least 2 blood glucose tests higher than 200 milligrams per deciliter (mg/dL).[18] We chose this conservative threshold to account for the possibility that the responders were not fasting before the blood test, although they were instructed to do so.

*Laboratory data for trajectory analyses.* To ensure sufficient measurements for the trajectory analysis, we restricted the sample to people with at least 4 measurements during the study period. Additionally, because this analysis focused on the investigation of worsening trajectories among individuals who had normal test values at baseline, we excluded responders with previously reported diabetes or hypertension, glucose greater than 140 mg/dL, or SBP greater than 130 millimeters of mercury (mm/Hg) at baseline. Finally, because glucose and SBP measurements were rare among people older than 75 years at baseline, we excluded these measurements to avoid bias.

### Exposures

We a priori selected environmental and psychological WTC exposures previously related to chronic health outcomes among responders.[11,12,19] We gathered exposure information via an exposure assessment questionnaire administered during the responders' first monitoring visit. The included exposures were the following:

1. Total number of hours on-site on 9/11,
2. Presence in Lower Manhattan on the day of the attack (yes/no),
3. Total number of days on-site October 2001 to June 2002,
4. Sustained injury (yes/no),
5. Witnessed horror (yes/no),
6. Lost someone (yes/no), and
7. WTC exposure index.

The WTC exposure index is a derived exposure variable that incorporates data on the overall time working at the

WTC site, exposure to the dust cloud, and direct work on the debris pile. The "low" category included responders who worked less than 40 days, were not exposed to the dust, and did not work directly on the pile. The "intermediate" category included responders who were not exposed to the cloud but worked 40 to 90 days or directly on the pile. The "high" category included responders who were directly exposed to the cloud or worked for more than 90 days.[17]

## Statistical Analysis

*Survival analyses.* We used separate single-exposure Cox proportional hazard regressions to study the association between each WTC exposure and each outcome (i.e., diabetes, hypertension, or coronary artery disease incidence). We adjusted the models for sociodemographic characteristics (i.e., age, sex, race, ethnicity, education, and marital status), body mass index, and census tract–level socioeconomic variables (i.e., percentage below poverty line, percentage of Black population, percentage with no high school diploma, and median household income) at the baseline visit.

*Trajectory analyses.* We categorized the trajectories of long-term glucose and SBP using latent class mixed models[20] and specified them as a function of the participant's age with adjustment for sex. We estimated the trajectories for each specification of trajectory shape, setting 2 to 4 groups. We used different functions to specify the random effect age distribution (i.e., linear, spline, and B) and the trajectory shapes (i.e., linear, quadratic, and cubic). The following criteria determined the best model fit: (1) smallest Bayesian information criterion, (2) no less than 2% membership in any single trajectory group, and (3) greater than 0.7 posterior probabilities in each group.[21] We achieved the best model fit for glucose by setting 3 trajectory groups (i.e., steady normal, normal to high, and normal to very high) using a B function for the trajectory shape. For SBP, we achieved the best model fit by setting 2 trajectory groups (normal to steady high and normal to very high) using a linear function for trajectory shape.

We assessed the associations between WTC exposures and glucose or SBP trajectory groups using logistic regressions. For SBP, we set the normal-to-steady-high group as a reference. For glucose, we set the steady-normal group as a reference. We conducted 2 separate models to assess the odds of assignment to the normal-to-high and normal-to-very-high categories compared with the reference group. We adjusted the models for the same set of confounders described in the survival analyses section.

*Sensitivity analyses.* First, because 40% of responders did not provide information regarding injuries and witnessing horror during the attack, we conducted a sensitivity analysis to ensure that this did not induce selection bias. We estimated the probability of having complete information in these variables using logistic regressions including sociodemographic characteristics (i.e., age, sex, race and ethnicity, education, and marital status), body mass index, and census tract–level socioeconomic variables (i.e., percentage below the poverty line, percentage of Black population, percentage with no high school diploma, and median household income) as predictors. Then, we incorporated the inverse probability weights into the main analyses to correct for the potential selection bias and ensure that the results did not change.

Second, we calculated the E-values for the statistically significant associations observed in the main analyses to evaluate the potential of confounding bias. The E-value is the minimum strength of association that an unmeasured confounder would need to have with both the exposure and the outcomes, conditional on the covariates, to fully explain away the associations found.[22]

# RESULTS

We included 47 795 responders, of whom 13% had diabetes, 30.75% had hypertension, and 3.19% had coronary artery disease. The average age at cohort entry was approximately 40 years; most were White, and almost 86% were male. The number of glucose and SBP measurements ranged from 4 to 16, with a mean number of 8 measurements per person. In the glucose trajectory analysis, we classified 90.38% as steady normal, 3.27% as normal to high, and 6.34% as normal to very high. In the SBP trajectory analysis, we classified 96.34% as normal to very high and the rest as normal to steady high (Table 1).

Approximately half of the responders were present in Lower Manhattan during the day of the attack. The responders spent 138 hours on-site in September on average and 54 days on average in the following 9 months. About 61% of the responders were exposed to the intermediate WTC exposure index category, followed by 15% in the high exposure category and 13% in the low exposure category. Finally, 14%

**TABLE 1— Descriptive Characteristics of World Trade Center Health Program General Responders in a Cardiometabolic Risk Study: New York City, 2003–2021**

| Variable | No. (%) or Mean ±SD |
| --- | --- |
| **Sociodemographic characteristics** | |
| Age at cohort entry, y | 40.6 ±8.8 |
| Marital status | |
| No | 13 018 (27.2) |
| Yes | 34 148 (71.4) |
| Unknown | 626 (1.3) |
| Race | |
| Black | 4 257 (8.9) |
| White | 25 008 (52.3) |
| Other | 5 282 (11.0) |
| Unknown | 12 916 (27.0) |
| Highest education level | |
| Elementary school | 3 144 (6.5) |
| High school | 9 240 (19.3) |
| Some college | 12 228 (25.5) |
| College graduate[a] | 19 388 (40.5) |
| Unknown | 3 792 (7.9) |
| Sex | |
| Male | 41 046 (85.8) |
| Female | 6 417 (13.4) |
| Body mass index, kg/m$^2$ | 30.20 ±4.4 |
| **Neighborhood characteristics** | |
| Black population, % | 0.8 ±1.5 |
| Under the poverty line, % | 9.3 ±7.6 |
| With no high school education, % | 3.9 ±3.4 |
| Median household income | 59 600 ±23 200 |
| **Outcomes** | |
| Diabetes | 6 027 (12.9) |
| Hypertension | 13 118 (30.7) |
| Coronary artery disease | 1 520 (3.1) |
| Glucose trajectory group | |
| Steady normal | 13 167 (90.3) |
| Normal to high | 477 (3.2) |
| Normal to very high | 924 (6.3) |
| SBP trajectory group | |
| Normal to steady high | 885 (3.6) |
| Normal to very high | 23 338 (96.3) |

*Note.* SBP = systolic blood pressure. The sample size was n = 47 795.
[a]Professional, bachelor's, or associate degree.

reported injuries, 52% lost someone they knew, and 26.12% reported witnessing horror (Table A, available as a supplement to the online version of this article at http://www.ajph.org). Elaborated descriptive statistics of population characteristics in each trajectory group are described in Tables B and C (available as a supplement to the online version of this article at http://www.ajph.org).

An interquartile range (IQR) increase in the number of days spent on-site during the 9 months following the attack was associated with increased diabetes (hazard ratio [HR] = 1.057; 95% confidence interval [CI] = 1.025, 1.089) and hypertension (HR = 1.035; 95% CI = 1.014, 1.057) risks. Diabetes risk was also associated with reported injuries (HR = 1.131; 95% CI = 1.040, 1.229). We also observed hypertension associations with reported injuries (HR = 1.123; 95% CI = 1.058, 1.192), the loss of someone (HR = 1.106; 95% CI = 1.063, 1.151), and exposure to the high WTC exposure index category (HR = 1.107; 95% CI = 1.036, 1.184). Finally, the associations with coronary artery disease were all positive but not statistically significant (Table 2).

The trajectory analyses included 14 178 people with glucose measurements and 27 455 people with SBP measurements. Figure 1 shows the mean glucose and SBP values by age in each trajectory group. In the steady-normal glucose trajectory group, glucose values did not exceed 110 mg/dL and remained within the normal range throughout the observation period. In the normal-to-high group, values reached as high as 175 mg/dL and then decreased, and in the normal-to-very-high group, values linearly increased with age. In the normal-to-steady-high SBP trajectory group, values gradually increased but did not exceed 135 mm/Hg. In the normal-to-very-high group, values increased linearly with age, exceeding 160 mm/Hg.

Compared with a steady-normal trajectory, an IQR increase in the total number of hours on-site during September 2001 (odds ratio [OR] = 1.040;

**TABLE 2— Associations Between World Trade Center Exposures and Cardiometabolic Disease Incidence: New York City, 2003–2021**

| Exposure | Diabetes, HR (95% CI) | Hypertension, HR (95% CI) | Coronary Artery Disease, HR (95% CI) |
|---|---|---|---|
| WTC exposure index[a] | | | |
| Low (Ref) | 1 | 1 | 1 |
| Intermediate | 0.98 (0.90, 1.06) | 1.00 (0.94, 1.06) | 1.18 (0.98, 1.42) |
| High | 0.98 (0.89, 1.08) | 1.10 (1.03, 1.18) | 1.20 (0.97, 1.48) |
| Hours on-site in Sep 2001 | 0.99 (0.94, 1.05) | 1.00 (0.96, 1.03) | 1.03 (0.93, 1.14) |
| Presence in Lower Manhattan | 1.02 (0.96, 1.08) | 1.02 (0.99, 1.06) | 1.07 (0.95, 1.20) |
| Days on-site (Oct 2001—Jun 2002) | 1.05 (1.02, 1.08) | 1.03 (1.01, 1.05) | 1.01 (0.95, 1.08) |
| Injuries | 1.13 (1.04, 1.22) | 1.12 (1.05, 1.19) | 1.15 (0.97, 1.37) |
| Lost someone | 1.01 (0.95 1.07) | 1.10 (1.06, 1.15) | 1.11 (0.99, 1.25) |
| Witnessed horror | 1.03 (0.96, 1.10) | 1.02 (0.97, 1.06) | 0.97 (0.85, 1.11) |

*Note.* CI = confidence interval; HR = hazard ratio; WTC = World Trade Center. We used the Cox proportional HR models to study the associations between each single WTC exposure and each outcome. We adjusted models for sex, age, race, education, marital status, body mass index, and neighborhood sociodemographic variables during the first year of follow-up. We weighted the models assessing the risks associated with having injuries and witnessing horror during the attack by the inverse probability of being included in the analytical data set to minimize selection bias attributable to/because of/owing to a high percentage of missing values. The associations with the total number of hours on-site in September 2001 and total number of days on-site during October 2001–June 2002 are presented per interquartile range increments (176 hours and 68 days). The sample size was n = 47 795.

[a]The low category includes responders who worked < 40 days, were not exposed to the dust, and did not work directly on the pile. The intermediate category includes responders who were not exposed to the cloud but worked 40–90 days or directly on the pile. The high category includes responders who were directly exposed to the cloud or worked for > 90 days.

AJPH July 2025, Vol. 115, No. 7

95% CI = 1.017, 1.064) and injuries (OR = 1.037; 95% CI = 1.003, 1.072) were associated with higher odds of a normal-to-very-high glucose trajectory (Table 3). Compared with a normal-to-steady-high trajectory, an IQR increase in the total number of hours on-site during September 2001 (OR = 1.006; 95% CI = 1.001, 1.010) and the loss of someone (OR = 1.006; 95% CI = 1.001, 1.011) were associated with higher odds of a normal-to-very-high SBP trajectory (Table 3).

The results obtained from the models, including inverse probability weights to account for incomplete injuries and witnessing horror information, were very similar to those of the main analyses (Figure A, available as a supplement to the online version of this article at http://www.ajph.org). Additionally, our E-value calculations show that the effects needed to completely explain our associations are relatively large. For example, the effect estimates needed to completely cancel out the association with diabetes and worse glucose trajectories were 1.515 for injuries and 1.161 for longer duration on-site in September 2001 (Table D, available as a supplement to the online version of this article at http://www.ajph.org).

## DISCUSSION

This study shows that WTC exposures are associated with increased cardiometabolic risk among responders more than the 20 years after 9/11. Specifically, our findings provide additional evidence of elevated diabetes and hypertension risk among responders with greater exposure to various WTC exposures. Longer on-site duration in the 9 months after the attack, injuries, and personal loss were associated with heightened risks of developing these conditions. To ensure the robustness of these findings, we examined time-varying clinical biomarkers of cardiometabolic risk. Our results show that extended hours on-site after the attack, injuries, and personal loss were also associated with worsening glucose and SBP trajectories.

Longer duration on-site was the most consistent predictor of cardiometabolic risk in our analysis. This WTC exposure was previously found to be associated with various health outcomes,[23] specifically respiratory symptoms[9] and cancer.[7] Duration on-site captures various aspects of the complex chemical and nonchemical exposures experienced by the responders. It represents a longer duration of exposure to the high levels of particulate matter pollution containing cement remnants, glass,

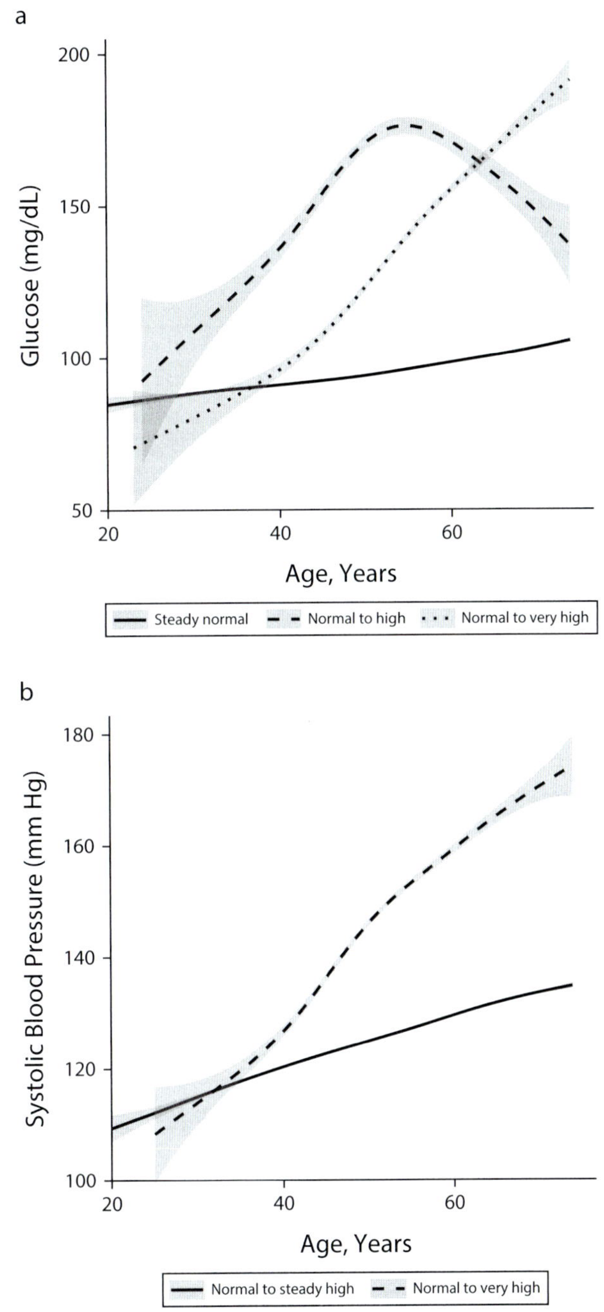


**FIGURE 1— Latent Class Mixed Model Categorization of Long-Term Trajectories of (a) Glucose and (b) Systolic Blood Pressure: New York City, 2003–2021**

*Note.* We categorized the trajectories of long-term glucose and systolic blood pressure (SBP) using latent class mixed models and specified as a function of the participant's age with adjustment for sex. For each specification of trajectory shape, we estimated the trajectories setting 2–4 groups. We used different functions to specify the random effect age distribution (i.e., linear, spline, and B) and the trajectory shapes (i.e., linear, quadratic, and cubic). The following criteria determined the best model fit: (1) smallest Bayesian information criterion, (2) ≥ 2% membership in any single trajectory group, and (3) > 0.7 posterior probabilities in each group. We achieved the best model fit for glucose by setting 3 trajectory groups (steady normal, normal to high, and normal to very high), using a B function for the trajectory shape. For SBP, we achieved the best model fit by setting 2 trajectory groups (normal to steady high and normal to very high), using a linear function for trajectory shape. Gray shading represents confidence intervals.

**TABLE 3— Associations Between World Trade Center Exposures and Glucose or Systolic Blood Pressure Trajectories: New York City, 2003–2021**

| Exposure | Glucose (n = 14 178) | | SBP (n = 27 455), Normal to Very High Exposure,[a] OR (95% CI) |
|---|---|---|---|
| | Normal to High Exposure,[a] OR (95% CI) | Normal to Very High Exposure,[a] OR (95% CI) | |
| WTC exposure index[b] | | | |
| Low (Ref) | 1 | 1 | 1 |
| Intermediate | 1.00 (0.99, 1.01) | 0.99 (0.95, 1.03) | 1.00 (0.99, 1.01) |
| High | 0.99 (0.98, 1.01) | 1.01 (0.96, 1.05) | 1.00 (0.99, 1.01) |
| Hours on-site (September 2001) | 1.00 (0.99, 1.01) | 1.04 (1.01, 1.06) | 1.006 (1.001, 1.010) |
| Presence in Lower Manhattan | 1.00 (0.99, 1.01) | 1.00 (0.98, 1.03) | 1.004 (0.999, 1.008) |
| Days on-site (October 2001–June 2002) | 1.00 (0.99, 1.004) | 1.00 (0.99, 1.02) | 1.002 (0.995, 1.009) |
| Injuries | 0.99 (0.99, 1.01) | 1.037 (1.003, 1.072) | 1.002 (0.995, 1.009) |
| Lost someone | 1.00 (0.99, 1.01) | 1.00 (0.97, 1.02) | 1.006 (1.001, 1.011) |
| Witnessed horror | 1.00 (0.99, 1.01) | 1.02 (0.93, 1.05) | 1.003 (0.997, 1.008) |

*Note.* CI = confidence interval; OR = odds ratio; SBP = systolic blood pressure; WTC = World Trade Center. We used logistic regressions to estimate the odds of being in each trajectory group compared with the normal-to-steady-high group. The glucose analysis included the 3 glucose trajectory groups. The SBP analysis included the 2 trajectory groups. We adjusted the models for sex, age, race, education, marital status, body mass index, and neighborhood sociodemographic variables during the first year of follow-up. We weighed the models assessing the risks associated with having injuries and witnessing horror during the attack by the inverse probability of being included in the analysis. The associations with the total number of hours on-site in September 2001 and total number of days on site during October 2001–June 2002 are presented per interquartile range increments (176 hours and 68 days).

[a]Steady normal is the reference.

[b]The low category includes responders who worked < 40 days, were not exposed to the dust, and did not work directly on the pile. The intermediate category includes responders who were not exposed to the cloud but worked 40–90 days or directly on the pile. The high category includes responders who where directly exposed to the cloud or worked for > 90 days.



asbestos, and many toxic metals and organics sustained in the air in the lower parts of Manhattan.[2] It also represents a higher probability of experiencing injuries and witnessing disturbing scenes, which can profoundly affect one's mental well-being. Finally, this measure is less affected by recall bias and possibly better captures the variation in WTC exposures.[24]

The epidemiological evidence and mechanistic underpinnings linking air pollution with cardiometabolic diseases have been reported in numerous studies, for example the 2024 review of Rajagopalan et al.[25] Our study found that a high WTC exposure index, indicative of dust exposure, is associated with an increased risk of hypertension but not diabetes, coronary artery disease, or cardiometabolic trajectories. Unlike our study, a recent analysis among the cohort responders showed elevated glucose and cholesterol levels associated with exposure to a higher WTC exposure index.[12] These mixed results may be related to the challenges in studying WTC-related health effects, especially dust-related effects, owing to the lack of nonexposed comparison groups, reliance on self-reported exposure questionnaires, and lack of direct dust exposure measurements.

Another interesting finding of our study is the consistently higher cardiometabolic disease risk associated with exposures that suggest intense stress (i.e., witnessing horror and the loss of someone). A large group of studies reported that a longer duration working at the site after the attack on the WTC is associated with an increased risk of posttraumatic stress disorder[26] and depression.[19] Studies also show that these mental health conditions are associated with an increased risk of diabetes[27,28] and hypertension.[29–31] The association with diabetes may be related to stress-induced cortisol secretion, which increases blood glucose levels and insulin resistance.[32] The association with blood pressure levels may be related to autonomic function dysregulation affecting heart rate.[33] To date, the links between mental health, trauma, and cardiovascular risk are unclear,[34] and further studies are needed to fully investigate these associations.

## Limitations

Our study has several limitations. First, the self-reported data may have been affected by recall bias. However, multiple studies have observed high levels of agreement between self-reported outcomes and medical records.[35] Moreover, the similar WTC exposure associations found with self-reported outcomes and clinical biomarkers support the robustness of our findings. Second, as in any epidemiologic study, our results may be biased because of residual confounding. However, our sensitivity analysis shows that the effect sizes needed to cancel out the associations observed in our study are very large and unlikely.

## Public Health Implications

Federally funded health care is provided to responders only for certified diseases related to 9/11 exposure, and cardiometabolic diseases are not currently certified. This has vast implications for health care costs and accessibility of treatment for WTC responders and survivors. By highlighting the elevated cardiometabolic risks linked to greater WTC-related exposures, this study contributes to the growing body of evidence needed to support the certification of these conditions.

## Conclusions

Our study indicates that prolonged on-site presence, injuries, and personal loss among WTC responders are associated with increased cardiometabolic risks in the years following 9/11. Linking WTC-related exposures to emerging diseases is critical, as the certification of these conditions has significant implications for health care costs and treatment accessibility for responders. AJPH

### ABOUT THE AUTHORS

Helena Krasnov, Pablo Knobel, Hsiao-Hsien Leon Hsu, Susan L. Teitelbaum, and Maayan Yitshak Sade are with the Department of Environmental Medicine, Icahn School of Medicine at Mount Sinai, New York, NY. Krupa Ambalal Patel is with the Graduate Program in Public Health, Icahn School of Medicine at Mount Sinai. Mary Ann McLaughlin is with the Department of Cardiology, Icahn School of Medicine at Mount Sinai. Allan C. Just is with the Department of Epidemiology, Brown University School of Public Health, Providence, RI.

### CORRESPONDENCE

Correspondence should be sent to Helena Krasnov, 17 E. 102nd St, CAM Building, 3 West, One Gustave L. Levy Place, Box 1057, New York, NY 10029 (e-mail: helena.furman@mssm.edu). Reprints can be ordered at https://www.ajph.org by clicking the "Reprints" link.

### PUBLICATION INFORMATION

Full Citation: Krasnov H, Patel KA, Knobel P, et al. World Trade Center (WTC) exposures and cardiometabolic risk among WTC Health Program general responders. *Am J Public Health*. 2025; 115(7):1120–1128.

Acceptance Date: February 16, 2025.

DOI: https://doi.org/10.2105/AJPH.2025.308079

ORCID iDs:

Helena Krasnov https://orcid.org/0000-0003-0230-3112

Hsiao-Hsien Leon Hsu https://orcid.org/0000-0001-8704-197X

Susan L. Teitelbaum https://orcid.org/0000-0002-2190-1575

Allan C. Just https://orcid.org/0000-0003-4312-5957

### CONTRIBUTORS

H. Krasnov performed the formal analyses, conducted the investigation, curated the data, created the analysis codes, and wrote the original draft of the article. K. A. Patel contributed to the investigation. P. Knobel contributed to the initial data curation. P. Knobel, H.-H. L. Hsu, S. L. Teitelbaum, M. McLaughlin, and M. Y. Sade wrote and edited the article. H.-H. L. Hsu, S. L. Teitelbaum, M. McLaughlin, and M. Y. Sade conceptualized the study and developed the methodology. A. C. Just supported software and code validation. M. Y. Sade supervised the study. All authors reviewed and approved the final version of the article.

### ACKNOWLEDGMENTS

This study was supported by the Centers for Disease Control and Prevention, National Institute for Occupational Safety and Health (cooperative agreements and contracts 200-2002-00384, U01-OH008216/23/25/32/39/75, 200-2011-39356/61/77/84/85/88,200-2017-93325 and 75D30122C15187). This study was also supported by the Mount Sinai Transdisciplinary Center On Early Environmental Exposures (grant P30 ES023515) and the National Institute of Environmental Health Sciences (grants R01ES034864, KL2TR004421).

We thank the staff of the World Trade Center (WTC) Workers and Volunteer Medical Screening, Medical Monitoring and Treatment, and Health Programs; the labor, community, and volunteer organization stakeholders; and the WTC rescue and recovery workers, who gave of themselves so readily in response to the WTC attacks and to whom the WTC Health Program is dedicated.

**Note.** The contents of this editorial are solely the responsibility of the authors and do not necessarily represent the official views of the Centers for Disease Control and Prevention, the National Institutes of Health, or the Mount Sinai Transdisciplinary Center On Early Environmental Exposures.

### CONFLICTS OF INTEREST

The authors have no conflicts of interest to disclose.

### HUMAN PARTICIPANT PROTECTION

This study was approved by the Mount Sinai School of Medicine institutional review board (STUDY-20-02018-MOD004), and consent for the secondary analysis was waived. We restricted the population to responders who consented to data aggregation for research (STUDY-11-02030, World Trade Center Health Program General Responder Data Center).

### REFERENCES

1. Farfel M, DiGrande L, Brackbill R, et al. An overview of 9/11 experiences and respiratory and mental health conditions among World Trade Center Health Registry enrollees. *J Urban Health*. 2008;85(6):880–909. https://doi.org/10.1007/s11524-008-9317-4
2. Lippmann M, Cohen MD, Chen L-C. Health effects of World Trade Center (WTC) dust: an unprecedented disaster with inadequate risk management. *Crit Rev Toxicol*. 2015;45(6):492–530. https://doi.org/10.3109/10408444.2015.1044601
3. Brackbill RM, Graber JM, Robison WAA. Editorial for "long-term health effects of the 9/11 disaster" in *International Journal of Environmental Research and Public Health*, 2019. *Int J Environ Res Public Health*. 2019;16(18):3289. https://doi.org/10.3390/ijerph16183289
4. Landrigan PJ, Lioy PJ, Thurston G, et al. Health and environmental consequences of the World Trade Center disaster. *Environ Health Perspect*. 2004;112(6):731–739. https://doi.org/10.1289/ehp.6702
5. Aldrich TK, Gustave J, Hall CB, et al. Lung function in rescue workers at the World Trade Center after 7 years. *N Engl J Med*. 2010;362(14):1263–1272. https://doi.org/10.1056/NEJMoa0910087
6. Cleven KL, Rosenzvit C, Nolan A, et al. Twenty-year reflection on the impact of World Trade Center exposure on pulmonary outcomes in Fire Department of the City of New York (FDNY) rescue and recovery workers. *Lung*. 2021;199(6):569–578. https://doi.org/10.1007/s00408-021-00493-z
7. Boffetta P, Hall CB, Todd AC, et al. Cancer risk among World Trade Center rescue and recovery workers: a review. *CA Cancer J Clin*. 2022;72(4):308–314. https://doi.org/10.3322/caac.21723

8. Yip J, Zeig-Owens R, Webber MP, et al. World Trade Center–related physical and mental health burden among New York City fire department emergency medical service workers. *Occup Environ Med.* 2016;73(1):13–20. https://doi.org/10.1136/oemed-2014-102601
9. Jordan HT, Osahan S, Li J, et al. Persistent mental and physical health impact of exposure to the September 11, 2001 World Trade Center terrorist attacks. *Environ Health.* 2019;18(1):12. https://doi.org/10.1186/s12940-019-0449-7
10. Liu B, Tarigan LH, Bromet EJ, Kim H. World Trade Center disaster exposure-related probable posttraumatic stress disorder among responders and civilians: a meta-analysis. *PLoS One.* 2014;9(7):e101491. https://doi.org/10.1371/journal.pone.0101491
11. Jordan HT, Stellman SD, Morabia A, et al. Cardiovascular disease hospitalizations in relation to exposure to the September 11, 2001 World Trade Center disaster and posttraumatic stress disorder. *J Am Heart Assoc.* 2013;2(5):e000431. https://doi.org/10.1161/JAHA.113.000431
12. Knobel P, Just AC, Colicino E, et al. Air pollution exposure and glucose and lipids levels among the World Trade Center Health Program general responder cohort. September 18, 2022. Available at: https://ehp.niehs.nih.gov/doi/10.1289/isee.2022.O-OP-002. Accessed April 12, 2025.
13. Colbeth HL, Zeig-Owens R, Hall CB, Webber MP, Schwartz TM, Prezant DJ. Mortality among fire department of the City of New York rescue and recovery workers exposed to the World Trade Center disaster, 2001–2017. *Int J Environ Res Public Health.* 2020;17(17):6266. https://doi.org/10.3390/ijerph17176266
14. Jordan HT, Stein CR, Li J, et al. Mortality among rescue and recovery workers and community members exposed to the September 11, 2001 World Trade Center terrorist attacks, 2003–2014. *Environ Res.* 2018;163:270–279. https://doi.org/10.1016/j.envres.2018.01.004
15. Moline JM, McLaughlin MA, Sawit ST, et al. The prevalence of metabolic syndrome among law enforcement officers who responded to the 9/11 World Trade Center attacks. *Am J Ind Med.* 2016;59(9):752–760. https://doi.org/10.1002/ajim.22649
16. Kim H, Kriebel D, Liu B, et al. Standardized morbidity ratios of four chronic health conditions among World Trade Center responders: comparison to the National Health Interview Survey. *Am J Ind Med.* 2018;61(5):413–421. https://doi.org/10.1002/ajim.22825
17. Wisnivesky JP, Teitelbaum SL, Todd AC, et al. Persistence of multiple illnesses in World Trade Center rescue and recovery workers: a cohort study. *Lancet.* 2011;378(9794):888–897. https://doi.org/10.1016/S0140-6736(11)61180-X
18. Buysschaert M, Medina J-L, Buysschaert B, Bergman M. Definitions (and current controversies) of diabetes and prediabetes. *Curr Diabetes Rev.* 2016;12(1):8–13. https://doi.org/10.2174/1573399811666150122150233
19. Santiago-Colón A, Daniels R, Reissman D, et al. World Trade Center Health Program: first decade of research. *Int J Environ Res Public Health.* 2020;17(19):7290. https://doi.org/10.3390/ijerph17197290
20. Proust-Lima C, Philipps V, Liquet B. Estimation of extended mixed models using latent classes and latent processes: the R package lcmm. *J Stat Softw.* 2017;78(2):1–56. https://doi.org/10.18637/jss.v078.i02
21. Yuan Z, Yang Y, Wang C, et al. Trajectories of long-term normal fasting plasma glucose and risk of coronary heart disease: a prospective cohort study. *J Am Heart Assoc.* 2018;7(4):e007607. https://doi.org/10.1161/JAHA.117.007607
22. Mathur MB, VanderWeele TJ. Sensitivity analysis for unmeasured confounding in meta-analyses. *J Am Stat Assoc.* 2020;115(529):163–172. https://doi.org/10.1080/01621459.2018.1529598
23. Webber MP, Moir W, Zeig-Owens R, et al. Nested case–control study of selected systemic autoimmune diseases in World Trade Center rescue/recovery workers. *Arthritis Rheumatol.* 2015;67(5):1369–1376. https://doi.org/10.1002/art.39059
24. Krayem Z, Hawila B, Al Barathie J, Karam E. Recall bias in trauma recollection. *Arab J Psychiatry.* 2021;32(2):112–123. https://doi.org/10.12816/0059211
25. Rajagopalan S, Brook RD, Salerno PR, et al. Air pollution exposure and cardiometabolic risk. *Lancet Diabetes Endocrinol.* 2024;12(3):196–208. https://doi.org/10.1016/S2213-8587(23)00361-3
26. Zvolensky MJ, Kotov R, Schechter CB, et al. Post-disaster stressful life events and WTC-related posttraumatic stress, depressive symptoms, and overall functioning among responders to the World Trade Center disaster. *J Psychiatr Res.* 2015;61:97–105. https://doi.org/10.1016/j.jpsychires.2014.11.010
27. Ducat L, Rubenstein A, Philipson LH, Anderson BJ. A review of the mental health issues of diabetes conference. *Diabetes Care.* 2015;38(2):333–338. https://doi.org/10.2337/dc14-1383
28. Miller-Archie SA, Jordan HT, Ruff RR, et al. Posttraumatic stress disorder and new-onset diabetes among adult survivors of the World Trade Center disaster. *Prev Med.* 2014;66:34–38. https://doi.org/10.1016/j.ypmed.2014.05.016
29. Gohardehi F, Seyedin H, Moslehi S. Prevalence rate of diabetes and hypertension in disaster-exposed populations: a systematic review and meta-analysis. *Ethiop J Health Sci.* 2020;30(3):439–448. https://doi.org/10.4314/ejhs.v30i3.15
30. Mendlowicz V, Garcia-Rosa ML, Gekker M, et al. Post-traumatic stress disorder as a predictor for incident hypertension: a 3-year retrospective cohort study. *Psychol Med.* 2023;53(1):132–139. https://doi.org/10.1017/S0033291721001227
31. Kibler JL, Ma M. Towards a better understanding of PTSD/hypertension associations: examining sociodemographic aspects. *Hearts.* 2021;2(1):149–155. https://doi.org/10.3390/hearts2010012
32. Golden SH. A review of the evidence for a neuroendocrine link between stress, depression and diabetes mellitus. *Curr Diabetes Rev.* 2007;3(4):252–259. https://doi.org/10.2174/157339907782330021
33. Grippo AJ, Johnson AK. Biological mechanisms in the relationship between depression and heart disease. *Neurosci Biobehav Rev.* 2002;26(8):941–962. https://doi.org/10.1016/S0149-7634(03)00003-4
34. Sumner JA, Maihofer AX, Michopoulos V, et al. Examining individual and synergistic contributions of PTSD and genetics to blood pressure: a trans-ethnic meta-analysis. *Front Neurosci.* 2021;15:678503. https://doi.org/10.3389/fnins.2021.678503
35. Jackson JM, DeFor TA, Crain AL, et al. Self-reported diabetes is a valid outcome in pragmatic clinical trials and observational studies. *J Clin Epidemiol.* 2013;66(3):349–350. https://doi.org/10.1016/j.jclinepi.2012.01.013

# Evaluating Algorithmic Approaches to Uncover Racial, Ethnic, and Gender Disparities in Scientific Authorship

Yimeng Song, PhD, Nabarun Dasgupta, PhD, MPH, and Michelle L. Bell, PhD

To explore the capabilities of race/ethnicity and gender prediction algorithms in uncovering patterns of authorship distribution in scientific paper submissions to a major peer-reviewed scientific journal (*AJPH*), we analyzed 17 667 manuscript submissions from the United States between 2013 and 2022. We used machine-learning algorithms to predict corresponding authors' race/ethnicity (Asian, Black, Hispanic, White) and gender categories based on name-derived probabilities to compare the predictive performance of these algorithms and their impact on disparity analysis.

Predicted White authors dominated submissions and had the highest acceptance rates (21.1%), while predicted Asian authors faced the lowest (14.9%). Predicted women, despite being the majority, had lower acceptance rates (17.9%) than men (20.5%), a trend consistent across most racial/ethnic groups. Different algorithms revealed similar disparities but were limited by biases and inaccuracies in predicting race and ethnicity.

Manuscript acceptance rates revealed disparities by race/ethnicity and gender; predicted White and male authors had the highest rates. While machine-learning algorithms can identify such patterns, their limitations necessitate combining them with self-identified demographic data for greater accuracy. (*Am J Public Health*. 2025;115(7):1129–1136. https://doi.org/10.2105/AJPH.2025.308017)

AJPH July 2025, Vol. 115, No. 7

The academic landscape in the United States is shaped by a complex interplay of socioeconomic and cultural factors, including both historical and contemporary issues related to racism and gender bias. These influences are evident in the demographic composition of the scientific community. Data from 2021 reveal significant racial/ethnic disparities among US tenure-track full-time faculty in degree-granting postsecondary institutions, with 5% Hispanic, 6% Black, 12% Asian, and 73% White achieving these coveted positions,[1] compared with being 19%, 14%, 6%, and 56% of the US population, respectively.[2] In addition, women are consistently underrepresented within these groups; in the United States, women constituted 46.7% of full-time faculty in 2018, up from 31.6% in 1991, reflecting significant progress yet still not achieving full parity despite constituting half of the overall adult population.[3] Moreover, research funding disparities, highlighted by 2019 National Science Foundation data, show a 22.7% funding rate for Asian and 26.5% for Black/African American principal investigators, compared with 31.3% for White principal investigators.[4] Along with disparities in faculty positions and funding, systematic biases are also evident in scientific publications,[5] underscoring the need to analyze authorship patterns for insights into inequities affecting academic visibility and representation.

While numerous studies have documented gender disparities in academic authorship, fewer have addressed racial/ethnic disparities. For example, studies have shown that women face significant barriers in publication and citation rates.[6–10] In 6 leading medical journals, female authorship grew from 5.9% to 29.3% for first authors and from 3.7% to 19.3% for senior authors between 1970 and 2004, yet women consistently lag behind their male counterparts.[6] Furthermore, female-authored works are cited less often, and men are more likely to engage in self-citation.[7] The COVID-19 pandemic has exacerbated these disparities, highlighting persistent structural challenges.[8–10] Regarding racial/ethnic disparities, research has revealed that Hispanic and Black individuals are underrepresented in doctoral degrees, academic employment, and publications.[11] Black scientists, for instance, have fewer publications and citations, contributing to funding gaps. Other studies have found that non-White scientists experience prolonged review times, receive fewer citations, and are underrepresented on editorial boards.[5,12,13] These patterns underscore systemic barriers limiting diversity in academic achievement and publishing.

The limited availability of data on authors' racial/ethnic identities has long hindered research on the racial/ethnic distribution of authors. While some journals, such as the *American Journal of Public Health* (*AJPH*) and *The BMJ*,[14] have begun collecting self-identified race/ethnicity data, the historical scarcity of such data poses challenges for analyzing trends. Advances in machine-learning algorithms, particularly natural language processing techniques, provide opportunities to estimate authors' race/ethnicity based on their names with increasing accuracy.[15–17] However, these methods have limitations. For instance, name-based prediction algorithms tend to underestimate Black authors while overestimating White authors, introducing biases that require careful validation and application.[18] Furthermore, while informative, no algorithm could predict race/ethnicity based on names with 100% accuracy. A systematic examination of these tools is necessary to better understand their potential and limitations in analyzing authorship disparities.

With this study, we aimed to explore the capabilities of race/ethnicity and gender prediction algorithms in uncovering patterns of authorship distribution. Leveraging manuscript submission data from *AJPH*, we evaluated the strengths and limitations of various machine-learning algorithms and used them to explore 3 key questions: (1) What are the racial/ethnic and gender disparities among authors? (2) What are the racial/ethnic and gender disparities in acceptance rates of submitted manuscripts? and (3) How have these disparities evolved over time?

# METHODS

We conducted a multistep analysis to examine disparities in authorship by race/ethnicity and gender using machine-learning prediction algorithms. The following methods detail the data sources, predictive models, and evaluation strategies applied in the study.

## Data Sets

We used *AJPH* manuscript submission data from January 1, 2013, to December 31, 2022, to investigate racial/ethnic and gender authorship differences when these variables were not self-identified. Each submission record includes the submission date, authors' names, the corresponding author's institutional affiliation and address (for submissions with multiple authors, only 1 corresponding author's address is provided), manuscript title, and the final decision status ("Accept," "Reject Without Peer Review," "Reject After Peer Review"). Notably, editors have access to the names and institutions of authors during the review process, but reviewers are masked and do not know the authors' identities.

Our analysis focused on corresponding authors and included only submissions from the United States. This was because the race/ethnicity prediction algorithms were trained on US data, and address information was only available for corresponding authors. The data set contains 17 667 unique submission records from the United States, representing 73.7% of all *AJPH* submissions worldwide from 2013 to 2022.

We used the L2 Inc voter registration data set (https://l2-data.com) as ground truth data to evaluate the performance of various race/ethnicity prediction algorithms. The data set, updated in November 2023, includes more than 187.3 million complete records from the 50 US states and the District of Columbia (DC). Each record contains the registrant's last name, first name, address, and self-identified race/ethnicity, categorized as Asian, Black, Hispanic, or White. We did not use the entire data set for the evaluation because of significant variation in the sizes of the L2 data records between states and differing algorithm accuracies across states (Table F, available as a supplement to the online version of this article at https://ajph.org). This data heterogeneity could introduce bias and affect the reliability of our analysis. To address this, we developed a sampling strategy to ensure a more balanced and representative evaluation. Specifically, we first divided the data into 51 regional groups based on the 50 states and DC. For each regional group, we randomly selected 1000 records from each of the 4 racial/ethnic categories, leading to a total of 4000 records per regional group. Each record represented a first–last name combination and associated self-identified racial identity. This process was repeated 5 times, creating 5 separate sample sets, each with a total of 204 000 records.

## Race/Ethnicity Prediction Algorithms

We used *pyethnicity* for the main analysis. The *pyethnicity* Python package (https://github.com/CangyuanLi/pyethnicity) was developed using the Bidirectional Long Short-Term Memory (BiLSTM) model and ensemble learning techniques.[17] BiLSTM is a type of recurrent neural network that has demonstrated state-of-the-art performance in many natural language processing tasks.[15] The *pyethnicity* was trained and validated using individuals' first and last names from the L2 voter registration data of all 50 US states.

We also explored 2 other algorithms, *rethnicity* and *predictrace*, for comparison. The *rethnicity* R package (https://github.com/fangzhou-xie/rethnicity), developed using the BiLSTM model,[15] was trained and validated on first and last names from Florida voter registration data. The *predictrace* R package (https://github.com/jacobkap/predictrace) was developed using a probabilistic model based on last names from Census data and a first name data set from Tzioumis.[19]

The racial/ethnic categories considered in this study were Asian, Black, Hispanic, and White, as all the algorithms used could differentiate among these 4 groups. We used the full-name model of each algorithm, taking first and last names as input. The output of the models is the probability of an individual being a particular racial/ethnic category. It is important to note that the algorithms predict the ethnic origin of names, which we use as a proxy for race/ethnicity. In the results, terms such as "White," "Asian," "Black," and "Hispanic" refer to these predicted categories rather than self-identified race/ethnicity.

We used a multiple imputation approach to account for uncertainty in the predicted race/ethnicity of authors. Based on the predicted probabilities generated by the model, we created 10 imputed data sets where each author's race/ethnicity was assigned probabilistically. For example, if the name "Samuel L. Jackson" generated probabilities of Asian: 0.017, Black: 0.890, Hispanic: 0.007, and White: 0.086, the imputation process assigned "Black" in most data sets, but occasionally assigned other groups based on their respective probabilities. Each data set was independently analyzed to calculate submission and acceptance rates for each racial/ethnic group. We aggregated the final results across the data sets and calculated 95% confidence intervals of mean probability to reflect the uncertainty from the imputation process (see "Method for Calculating 95% Confidence Intervals," available as a supplement to the online version of this article at https://ajph.org).

## Gender Prediction Algorithm

We classified the gender of authors by using an algorithm by an online platform of Gender API, which had been adopted in our previous work.[7] The algorithm was developed using multiple publicly available government and social network data sources. Based on first name and country-of-origin inputs for each individual, the algorithm generated an estimate of whether the individual was male or female, along with a probability. For example, the input of "Karen" and "United States" provides an estimate of female with estimated 0.99 probability. Gender classifications with probability of less than 50% were categorized by the algorithm as unknown. Similar to race/ethnicity prediction, these predictions rely on name-derived probabilities, which we used as a proxy for gender. In the results, "male" and "female" were used to indicate these predicted classifications. We also adopted the multiple imputation approach described previously to incorporate the uncertainty in gender prediction.

## Evaluating Predictive Performance

We used 5 metrics to evaluate and compare the performance of selected algorithms: accuracy, precision, recall, f1-score, and coverage (see "Evaluation Metrics," available as a supplement to the online version of this article at https://ajph.org). All these metrics take values between 0 and 1, with higher values indicating better performance on the corresponding dimension in prediction. We averaged the final score of each metric from the scores of all the 5 sample sets of ground truth data. In addition, we performed a sensitivity analysis on *pyethnicity* predictions to assess how varying probability thresholds impacted acceptance rates for racial/ethnic groups, evaluating the stability and implications of these predictions.

## RESULTS

We first analyzed submission proportions and acceptance rates by race/ethnicity and gender of authors using *pyethnicity* and Gender API (Table 1).

**TABLE 1— Submission and Acceptance Rates by Race/Ethnicity and Gender for Corresponding US Authors in *AJPH*: 2013–2022**

| Race/Ethnicity and Gender | Overall Submissions (n = 17 667) | | Accepted Submissions (n = 3 352) | | Acceptance Rate, % (95% CI) |
|---|---|---|---|---|---|
| | No. (95% CI) | % (95% CI) | No. (95% CI) | % (95% CI) | |
| Race/ethnicity classified as | | | | | |
| Asian | 3 955 (3 938, 3 971) | 22.38 (22.29, 22.48) | 588 (581, 594) | 17.53 (17.33, 17.73) | 14.86 (14.71, 15.01) |
| Black | 2 494 (2 476, 2 512) | 14.12 (14.01, 14.22) | 453 (442, 463) | 13.50 (13.19, 13.81) | 18.14 (17.75, 18.53) |
| Hispanic | 1 573 (1559, 1586) | 8.9 (8.82, 8.98) | 274 (268, 279) | 8.16 (8.01, 8.31) | 17.39 (17.08, 17.70) |
| White | 9 646 (9 622, 9 670) | 54.6 (54.46, 54.74) | 2 038 (2 024, 2 052) | 60.81 (60.40, 61.21) | 21.13 (20.99, 21.27) |
| Gender classified as | | | | | |
| Woman | 10 142 (10 124 10 160) | 57.41 (57.30, 57.51) | 1 810 (1 803, 1 817) | 54.00 (53.80, 54.20) | 17.85 (17.79, 17.90) |
| Man | 7 525 (7 507, 7 543) | 42.59 (42.49, 42.70) | 1 542 (1 535, 1 549) | 46.00 (45.80, 46.20) | 20.49 (20.41, 20.57) |
| Race/ethnicity and gender classified as | | | | | |
| Asian woman | 2 333 (2 318, 2 348) | 13.21 (13.12, 13.29) | 350 (344, 357) | 10.45 (10.26, 10.64) | 15.01 (14.79, 15.23) |
| Asian man | 1 617 (1 607, 1 628) | 9.15 (9.09, 9.22) | 239 (234, 244) | 7.14 (6.99, 7.28) | 14.79 (14.51, 15.07) |
| Black woman | 1 446 (1 434, 1 458) | 8.19 (8.12, 8.25) | 237 (232, 242) | 7.07 (6.93, 7.22) | 16.39 (16.10, 16.69) |
| Black man | 1 016 (1 005, 1 027) | 5.75 (5.69, 5.81) | 202 (193, 212) | 6.03 (5.75, 6.31) | 19.89 (19.09, 20.69) |
| Hispanic woman | 958 (947, 969) | 5.42 (5.36, 5.49) | 157 (151, 162) | 4.67 (4.52, 4.83) | 16.36 (15.80, 16.92) |
| Hispanic man | 615 (607, 624) | 3.48 (3.43, 3.53) | 112 (108, 116) | 3.35 (3.22, 3.47) | 18.24 (17.54, 18.93) |
| White woman | 5 419 (5 400, 5 439) | 30.68 (30.57, 30.78) | 1 074 (1 067, 1 082) | 32.05 (31.84, 32.26) | 19.82 (19.73, 19.92) |
| White man | 4 261 (4 246, 4 277) | 24.12 (24.03, 24.21) | 980 (967, 993) | 29.23 (28.84, 29.62) | 22.99 (22.72, 23.27) |

*Note.* CI = confidence interval. Results classified using *pyethnicity* and Gender API.

Among the 17 667 submissions, 54.6% were authored by individuals classified as White, who had the highest acceptance rate at 21.1%. Asian authors contributed 22.4% of submissions but had the lowest acceptance rate at 14.9%. Black and Hispanic authors, contributing fewer papers, had acceptance rates of 18.1% and 17.4%, respectively.

Gender analysis revealed that women authored 57.4% of submissions but had a lower acceptance rate (17.9%) compared with men (20.5%). An examination of race/ethnicity and gender shows that women submitted more papers than men across all racial/ethnic categories. However, women generally had lower acceptance rates than men, except for Asian women, whose acceptance rate was slightly higher than that of Asian men.

We also categorized rejected submissions as either rejected without peer review or rejected after peer review to detail the pattern of rejection (Table A, available as a supplement to the online version of this article at https://ajph.org). White authors were less likely to have their submissions rejected without review (70.6% of submitted articles) compared with Black (74%), Hispanic (74.2%), and Asian (78%) authors. However, White authors experienced a post–peer review rejection rate of 7.8%, higher than Black (7.5%) and Asian (6.9%) authors.

For annual submissions distribution by race/ethnicity (Figure 1a), there is a very consistent ranking for each year, with most articles being submitted by White authors and the fewest by Hispanic authors. For annual acceptance rates by race/ethnicity (Figure 1b), the general temporal trend shows that White authors consistently had the highest acceptance rates over the 10 years studied, followed by Black authors and Asian authors. In contrast, the acceptance rates for Hispanic authors exhibited greater variability over time, with no consistent trend observed.

Upon repeating our analysis using the *rethnicity* and *predictrace* algorithms, similar patterns of disparity were observed (Tables B and C, available as supplements to the online version of this article at https://ajph.org). White authors continued to contribute the most submissions and had the highest acceptance rates. In contrast, Asian authors, despite submitting the second-highest number of papers,

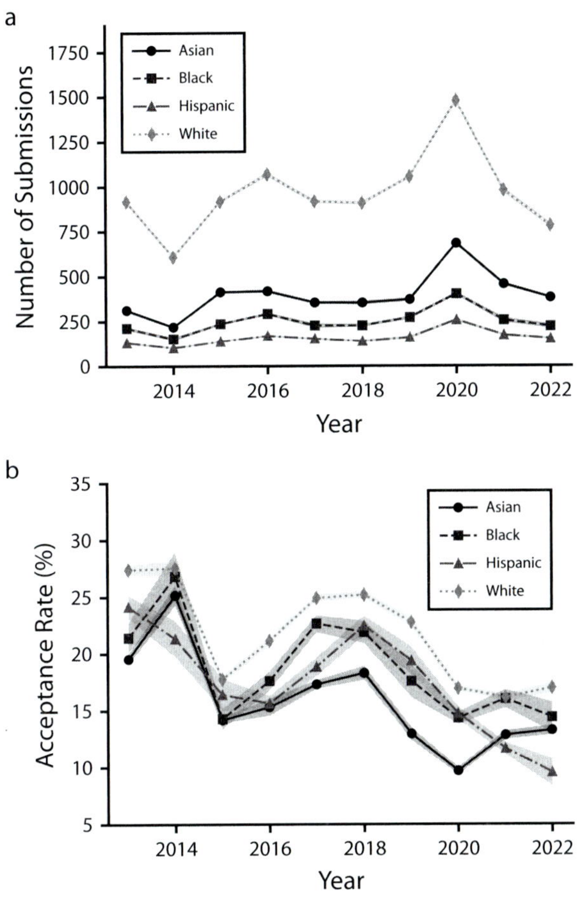


**FIGURE 1— Annual (a) Submissions and (b) Acceptance Rates Over Time by Race/Ethnicity for Corresponding US Authors in *AJPH*, With 95% Confidence Intervals: 2013–2022**

faced the lowest acceptance rates. Black and Hispanic authors contributed the fewest papers and had lower acceptance rates than White authors. In addition, the trend of women submitting more papers but having lower acceptance rates than men persisted across most racial/ethnic groups using the alternate algorithms.

## Algorithm Accuracy

We evaluated race/ethnicity prediction algorithms using L2 data. All algorithms were less effective at predicting Black and White races compared with Asian and Hispanic race/ethnicities (Table D, available as a supplement to the online version of this article at https://ajph.org). *pyethnicity* performed best with high accuracy and precision rates: 0.975 and 0.969, respectively, for Hispanic; 0.952 and 0.967, respectively, for Asian; 0.882 and 0.810, respectively, for Black; and 0.853 and 0.656, respectively, for White. *rethnicity* and *predictrace* showed varying performance across racial/ethnic groups, with lower and less consistent accuracy and precision compared with *pyethnicity*. *predictrace* also had a major issue with coverage, failing to provide predictions for all names.

We found that *pyethnicity* had higher probability scores for its predictions (Figure A, available as a supplement to the online version of this article at https://ajph.org). For the 17 667 submissions analyzed, *pyethnicity* provided 14 466 predictions with probabilities greater than 0.7 and 12 314 with probabilities greater than 0.8, higher than *predictrace* (9644 and 6921) and *rethnicity* (11 901 and 9991). Higher probabilities usually mean higher accuracy and lower uncertainty (Table E, available as a supplement to the online version of this article at https://ajph.org).

We then conducted a sensitivity analysis on *pyethnicity* predictions focusing on probability thresholds and their impact on acceptance rates for various racial/ethnic groups (Table 2). We observed stable acceptance rates for Asian and Hispanic submissions at around 14.4% and 17.0%, respectively. However, as the probability threshold increased, the acceptance rate for White authors rose, while that for Black authors decreased. At a threshold of 0.9 or higher, the acceptance rate for Black submissions was the lowest at 14.5%, while that for White authors increased to 23.5%.

# DISCUSSION

Science is strengthened by diversity of thought, and academic publishing is critical to shaping scientific knowledge. However, in this sample of *AJPH* articles, 61 out of every 100 published articles were from White corresponding authors, while only 8 were from Hispanic authors. Academic publishing remains an overwhelmingly White enterprise by volume. We encourage entities in scientific publishing to make serious assessments of how to ameliorate these fundamental inequities.

We drew 3 conclusions from our findings. First, the absolute volume of submissions from racially minoritized authors was considerably lower

**TABLE 2— Acceptance Rates of US Authors in *AJPH* by Race/Ethnicity Across Different Probability Thresholds: 2013–2022**

| Probability ≥ | Classified as White, % (95% CI) | Classified as Asian, % (95% CI) | Classified as Black, % (95% CI) | Classified as Hispanic, % (95% CI) |
|---|---|---|---|---|
| 0.27 | 21.13 (20.99, 21.27) | 14.86 (14.71, 15.01) | 18.14 (17.75, 18.53) | 17.39 (17.08, 17.70) |
| 0.4 | 21.24 (21.13, 21.35) | 14.73 (14.51, 14.94) | 18.19 (17.94, 18.44) | 17.16 (16.84, 17.49) |
| 0.5 | 21.34 (21.24, 21.44) | 14.81 (14.61, 15.02) | 18.02 (17.85, 18.19) | 16.96 (16.60, 17.32) |
| 0.6 | 21.42 (21.34, 21.49) | 14.84 (14.69, 14.99) | 17.52 (17.14, 17.91) | 16.78 (16.44, 17.11) |
| 0.7 | 21.84 (21.78, 21.90) | 14.84 (14.71, 14.96) | 17.64 (17.46, 17.82) | 17.04 (16.68, 17.40) |
| 0.8 | 23.72 (23.58, 23.86) | 13.97 (13.88, 14.05) | 14.59 (14.18, 14.99) | 16.93 (16.73, 17.14) |
| 0.9 | 23.46 (23.34, 23.59) | 14.23 (14.12, 14.34) | 14.53 (14.22, 14.84) | 17.13 (16.91, 17.35) |

*Note.* CI = confidence interval. Results classified using *pyethnicity*.

than their composition in the general population of the United States. This highlights the need for policies that actively encourage submissions from underrepresented, racially minoritized authors and address the racial/ethnic composition of scientists.

Second, the acceptance rates were highest for White authors (21.1%) and lowest for Asian authors (14.9%), showing a considerable gap between the groups. This study is not able to establish root causes for this discrepancy, but our findings warrant further examination. Within academia, upstream mentorship, funding, and research opportunities could have roles to play.

Third, while overall acceptance rates were lower for racially minoritized authors, it is important to note that post–peer review rejection rates were slightly higher for White authors than for Asian and Black authors. Within academic publishing, the longstanding belief has been that science should stand on its own merits, regardless of authorship. This is the core belief justifying masked peer review (historically called "blinded"), where the authors' names are withheld from the reviewers. We concur with others involved in academic publishing in the domains of health[20,21] and psychology[13] who have called for a re-examination of representation by racially minoritized authors in the literature.

Consider, also, that others have found that racially minoritized authors are cited less frequently than White scholars.[5] When less than 40% of published articles are from racially minoritized authors, and those articles are also less frequently cited, the impact of such science is comparatively limited. Taken together, our findings and previous studies suggest that the issues are not merely stochastic; academic social networks, hiring policies, funding, and many other factors may have led to inequities in scientific publishing. We provide 1 quantitative perspective, but clearly, more difficult questions and in-depth research into social and structural determinants are imperative.

These disparities underscore the need to address underlying causes. A recent study found that 77.2% of editors at leading medical and scientific journals were White, 14.9% Asian, 3.8% Hispanic, and 1.1% Black.[22] In addition, faculty of color and women faculty often shoulder more nonresearch duties, such as advising and committee work, which are less recognized in tenure evaluations, potentially hindering career progress and research output.[23,24] They also frequently face racial bias and discrimination, including microaggressions and a lack of colleague support.[25] Minoritized medical school faculty in the United States are promoted at lower rates than their White counterparts, with significantly fewer advancing from assistant or associate professor positions.[26]

We encourage continued review of the existing literature and future research on structural racism and gender discrimination in academia and administrative policies that may perpetuate or mitigate such disparities. Access to financial resources, support networks, and mentorship are likely significant factors affecting these outcomes. The complex dynamics before the submission of a scientific article play a crucial role in determining whose work is submitted and ultimately accepted.

Although our work is one of the few studies to examine racial bias in scientific publishing, we note that it represents only the experience from 1 journal and has inherent limitations. The use of only the corresponding author could also favor White authorship, because corresponding authors tend to have seniority within academic institutions and are often selected as corresponding authors because they have tenure, name recognition, or long-term job stability. In this way, the use of the corresponding author is a proxy for prestige and favored academic positions. Our analysis cannot evaluate the impact of the quality of submitted manuscripts; however, this could also be impacted by systematic inequities, such as unequal access to mentorship, funding, writing and language assistance, or research opportunities.

Our findings showed differences in the performance of the 3 algorithms used for race/ethnicity prediction. *pyethnicity* outperformed *rethnicity* and *predictrace*, achieving higher accuracy and precision, particularly for Asian and Hispanic categories. However, prediction accuracy was lower for Black and White categories across all algorithms, reflecting challenges in accurately classifying these groups. *predictrace* also faced significant coverage issues, failing to provide predictions for some names. These differences highlight the importance of algorithm design, including the quality and diversity of training data, and underscore the need for careful validation to ensure these tools do not amplify existing disparities or perpetuate inequities.

Several limitations of the algorithms could have impacted the observed results. First, all the algorithms were trained using US election data, with accuracy varying across states (Table F, available as a supplement to the online version of this article at https://ajph.org). This variation introduces uncertainty when predicting on a global scale. While we analyzed only US submissions, many authors could be from outside the United States. Second, our data may not capture surname changes from marriage, leading to discrepancies in predicted versus actual racial/ethnic identities, especially for female authors. Third, the race/ethnicity categories used (White, Asian, Black, Hispanic) do not capture other races/ethnicities such as Native American peoples; differences among Native Americans (e.g., Cherokee, Lumbee), Hispanics (e.g., Mexican, Cuban), or Asians (e.g., Indian, Chinese); further cultural and societal differences within these subcategories; or multiracial identities. Similarly, the gender identification algorithm only considers male and female categories, ignoring other gender identities like nonbinary. Furthermore, the similar disparity patterns observed across algorithms may reflect shared biases in their design or training data, such as overrepresentation or underrepresentation of certain groups, which could influence the results.

Our sensitivity analysis further revealed that varying probability thresholds influence the estimated acceptance rates across racial/ethnic groups. Higher thresholds resulted in estimates of a higher acceptance rate for White authors and a lower rate for Black authors, suggesting that acceptance rates for Black authors may be overestimated while those for White authors may be underestimated. These findings underscore the uncertainty in predictions for these groups and highlight the risks of relying solely on algorithmic predictions without addressing their inherent biases.

Despite these limitations, our analysis identified consistent trends. Most submissions came from White authors, who also had the highest acceptance rates. Women, while submitting more papers overall, had lower acceptance rates than men across most racial/ethnic groups. These disparities align with existing literature and underscore systemic inequities in academic publishing.

To address these issues, future studies would benefit from incorporating self-identified data on race/ethnicity and gender. Some journals have begun collecting such data voluntarily, which could improve analysis precision and provide deeper insights into disparities. These efforts, combined with continued refinement of prediction algorithms, are critical for developing strategies to promote equity in scholarly publishing. AJPH

## ABOUT THE AUTHORS

Yimeng Song is with the School of the Environment, Yale University, New Haven, CT. Nabarun Dasgupta is with the Gillings School of Global Public Health, University of North Carolina at Chapel Hill. Michelle L. Bell is with the School of the Environment, Yale University, New Haven, CT, and the School of Health Policy and Management, College of Health Sciences, Korea University, Seoul, Republic of Korea.

## CORRESPONDENCE

Correspondence should be sent to Yimeng Song, Yale University, School of the Environment, 195 Prospect St, New Haven, CT 06511 (e-mail: yimeng.song@yale.edu). Reprints can be ordered at https://www.ajph.org by clicking the "Reprints" link.

## PUBLICATION INFORMATION

Full Citation: Song Y, Dasgupta N, Bell ML. Evaluating algorithmic approaches to uncover racial, ethnic, and gender disparities in scientific authorship. *Am J Public Health*. 2025;115(7):1129–1136.

Acceptance Date: January 2, 2025.

DOI: https://doi.org/10.2105/AJPH.2025.308017

ORCID iD:

Yimeng Song https://orcid.org/0000-0001-9558-1220

## CONTRIBUTORS

Y. Song and M. L. Bell originated and developed the study's concept and hypothesis, conducted the analysis, and contributed to the overall conceptual framework and interpretation of the results. Y. Song, N. Dasgupta, and M. L. Bell contributed to the conclusions and preparation of the article.

## ACKNOWLEDGMENTS

We thank Meredith Loui for helping prepare the data set and Alfredo Morabia for valuable insights.

## CONFLICTS OF INTEREST

The authors have no conflicts of interest to report.

## HUMAN PARTICIPANT PROTECTION

Yale University's institutional review boards approved this project on May 31, 2023 (IRB-2000035422).

## REFERENCES


1. National Center for Education Statistics. Characteristics of postsecondary faculty. US Department of Education, Institute of Education Sciences. 2024. Available at: https://nces.ed.gov/programs/coe/indicator/csc. Accessed August 30, 2023.
2. US Census Bureau. Population estimates, July 1, 2023 (V2023). 2023. Available at: https://www.census.gov/quickfacts/fact/table/US/PST045221. Accessed August 30, 2023.
3. Colby G, Fowler C. Data snapshot: IPEDS data on full-time women faculty and faculty of color. American Association of University Professors. 2020. Available at: https://www.aaup.org/news/data-snapshot-full-time-women-faculty-and-faculty-color#.Y_MVrdVByUI. Accessed August 30, 2023.
4. Chen CY, Kahanamoku SS, Tripati A, et al. Systemic racial disparities in funding rates at the National Science Foundation. *eLife*. 2022;11:e83071. https://doi.org/10.7554/eLife.83071
5. Liu F, Rahwan T, AlShebli B. Non-White scientists appear on fewer editorial boards, spend more time under review, and receive fewer citations. *Proc Natl Acad Sci USA*. 2023;120(13):e2215324120. https://doi.org/10.1073/pnas.2215324120
6. Jagsi R, Guancial EA, Worobey CC, et al. The "gender gap" in authorship of academic medical literature—a 35-year perspective. *N Engl J Med*. 2006;355(3):281–287. https://doi.org/10.1056/NEJMsa053910
7. Bell ML, Fong KC. Gender differences in first and corresponding authorship in public health research submissions during the COVID-19 pandemic. *Am J Public Health*. 2021;111(1):159–163. https://doi.org/10.2105/AJPH.2020.305975
8. Bendels MHK, Müller R, Brueggmann D, Groneberg DA. Gender disparities in high-quality research revealed by Nature Index journals. *PLoS One*. 2018;13(1):e0189136. https://doi.org/10.1371/journal.pone.0189136
9. Andersen JP, Schneider JW, Jagsi R, Nielsen MW. Gender variations in citation distributions in medicine are very small and due to self-citation and journal prestige. *eLife*. 2019;8:e45374. https://doi.org/10.7554/eLife.45374
10. King MM, Bergstrom CT, Correll SJ, Jacquet J, West JD. Men set their own cites high: gender and self-citation across fields and over time. *Socius*. 2017;3:2378023117738903. https://doi.org/10.1177/2378023117738903
11. Hopkins AL, Jawitz JW, McCarty C, Goldman A, Basu NB. Disparities in publication patterns by gender, race and ethnicity based on a survey of a random sample of authors. *Scientometrics*. 2013;96(2):515–534. https://doi.org/10.1007/s11192-012-0893-4
12. Ginther DK, Basner J, Jensen U, Schnell J, Kington R, Schaffer WT. Publications as predictors of racial and ethnic differences in NIH research awards. *PLoS One*. 2018;13(11):e0205929. https://doi.org/10.1371/journal.pone.0205929
13. Roberts SO, Bareket-Shavit C, Dollins FA, Goldie PD, Mortenson E. Racial inequality in psychological research: trends of the past and recommendations for the future. *Perspect Psychol Sci*. 2020;15(6):1295–1309. https://doi.org/10.1177/1745691620927709
14. Richards M. BMJ journals collect gender, race, and ethnicity data on submissions. *BMJ*. 2022;379:o2542. https://doi.org/10.1136/bmj.o2542
15. Xie F. rethnicity: An R package for predicting ethnicity from names. *SoftwareX*. 2022;17:100965. https://doi.org/10.1016/j.softx.2021.100965
16. predictrace: Predict the Race and Gender of a Given Name Using Census and Social Security Administration Data. Version 1.7.1. 2023. Available at: https://github.com/jacobkap/predictrace. Accessed August 30, 2023.
17. Li C. Can we trust race prediction? Preprint. Posted online July 17, 2023. arXiv 230708496. https://doi.org/10.48550/arXiv.2307.08496
18. Kozlowski D, Murray DS, Bell A, et al. Avoiding bias when inferring race using name-based approaches. *PLoS One*. 2022;17(3):e0264270. https://doi.org/10.1371/journal.pone.0264270
19. Tzioumis K. Demographic aspects of first names. *Sci Data*. 2018;5(1):180025. https://doi.org/10.1038/sdata.2018.25
20. Watts V. Dismantling racism in scholarly publishing, intentionally and unapologetically. *Health Affairs Forefront*. January 26, 2021. https://doi.org/10.1377/forefront.20210125.666787
21. Boyd RW, Lindo EG, Weeks LD, McLemore MR. On racism: a new standard for publishing on racial health inequities. *Health Affairs Forefront*. July 2, 2020. https://doi.org/10.1377/forefront.20200630.939347
22. Salazar JW, Claytor JD, Habib AR, Guduguntla V, Redberg RF. Gender, race, ethnicity, and sexual orientation of editors at leading medical and scientific journals: a cross-sectional survey. *JAMA Intern Med*. 2021;181(9):1248–1251. https://doi.org/10.1001/jamainternmed.2021.2363
23. Misra J, Lundquist JH, Holmes E, Agiomavritis S. The ivory ceiling of service work. *Academe*. 2011;97(1):22–26.
24. Griffin KA, Reddick RJ. Surveillance and sacrifice: gender differences in the mentoring patterns of Black professors at predominantly White research universities. *Am Educ Res J*. 2011;48(5):1032–1057. https://doi.org/10.3102/0002831211405025
25. Garcia GA, Johnston-Guerrero MP. Challenging the utility of a racial microaggressions framework through a systematic review of racially biased incidents on campus. *J Crit Scholarship Higher Educ Student Aff*. 2015;2(1):48–66.
26. Fang D, Moy E, Colburn L, Hurley J. Racial and ethnic disparities in faculty promotion in academic medicine. *JAMA*. 2000;284(9):1085–1092. https://doi.org/10.1001/jama.284.9.1085

# Adverse Childhood Experiences Among LGBTQ+ High School Students: National Evidence From the 2023 Youth Risk Behavior Survey

Joel Mittleman, PhD

See also Cimpian and McQuillan, p. 982.

**Objectives.** To provide population-representative estimates of US high school students' exposure to adverse childhood experiences (ACEs), separately by sexual orientation, gender identity, and 3 demographic moderators: sex assigned at birth, race/ethnicity, and age.

**Methods.** Using data from the 2023 US National Youth Risk Behavior Survey (n = 12 131), this cross-sectional study calculated descriptive statistics, estimated multivariable regressions, and screened for mischievous respondents.

**Results.** Lesbian, gay, bisexual, transgender, and questioning (LGBTQ+) students reported elevated exposure to 8 separate ACEs, with a cumulative ACE score of 3.0 (95% confidence interval [CI] = 2.9, 3.1), compared with 1.8 (95% CI = 1.7, 1.9) among cisgender-heterosexual (cishet) students. This pattern held across all demographic subgroups and could not be explained by mischievous responders. Nearly half (46.1%; 95% CI = 39.7, 52.5) of all gender minorities reported 4 or more ACEs, compared with 34.5% (95% CI = 30.9, 38.0) of cisgender sexual minorities and 15.4% (95% CI = 14.2, 16.7) of cishet students.

**Conclusions.** The first national ACE prevalence data for US high school students show that LGBTQ+ youths—particularly transgender youths—face far greater levels of abuse, neglect, and other adversities than cishet youths. (*Am J Public Health*. 2025;115(7):1137–1145. https://doi.org/10.2105/AJPH.2025.308094)

AJPH July 2025, Vol. 115, No. 7

Adverse childhood experiences (ACEs) are potentially traumatic events or conditions occurring before adulthood, such as abuse (physical, emotional, or sexual), neglect, and the experience of household challenges, such as intimate partner violence or parental incarceration. Although experiencing any single ACE can be detrimental, the negative effects of ACEs rise sharply as children's total number of ACEs increases. A large body of research demonstrates a graded, dose–response relationship between cumulative ACE counts and increasingly negative health outcomes across the lifespan,[1–3] including early mortality.[4] The magnitude of these effects is often quite large. For instance, a 2016 meta-analysis estimated that, compared with those with no ACE exposure, adults who had experienced 4 or more ACEs had 2.3 times greater odds of being diagnosed with cancer, 10.2 times greater odds of developing a substance use disorder, and 30.1 times greater odds of attempting suicide.[2] Research suggests that these negative effects result not only from maladaptive coping behaviors, but also from more fundamental changes in the nervous, endocrine, and immune systems triggered by chronic, toxic stress.[5,6]

Although all children may be exposed to ACEs, the burden of ACE exposure is unequally distributed. Recent Centers for Disease Control and Prevention (CDC) estimates suggest that about 17% of American adults have experienced 4 or more ACEs, with higher levels of exposure among females (19%), lower-income households (24%), and certain minoritized groups, such as American Indians and Alaska Natives (32%).[7] Given ACEs' wide-ranging consequences as well as their unequal distribution, there is growing interest in preventing ACEs as a way to target population health disparities.[8,9]

One group that has attracted particular concern with respect to ACEs exposure is lesbian, gay, bisexual, transgender, and queer or questioning (LGBTQ+) youths. Research using in-depth interviews,[10] community-based surveys,[11] and online nonprobability samples[12,13] consistently finds that LGBTQ+ individuals report having experienced high levels of ACE exposure. For instance, in a large nonprobability sample of LGBTQ+ adolescents, 41% of all respondents reported experiencing 4 or more ACEs.[13]

Although studies like these play a vital role in illustrating the impact of ACEs for many LGBTQ+ young people, they cannot establish the full prevalence of ACE exposure within the population of LGBTQ+ youths at large. Population-representative research on ACE exposure among US LGBTQ+ individuals has primarily analyzed retrospective reports from LGBTQ+ adults,[14–20] whose experiences with families of origin may have been very different from those faced by LGBTQ+ youths today. When population-based studies have examined direct reports from LGBTQ+ youths themselves, they have been limited to individual states.[21,22] Moreover, much of the existing population-based research has been unable to specifically identify gender minorities[17–21] or has only analyzed them as part of a broader LGBTQ+ group.[15]

For all of these reasons, research is needed to document the extent of ACE exposure among contemporary LGBTQ+ youths. Drawing on a nationally representative survey of US high school students, the current study aimed to provide new population estimates of ACE exposure by sexual orientation and gender identity as well as 3 potentially important demographic moderators: sex assigned at birth, race/ethnicity, and age.

## METHODS

The current cross-sectional study took advantage of the important new possibilities created by the 2023 National Youth Risk Behavior Survey (YRBS). A biennial system of surveys sponsored by the CDC, the YRBS has tracked the health behaviors and experiences of US high school students since 1991. Employing a 3-stage cluster sampling design, the National YRBS is designed to generate a representative sample of students in grades 9 through 12 enrolled in public and private schools in all 50 states and the District of Columbia.[23] The 2023 National YRBS consisted of 107 questions and was completed anonymously by students on provided tablet devices in the spring of 2023.[23]

For the purposes of examining LGBTQ+ students' exposure to ACEs, the 2023 National YRBS marks a critical opportunity in 2 important regards. First, the 2023 survey introduced a new ACEs module designed to provide the first national prevalence estimates of self-reported ACEs among US high school students.[23] Second, beyond these historic data on ACEs, 2023 was also the first year that the National YRBS assessed gender identity, generating the first nationally representative sample of transgender high school students in the United States.[23] Together, these 2 new sets of items offer a unique opportunity to document ACE exposure among contemporary LGBTQ+ youths.

### Measures

*Adverse childhood experiences.* This study analyzed responses to a set of 8 questions assessing lifetime exposure to ACEs. Designed to measure the same domains as the original ACEs study,[1] the 2023 National YRBS ACEs module included 3 questions on abuse (physical, emotional, and sexual) by parents or other adults, 1 question on neglect (the absence of an adult working to meet the child's basic needs), and 4 questions on household challenges (intimate partner violence, caregiver substance abuse, caregiver mental health challenges, and caregiver incarceration or detention). Physical abuse was assessed as whether "a parent or other adult in your home hit, beat, kicked, or physically hurt you in any way," emotional abuse as whether "a parent or other adult in your home insulted you or put you down," and sexual abuse as whether "an adult or person at least 5 years older than you made you do sexual things that you did not want to do." Complete question wordings for all ACE items are provided in Appendix Table A (available as a supplement to the online version of this article at http://www.ajph.org). Notably, the YRBS did not assess 2 additional ACEs commonly included in ACE scales—parental separation or divorce and emotional neglect—nor did it assess any of the expanded ACE items recently designed to capture childhood adversities rooted in structural racism[24,25] and cisheterosexism.[26,27]

Four of the ACE questions assessed the frequency of exposure and 4 only offered yes/no response options.

To maintain consistency with prior ACE research, I dichotomized all items into binary indicators of any exposure or none. In addition to analyzing each exposure separately, I calculated students' cumulative ACE scores and summarized them using the established cutoffs in this literature: zero, 1, 2 to 3, and 4 or more.

*Sexual orientation and gender identity.* I identified LGBTQ+ students using 2 separate survey items assessing sexual orientation and gender identity. For sexual orientation, students were asked, "Which of the following best describes you?" and provided with the following response options: "heterosexual (straight); gay or lesbian; bisexual; I describe my sexual identity some other way; I am not sure about my sexual identity (questioning)." For gender identity, students were given a definition of the word transgender and asked, "Are you transgender?" with the following response options: "no, I am not transgender; yes, I am transgender; I am not sure if I am transgender." Both items also included the response option, "I do not know what this question is asking."

The current study's primary comparisons were between cisgender heterosexual (cishet) students—those who selected "heterosexual (straight)" and "no, I am not transgender"—and LGBTQ+ students—those who selected any other combination of sexual orientation and gender identity options, excluding those who selected "I do not know what this question is asking." For space, results for students who answered "I do not know what this question is asking" are presented in the Appendix.

In addition to examining LGBTQ+ students overall, this study also documented the distinct experiences of cisgender sexual minorities and transgender or gender questioning students of all sexual identities. As shown in the Appendix, students who answered "Yes, I am transgender" and students who answered "I am not sure if I am transgender" reported ACE exposures that were statistically indistinguishable from one another; therefore, to maximize sample sizes and simplify the presentation of results, this study combined them into a single gender minority group. By separately analyzing cisgender sexual minorities and gender minorities in this way, this study followed the approach taken in prior research.[11,12,14,22]

*Demographic controls and moderators.* This study's regression analyses control for 3 demographic characteristics of students: their sex assigned at birth, race/ethnicity, and age. To avoid sparse cell counts, I operationalized age in 3 categories—12 through 14, 15 and 16, and 17 years and older—and race/ethnicity in 6 categories—White (non-Hispanic), Black or African American, Asian and Pacific Islander, Hispanic or Latino, American Indian or Alaska Native, and Multiracial. Sex was assessed with the item, "What is your sex? Female; Male." Although this item is imprecise in its wording, I interpret it as a measure of sex assigned at birth. After primary analyses that control for student demographics, this study also tested whether LGBTQ+ students' ACE exposure varies across demographic groups, interacting LGBTQ+ identification and each demographic characteristic.

## Statistical Analysis

Of the 20 103 students who participated in the 2023 National YRBS, 2166 did not answer the sexual orientation or gender identity items. Excluding these observations as well as those who didn't report their age, race/ethnicity, or sex (n = 280) yields an initial analytic sample of 17 566 students. Within this sample, 69% (n = 12 131) provided complete responses for all ACE items. This degree of missingness on ACE questions is consistent with that found in nonprobability samples of LGBTQ+ adolescents[12] and is only somewhat higher than that found among representative surveys of US adults.[15]

Analyzing the 12 131 students who provided complete data, this study reported descriptive statistics, calculated adjusted risk ratios using log-binomial regressions, and calculated adjusted ACE scores using Poisson regressions. To account for the multiple outcomes and comparison groups being analyzed in these regressions, a Bonferroni correction was applied and a new statistical significance cutoff of $P < .001$ was set. All results were calculated using CDC-provided weights to account for the YRBS's complex sampling design and adjusted for school and student nonresponse.[23]

To adjust for potential mischievous respondents in the data,[28–30] this study adopted Cimpian, Timmer, and Kim's screening and reweighting approach.[30] This approach, described more fully in the Appendix, trains a boosted logistic regression to predict students' likelihood of mischievously identifying as LGBTQ+ based on their responses to 6 screener items. Unlike earlier approaches, which removed possible mischievous responders above a given threshold,[28,29] this approach retains all observations but reweights LGBTQ+ students' responses by their inverse probability of mischievous response.[30] Raw results, unadjusted for mischievous response, are substantively similar and presented in the Appendix.

## RESULTS

Table 1 reports the demographic characteristics of the sample. Overall, 24.2% (unweighted n = 2926) of students identified as LGBTQ+, with 19.3% (n = 2305) identifying as cisgender sexual minorities and 4.9% (n = 621) identifying as transgender or gender questioning. When demographic characteristics of LGBTQ+ students and cishet students were compared, the most pronounced difference was in sex assigned at birth. Consistent with prior years of the YRBS,[31] LGBTQ+ identification was more common among those who reported that their sex was female. In an overall sample in which 47.7% of students reported being female, female students constituted 73.9% of the LGBTQ+ sample but only 39.7% of the cishet sample. These and other demographic differences across groups illustrate the potential importance of adjusting for demographic characteristics when estimating LGBTQ+ and cishet students' patterns of ACE exposure.

Table 2 presents descriptive statistics on the estimated lifetime prevalence of ACE exposure across groups. In every category of ACE exposure, LGBTQ+ students reported experiencing greater adversity than cishet students. Although both cisgender sexual minorities and gender minorities reported an elevated prevalence of ACEs, ACE exposure was consistently highest among gender minority students. For instance, the estimates in Table 2 imply that nearly half (46.1%) of all transgender or gender questioning high school students in the United States had experienced 4 or more ACEs by the spring of 2023, compared with 34.5% of cisgender sexual minorities and 15.4% of cishet students.

Focusing specifically on experiences of abuse underscores the magnitude of ACE exposure among contemporary LGBTQ+ high school students. Emotional abuse was reported by 81.6% of LGBTQ+ students compared with 56.2% of cishet students. Among gender minority students, emotional abuse was a nearly universal experience, reported by 91.7% of all respondents.

**TABLE 1— Demographic Characteristics of the Analytic Sample: United States, National Youth Risk Behavior Survey, 2023**

| | Overall Sample, No. (%) | Cisgender Heterosexual, No. (%) | LGBTQ+, No. (%) | Cisgender Sexual Minority, No. (%) | Transgender and Gender Questioning, No. (%) |
|---|---|---|---|---|---|
| Age, y | | | | | |
| 12–14 | 1461 (12.7) | 1058 (12.6) | 360 (13.0) | 287 (13.4) | 73 (11.5) |
| 15–16 | 6391 (50.4) | 4664 (50.6) | 1561 (49.7) | 1209 (49.5) | 352 (50.5) |
| ≥ 17 | 4279 (36.9) | 3144 (36.8) | 1005 (37.3) | 809 (37.1) | 196 (37.9) |
| Assigned sex | | | | | |
| Female | 5986 (47.7) | 3659 (39.7) | 2214 (73.9) | 1803 (75.6) | 411 (67.1) |
| Male | 6145 (52.3) | 5207 (60.3) | 712 (26.1) | 502 (24.4) | 210 (32.9) |
| Race/ethnicity | | | | | |
| Black or African American | 1439 (15.4) | 1031 (15.3) | 369 (15.8) | 322 (17.6) | 47 (8.6) |
| Hispanic | 593 (7.4) | 468 (8.2) | 99 (4.6) | 83 (5.1) | 16 (2.8) |
| White | 5616 (47.2) | 1348 (46.9) | 1348 (49.6) | 1001 (47) | 347 (59.7) |
| Asian American and Pacific Islander | 603 (4.4) | 455 (4.6) | 122 (3.3) | 101 (3.3) | 21 (3.3) |
| American Indian or Alaska Native | 847 (0.3) | 617 (0.2) | 182 (0.4) | 147 (0.4) | 35 (0.4) |
| Multiracial | 3033 (25.3) | 2138 (24.8) | 806 (26.2) | 651 (26.5) | 155 (25.2) |
| Unweighted sample size (weighted %) | 12131 (100.0) | 8866 (73.2) | 2926 (24.2) | 2305 (19.3) | 621 (4.9) |

*Note.* Data are from the 2023 National Youth Risk Behavior Survey. LBGTQ+ = lesbian, gay, bisexual, transgender, "I describe my sexual identity some other way," or questioning sexual orientation/gender identity. Results for students who answered "I do not know what this question is asking" for sexual orientation or gender identity (n = 339) are presented in the Appendix (available as a supplement to the online version of this article at http://www.ajph.org). All percentages are calculated using Centers for Disease Control and Prevention–provided sampling weights that adjust for complex sampling design as well as school and student nonresponse.

**TABLE 2— Prevalence of Adverse Childhood Experiences (ACEs) Among High School Students: United States, National Youth Risk Behavior Survey, 2023**

| | Overall Sample | Cisgender Heterosexual | LGBTQ+ | Cisgender Sexual Minority | Transgender and Gender Questioning |
|---|---|---|---|---|---|
| Physical abuse, % (95% CI) | 31.8 (29.7, 33.8) | 28.1 (26, 30.2) | 43.9 (41.4, 46.3) | 41.3 (38.4, 44.3) | 54.1 (48.6, 59.5) |
| Emotional abuse, % (95% CI) | 61.9 (59.3, 64.5) | 56.2 (53.7, 58.6) | 81.6 (78.9, 84.3) | 79.1 (76.3, 81.9) | 91.7 (88.1, 95.2) |
| Sexual abuse, % (95% CI) | 7.0 (6.1, 7.9) | 4.1 (3.4, 4.7) | 15.9 (12.9, 18.9) | 14.7 (11.5, 17.9) | 20.6 (15.2, 26) |
| Physical neglect, % (95% CI) | 23.3 (21.8, 24.9) | 20.7 (19, 22.3) | 29.7 (27.1, 32.2) | 27.8 (25.3, 30.3) | 37.3 (32.7, 41.9) |
| Witnessed intimate partner violence, % (95% CI) | 17.6 (16.4, 18.7) | 14.7 (13.5, 15.9) | 26.8 (24, 29.6) | 26.6 (23.5, 29.7) | 27.6 (22.8, 32.3) |
| Household substance use, % (95% CI) | 24.4 (22.3, 26.4) | 20.3 (18.4, 22.1) | 36.8 (33.3, 40.2) | 35.5 (32, 39) | 42 (36.7, 47.3) |
| Household poor mental health, % (95% CI) | 28.8 (26.5, 31.1) | 22.6 (20.8, 24.4) | 48.2 (44.4, 52.1) | 46.3 (42.2, 50.3) | 56.3 (49.7, 62.9) |
| Parent or guardian incarcerated or detained, % (95% CI) | 13.3 (11.8, 14.9) | 11.7 (10.2, 13.3) | 18.0 (15, 20.9) | 18.6 (15.3, 21.8) | 15.6 (10.8, 20.5) |
| No ACEs, % (95% CI) | 22.3 (20.5, 24.1) | 26.6 (24.8, 28.4) | 8.7 (7.3, 10.1) | 10 (8.4, 11.6) | 3.6 (1.8, 5.4) |
| 1 ACE, % (95% CI) | 24.1 (23.2, 24.9) | 26.0 (25.0, 27.1) | 17.6 (16, 19.2) | 18.1 (16.6, 19.6) | 15.6 (11.5, 19.6) |
| 2 or 3 ACEs, % (95% CI) | 32.8 (31.1, 34.6) | 32.0 (30.3, 33.6) | 36.9 (33.8, 39.9) | 37.4 (33.9, 40.9) | 34.7 (29.5, 40) |
| ≥4 ACEs, % (95% CI) | 20.8 (19.2, 22.3) | 15.4 (14.2, 16.7) | 36.8 (33.4, 40.1) | 34.5 (30.9, 38) | 46.1 (39.7, 52.5) |
| Cumulative ACE score, mean (95% CI) | 2.1 (2, 2.2) | 1.8 (1.7, 1.9) | 3 (2.9, 3.1) | 2.9 (2.8, 3) | 3.5 (3.2, 3.7) |

*Note.* Data are from the 2023 National Youth Risk Behavior Survey. LBGTQ+ = lesbian, gay, bisexual, transgender, "I describe my sexual identity some other way," or questioning sexual orientation/gender identity. Results for students who answered "I do not know what this question is asking" for sexual orientation or gender identity are presented in the Appendix (available as a supplement to the online version of this article at http://www.ajph.org). All estimates calculated using Centers for Disease Control and Prevention–provided sampling weights that adjust for complex sampling design as well as school and student nonresponse. LGBTQ+, cisgender sexual minority, and transgender/gender questioning students' responses are weighted by the inverse probability of mischievous response; further details and unweighted responses provided in the Appendix.

Although emotional abuse was the most common form of abuse reported, experiences of physical and sexual abuse were also widespread. For instance, over half (54.1%) of all gender minority students reported physical abuse, compared with 41.3% of cisgender sexual minorities and 28.1% of cishet students.

To test whether these disparities were driven, in part, by compositional differences between those who did or did not identify as LGBTQ+ on this survey, Table 3 reports the results of log-binomial regressions controlling for students' assigned sex, race/ethnicity, and age. In every ACE category, LGBTQ+ students were significantly ($P<.001$) more likely to report ACE exposure.

Of all forms of ACE exposure, sexual abuse stands out as exhibiting the largest disparities between cishet and LGBTQ+ students. Compared with demographically similar cishet students, LGBTQ+ students were an estimated 2.71 times as likely to report having experienced sexual abuse. Here, too, gender minority students faced the most pronounced disparities. Compared with demographically similar cishet students, gender minorities were an estimated 3.69 times as likely to report sexual abuse.

Whereas the results in Table 3 controlled for student demographic characteristics, it is also possible that LGBTQ+ students' risk for ACEs may vary across demographic groups.

To explore this possibility, Figure 1 presents the results of 3 separate Poisson regressions modeling students' cumulative ACE counts, allowing the effect of LGBTQ+ identity to vary by each demographic characteristic. Sample size constraints prevented an analysis of interaction effects among cisgender sexual minorities and gender minorities separately.

Figure 1 illustrates that LGBTQ+ students experienced a greater cumulative total of ACEs within every demographic group analyzed. Even so, there is variation in ACE counts across groups, particularly by race/ethnicity. Consistent with recent CDC estimates for the US adult population overall,[7] Figure 1 shows that the cumulative burden of

AJPH July 2025, Vol. 115, No. 7

**TABLE 3— Regression Adjusted Risk Ratios for Adverse Childhood Experiences (ACEs) Exposure Among High School Students: United States, National Youth Risk Behavior Survey, 2023**

| | LGBTQ+ vs Cisgender Heterosexual, ARR (99.9% CI) | Cisgender Sexual Minority vs Cisgender Heterosexual, ARR (99.9% CI) | Transgender and Gender Questioning vs Cisgender Heterosexual, ARR (99.9% CI) |
|---|---|---|---|
| Physical abuse | 1.57 (1.38, 1.77) | 1.46 (1.27, 1.68) | 2.00 (1.61, 2.48) |
| Emotional abuse | 1.37 (1.28, 1.46) | 1.33 (1.23, 1.43) | 1.53 (1.42, 1.65) |
| Sexual abuse | 2.71 (1.64, 4.47) | 2.48 (1.43, 4.28) | 3.69 (2.07, 6.59) |
| Physical neglect | 1.43 (1.18, 1.72) | 1.33 (1.11, 1.59) | 1.85 (1.39, 2.47) |
| Witnessed intimate partner violence | 1.63 (1.28, 2.08) | 1.60 (1.24, 2.07) | 1.75 (1.20, 2.56) |
| Household substance use | 1.61 (1.32, 1.97) | 1.57 (1.28, 1.93) | 1.76 (1.35, 2.28) |
| Household poor mental health | 1.90 (1.64, 2.19) | 1.83 (1.57, 2.13) | 2.14 (1.70, 2.70) |
| Parent incarcerated or detained | 1.49 (1.12, 1.98) | 1.53 (1.12, 2.08) | 1.35 (0.79, 2.29) |
| No ACEs | 0.37 (0.27, 0.49) | 0.42 (0.31, 0.57) | 0.15 (0.06, 0.35) |
| 1 ACE | 0.68 (0.57, 0.80) | 0.70 (0.60, 0.82) | 0.59 (0.38, 0.93) |
| 2 or 3 ACEs | 1.16 (1.01, 1.33) | 1.17 (1.00, 1.38) | 1.10 (0.85, 1.42) |
| ≥4 ACEs | 2.12 (1.74, 2.58) | 1.98 (1.62, 2.43) | 2.66 (1.94, 3.65) |

*Note.* ARR = adjusted risk ratio; CI = confidence interval; LBGTQ+ = lesbian, gay, bisexual, transgender, "I describe my sexual identity some other way," or questioning sexual orientation/gender identity. Statistical significance cutoffs were established applying Bonferroni correction for multiple comparisons. All estimates are exponentiated coefficients from log-binominal regressions controlling for students' sex, race/ethnicity, and age, calculated using Centers for Disease Control and Prevention–provided sampling weights that adjust for complex sampling design as well as school and student nonresponse. LGBTQ+, cisgender sexual minority, and transgender/gender questioning students' students' responses are weighted by the inverse probability of mischievous response; further details and unweighted responses provided in the Appendix (available as a supplement to the online version of this article at http://www.ajph.org). Results for students who answered "I do not know what this question is asking" for sexual orientation or gender identity are presented in the Appendix.

ACE exposure was highest among American Indian or Alaska Native students. The estimates in Figure 1 imply that American Indian or Alaska Native high school students who identified as LGBTQ+ had experienced, on average, 3.5 ACEs by the spring of 2023. Notably, these estimates revealing the distinctly high burden of ACEs among LGBTQ+ American Indian or Alaska Native students were made possible by the fact that the 2023 National YRBS was the first ever to include a large oversample of American Indian or Alaska Native students.[23]

## DISCUSSION

Drawing on the first CDC data designed to provide national prevalence estimates of self-reported ACEs among American high school students,[23] this study documented that LGBTQ+ students face substantially greater exposure to ACEs than their cishet peers. LGBTQ+ students reported a higher prevalence on all 8 items in the YRBS ACEs module, cumulatively reporting an ACE score of 3.0 compared with the 1.8 reported by cishet students. LGBTQ+ students' elevated exposure to ACEs was reported across all demographic subgroups, with the highest ACE scores being reported by LGBTQ+ American Indians and Alaska Natives. With nearly 1 in 4 students in this sample identifying as LGBTQ+, these widespread ACE exposures could forebode substantial population health challenges as this cohort ages into adulthood.

Although elevated levels of ACE exposure were reported by both cisgender sexual minorities and gender minorities, gender minorities consistently reported the highest levels of ACEs of all groups. In analyses made possible by the first gender identity item ever included in a nationally representative survey of current US high school students,[23] this study underscored the importance of analyzing the distinct experiences of gender minorities over and above those of LGBTQ+ youths overall.

Troublingly, the levels of abuse reported by LGBTQ+ high school students in this nationally representative sample surpass those previously reported in nonprobability samples of LGBTQ+ adolescents.[12,13] For instance, in a sample of adolescents recruited through social media and community organizations, Thoma et al.[12] found that 71% of gender minorities reported emotional abuse, 40% reported physical

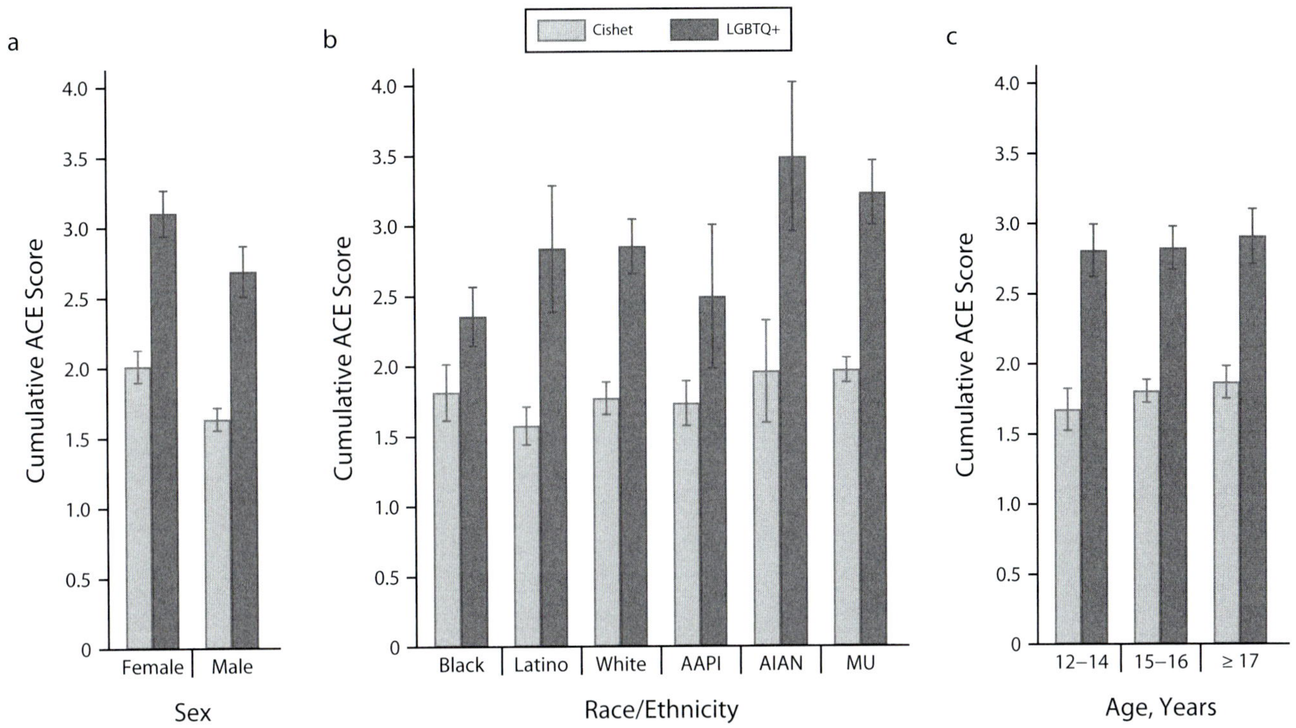


**FIGURE 1— Regression Adjusted Cumulative Adverse Childhood Experiences (ACE) Scores Across Demographic Subgroups: United States, National Youth Risk Behavior Survey, 2023**

*Note.* AAPI = Asian American or Pacific Islander; AIAN = American Indian and Alaska Native; Black = Black or African American; Cishet = cisgender and heterosexual; Latino = Latino or Hispanic; LBGTQ+ = lesbian, gay, bisexual, transgender, "I describe my sexual identity some other way," or questioning sexual orientation/gender identity; MU = Multiracial. Estimates from 3 separate Poisson regressions, interacting LGBTQ+ identity with highlighted demographic characteristic, controlling for the other 2 demographic characteristics, calculated using Centers for Disease Control and Prevention–provided sampling weights that adjust for complex sampling design as well as school and student nonresponse. LGBTQ+ students' responses are weighted by the inverse probability of mischievous response; further details and unweighted responses provided in the Appendix (available as a supplement to the online version of this article at http://www.ajph.org).

abuse, and 19% reported sexual abuse. By contrast, in the 2023 National YRBS, 92% of gender minorities reported emotional abuse, 54% reported physical abuse, and 21% reported sexual abuse. As such, the United States' first nationally representative sample of gender minority high school students didn't just affirm the results of prior nonprobability samples; if anything, it indicated that prior samples had underestimated the full extent of abuse that gender minority youths face.

These results have important implications for broader understandings of LGBTQ+ health and well-being. They suggest that many LGBTQ+ population health disparities may reflect not just minority stress and discrimination experienced in adulthood, but also the longer shadow of adversities endured in childhood. Indeed, it is notable that LGBTQ+ students' ACE scores increased only slightly across age groups, with large disparities already firmly established among those aged 12 to 14 years. This fact emphasizes the importance of understanding LGBTQ+ youths' earliest experiences, identifying common sensitive periods when intervention could occur. This study's results also underscore the central role of families of origin in shaping LGBTQ+ well-being.[32] The widespread abuse and disproportionate exposure to household challenges reported by the LGBTQ+ youths in this study illustrate the necessity of analyzing the family as a key social institution implicated in the production of LGBTQ+ health disparities, alongside other institutions like schools, health care providers, and religious institutions.

## Limitations

Despite the unique strengths of the 2023 National YRBS data, this study's conclusions come with important limitations.

First, although the amount of missing data in this study is consistent with that found in other research on LGBTQ+ ACE exposure,[12,15] the overall reduction in sample size makes it difficult to be certain how the results reported here would generalize to the full population of US high school students. Moreover, even if this study's sample were to be representative of all US high school students, the YRBS is not designed to be representative of all US adolescents more broadly. To the extent that LGBTQ+ youths—particularly those experiencing high levels of ACEs—are less stably connected to school attendance, this study's sample will systematically understate the true prevalence of ACEs among LGBTQ+ youths in the United States.

Second, and relatedly, although this study analyzed students' responses to every survey question included in the YRBS ACEs module, these items do not exhaust the traumatic stressors to which LGBTQ+ youths are disproportionately exposed. As emphasized by the sexual and gender minority ACEs framework,[26,27] there are many LGBTQ+ specific adversities—such as "conversion therapy" and homophobic or transphobic religious teachings—that affect LGBTQ+ well-being over and above traditional ACEs. In this regard as well, this study's results reflect a lower bound estimate on the full burden of ACEs among contemporary LGBTQ+ youths.

Third, although the inclusion of a gender identity item in the 2023 National YRBS marks a critical milestone in the recognition of transgender students, the item itself may fail to capture gender diverse students who did not identify with the specific term "transgender." This study's results for transgender and gender questioning students cannot be assumed to reflect the potentially distinct experiences of gender nonbinary, genderfluid, or genderqueer students.[33]

Finally, although the YRBS data allow for new estimates of ACE prevalence, the YRBS is unable to address the specific mechanisms through which LGBTQ+ youths come to experience ACEs. No research has found that ACEs "cause" LGBTQ+ identities.[17,19] However, more research is needed to explore how LGBTQ+ youths come to experience, for example, elevated levels of parental incarceration or detention. Understanding the specific social processes by which LGBTQ+ youths come to face higher levels of ACEs—particularly household challenge ACEs—should be an important priority for future research.

## Public Health Implications

The results reported in this study emphasize the importance of working to prevent, monitor, and mitigate the impact of ACEs in the United States. Although there is debate regarding the wisdom of universal ACE screening by pediatric care providers,[34] the historic inclusion of an ACEs module in the 2023 National YRBS illustrates the viability and value of large-scale public surveillance efforts in this area. To track trends and allow comparisons across contexts, ACE items should become an ongoing component of existing national, state, and local public health surveillance systems. Amid a political and policy environment that is growing increasingly hostile to LGBTQ+ youths, monitoring LGBTQ+ youths' exposure to abuse is likely to become even more important in the years to come.

The breadth of ACEs reported by the LGBTQ+ youths in this study indicates that the particular needs of this population must be an essential part of any broader strategy for addressing ACEs in the United States. With 37% of all LGBTQ+ students enrolled in US high schools currently reporting 4 or more ACEs, this study's results emphasize the importance of preventing ACEs as a way to address LGBTQ+ population health disparities. This study's results also underscore the importance of a trauma-informed approach to care and services for LGBTQ+ populations, particularly gender minority populations.[35] AJPH

### ABOUT THE AUTHOR

Joel Mittleman is with the Department of Sociology and the Population Studies Center, University of Pennsylvania, Philadelphia.

### CORRESPONDENCE

Correspondence should be sent to Joel Mittleman, University of Pennsylvania, 274 McNeil Building, Philadelphia, PA 19104 (e-mail: jmittlem@sas.upenn.edu). Reprints can be ordered at https://www.ajph.org by clicking the "Reprints" link.

### PUBLICATION INFORMATION

Full Citation: Mittleman J. Adverse childhood experiences among LGBTQ+ high school students: national evidence from the 2023 Youth Risk Behavior Survey. *Am J Public Health*. 2025; 115(7):1137–1145.

Acceptance Date: February 19, 2025.

DOI: https://doi.org/10.2105/AJPH.2025.308094

ORCID iD:

Joel Mittleman https://orcid.org/0000-0001-6353-7890

### ACKNOWLEDGMENTS

This study was supported through the University of Pennsylvania's Population Studies Center, National Institute of Child Health and Human Development (grant P2CHD044964).

I thank 3 anonymous reviewers for their insightful feedback and recommendations.

### CONFLICTS OF INTEREST

The author has no conflicts of interest to disclose.

### HUMAN PARTICIPANT PROTECTION

Because it used de-identified, publicly available data, this study was deemed exempt by the institutional review board of the University of Pennsylvania.

### REFERENCES

1. Felitti VJ, Anda RF, Nordenberg D, et al. Relationship of childhood abuse and household dysfunction to many of the leading causes of death in adults. The Adverse Childhood Experiences (ACE)

Study. *Am J Prev Med.* 1998;14(4):245–258. https://doi.org/10.1016/S0749-3797(98)00017-8

2. Hughes K, Bellis MA, Hardcastle KA, et al. The effect of multiple adverse childhood experiences on health: a systematic review and meta-analysis. *Lancet Public Health.* 2017;2(8):e356–e366. https://doi.org/10.1016/S2468-2667(17)30118-4
3. Merrick MT, Ford DC, Ports KA, et al. Vital signs: estimated proportion of adult health problems attributable to adverse childhood experiences and implications for prevention—25 states, 2015–2017. *MMWR Morb Mortal Wkly Rep.* 2019; 68(44):999–1005. https://doi.org/10.15585/mmwr.mm6844e1
4. Brown DW, Anda RF, Tiemeier H, et al. Adverse childhood experiences and the risk of premature mortality. *Am J Prev Med.* 2009;37(5):389–396. https://doi.org/10.1016/j.amepre.2009.06.021
5. Danese A, McEwen BS. Adverse childhood experiences, allostasis, allostatic load, and age-related disease. *Physiol Behav.* 2012;106(1): 29–39. https://doi.org/10.1016/j.physbeh.2011.08.019
6. Pechtel P, Pizzagalli DA. Effects of early life stress on cognitive and affective function: an integrated review of human literature. *Psychopharmacology (Berl).* 2011;214(1):55–70. https://doi.org/10.1007/s00213-010-2009-2
7. Swedo EA, Aslam MV, Dahlberg LL, et al. Prevalence of adverse childhood experiences among US adults—Behavioral Risk Factor Surveillance System, 2011. *MMWR Morb Mortal Wkly Rep.* 2023;72(26):707–715. https://doi.org/10.15585/mmwr.mm7226a2
8. Jones CM, Merrick MT, Houry DE. Identifying and preventing adverse childhood experiences: implications for clinical practice. *JAMA.* 2020; 323(1):25–26. https://doi.org/10.1001/jama.2019.18499
9. Guinn AS, Ottley PG, Anderson KN, Oginga ML, Gervin DW, Holmes GM. Leveraging surveillance and evidence: preventing adverse childhood experiences through data to action. *Am J Prev Med.* 2022;62(6 suppl 1):S24–S30. https://doi.org/10.1016/j.amepre.2021.12.003
10. Stone AL, Nimmons E, Salcido R. Refusing gender: intimate (mis)recognition of gender identity and its relation to family instabilities. *Gend Soc.* 2024;38(5):788–815. https://doi.org/10.1177/08912432241277218
11. Schnarrs PW, Stone AL, Salcido R Jr, Baldwin A, Georgiou C, Nemeroff CB. Differences in adverse childhood experiences (ACEs) and quality of physical and mental health between transgender and cisgender sexual minorities. *J Psychiatr Res.* 2019;119:1–6. https://doi.org/10.1016/j.jpsychires.2019.09.001
12. Thoma BC, Rezeppa TL, Choukas-Bradley S, Salk RH, Marshal MP. Disparities in childhood abuse between transgender and cisgender adolescents. *Pediatrics.* 2021;148(2):e2020016907. https://doi.org/10.1542/peds.2020-016907
13. Craig SL, Austin A, Levenson J, Leung VWY, Eaton AD, D'Souza SA. Frequencies and patterns of adverse childhood events in LGBTQ+ youth. *Child Abuse Negl.* 2020;107:104623. https://doi.org/10.1016/j.chiabu.2020.104623
14. Solberg MA, Blair LM, Schlegel EC, Kurzer JAMJ. Health disparities among sexual and gender minorities with adverse childhood experiences: insights from the 2021 Behavioral Risk Factor Surveillance System Data. *Am J Public Health.* 2023;113(12):1343–1351. https://doi.org/10.2105/AJPH.2023.307420
15. Hughes PM, Ostrout TL, Pérez Jolles M, Thomas KC. Adverse childhood experiences across birth generation and LGBTQ+ identity, Behavioral Risk Factor Surveillance System, 2019. *Am J Public Health.* 2022;112(4):662–670. https://doi.org/10.2105/AJPH.2021.306642
16. Tran NM, Mann S, Cortez MG, Harrell B, Nettuno L. Adverse childhood experiences (ACEs) and mental health by gender identity in the United States, 2019–2021. *Prev Med.* 2023;175:107705. https://doi.org/10.1016/j.ypmed.2023.107705
17. Giano Z, Wheeler DL, Hubach RD. The frequencies and disparities of adverse childhood experiences in the US. *BMC Public Health.* 2020;20(1): 1327. https://doi.org/10.1186/s12889-020-09411-z
18. Austin A, Herrick H, Proescholdbell S. Adverse childhood experiences related to poor adult health among lesbian, gay, and bisexual individuals. *Am J Public Health.* 2016;106(2):314–320. https://doi.org/10.2105/AJPH.2015.302904
19. Tran NM, Henkhaus LE, Gonzales G. Adverse childhood experiences and mental distress among US adults by sexual orientation. *JAMA Psychiatry.* 2022;79(4):377–379. https://doi.org/10.1001/jamapsychiatry.2022.0001
20. Mersky JP, Lee CP, Hami D. Adverse childhood experiences and sexual orientation: an intersectional analysis of nationally representative data. *Am J Prev Med.* 2024;66(3):483–491. https://doi.org/10.1016/j.amepre.2023.10.015
21. Clements-Nolle K, Lensch T, Baxa A, Gay C, Larson S, Yang W. Sexual identity, adverse childhood experiences, and suicidal behaviors. *J Adolesc Health.* 2018;62(2):198–204. https://doi.org/10.1016/j.jadohealth.2017.09.022
22. Baams L. Disparities for LGBTQ and gender nonconforming adolescents. *Pediatrics.* 2018;141(5): e20173004. https://doi.org/10.1542/peds.2017-3004
23. Brener ND, Mpofu JJ, Krause KH, et al. Overview and methods for the Youth Risk Behavior Surveillance System—United States, 2023. *MMWR Suppl.* 2024;73(4):1–12. https://doi.org/10.15585/mmwr.su7304a1
24. Bernard DL, Calhoun CD, Banks DE, Halliday CA, Hughes-Halbert C, Danielson CK. Making the "C-ACE" for a culturally-informed adverse childhood experiences framework to understand the pervasive mental health impact of racism on black youth. *J Child Adolesc Trauma.* 2020;14(2): 233–247. https://doi.org/10.1007/s40653-020-00319-9
25. Zhen-Duan J, Colombo D, Alvarez K. Inclusion of expanded adverse childhood experiences in research about racial/ethnic substance use disparities. *Am J Public Health.* 2023;113(S2):S129–S132. https://doi.org/10.2105/AJPH.2023.307220
26. Schnarrs PW, Dorri AA, Yockey RA, Stone AL, Russell ST, Rosenberger JG. The Sexual and Gender Minority Adverse Childhood Experiences Scale. *Am J Prev Med.* 2023;65(6):1050–1058. https://doi.org/10.1016/j.amepre.2023.08.006
27. Kennedy KS, Johns MM, Schnarrs PW, Russell ST. Cisheterosexism as childhood adversity: implications for sexual and gender minority health. *Am J Prev Med.* 2025;68(4):824–827. https://doi.org/10.1016/j.amepre.2024.12.015
28. Cimpian JR, Timmer JD, Birkett MA, Marro RL, Turner BC, Phillips GL 2nd. Bias from potentially mischievous responders on large-scale estimates of lesbian, gay, bisexual, or questioning (LGBQ)-heterosexual youth health disparities. *Am J Public Health.* 2018;108(S4):S258–S265. https://doi.org/10.2105/AJPH.2018.304407
29. Cimpian JR, Timmer JD. Large-scale estimates of LGBQ-heterosexual disparities in the presence of potentially mischievous responders: a preregistered replication and comparison of methods. *AERA Open.* 2019;5(4):2332858419888892. https://doi.org/10.1177/2332858419888892
30. Cimpian JR, Timmer JD, Kim TH. Mitigating invalid and mischievous survey responses: a registered report examining risk disparities between heterosexual and lesbian, gay, bisexual, or questioning youth. *Child Dev.* 2023;94(5):1136–1161. https://doi.org/10.1111/cdev.13957
31. Mittleman J. Stable and shifting sexualities among American high school students, 2015 to 2021. *Socius.* 2023;9:23780231231196012. https://doi.org/10.1177/23780231231196012
32. Reczek R, Bosley-Smith E. *Families We Keep: LGBTQ People and Their Enduring Bonds With Parents.* New York, NY: New York University Press; 2022.
33. Scandurra C, Mezza F, Maldonato NM, et al. Health of non-binary and genderqueer people: a systematic review. *Front Psychol.* 2019;10:1453. https://doi.org/10.3389/fpsyg.2019.01453
34. Finkelhor D. Screening for adverse childhood experiences (ACEs): cautions and suggestions. *Child Abuse Negl.* 2018;85:174–179. https://doi.org/10.1016/j.chiabu.2017.07.016
35. Levenson JS, Craig SL, Austin A. Trauma-informed and affirmative mental health practices with LGBTQ+ clients. *Psychol Serv.* 2023;20(suppl 1): 134–144. https://doi.org/10.1037/ser0000540

# COVID-19 Vaccine Mandate and Vaccination Rates in the US Military, 2020–2022

Elizabeth J. Dullea, Angelia A. Eick-Cost, PhD, Cara H. Olsen, DrPH, and James D. Mancuso, MD, DrPH

See also Hodge, p. 985.

**Objectives.** To assess the effect of the vaccination mandate on COVID-19 vaccination rates and identify independent factors associated with lack of postmandate vaccination among service members.

**Methods.** We assessed all active component service members for COVID-19 vaccination status from December 11, 2020, to January 1, 2022. We used comparative interrupted time series analysis and logistic regression to compare pre- and postmandate completion of the vaccine series between the US military and the US general population.

**Results.** Previous documented infection with severe acute respiratory syndrome coronavirus 2 (SARS-CoV-2), lower rank, and non-Hispanic Black race were associated with lower premandate vaccination. Postmandate vaccination rates were significantly higher in the active component population ($P < .001$) compared with the premandate period and the US population. Also notable was the higher incidence of postmandate vaccination among those who were non-Hispanic Black or of lower rank.

**Conclusions.** The US military's COVID-19 vaccination mandate was effective at both increasing overall vaccination rates and reducing disparities in vaccination, including race and ethnicity and rank. Vaccine mandates increase the receipt of vaccines and promote health, readiness, and equity within the US military. (*Am J Public Health*. 2025;115(7):1146–1156. https://doi.org/10.2105/AJPH.2025.308120)

AJPH July 2025, Vol. 115, No. 7

Severe acute respiratory syndrome coronavirus 2 (SARS-CoV-2), the causative agent of COVID-19, has infected more than 95 000 000 people and caused more than 1.2 million deaths in the United States alone.[1] SARS-CoV-2 continues to be a major health threat in the United States, causing an estimated 2.5 to 4.4 million infections, 72 000 to 120 000 hospitalizations, and 8200 to 13 000 deaths between October 1 and December 7, 2024.[2] The pandemic has also had a substantial impact on the health and readiness of the US military, resulting in 2741 hospitalizations and 96 deaths among military service members as of December 2022 and disrupting almost every facet of military life from recruit training to routine sea- and land-based missions.[3–5] For example, the USS Theodore Roosevelt was diverted from its assigned mission for 10 weeks and had more than 1000 infections and 1 death.[4] Non-Hispanic Black and Hispanic service members have been shown to have higher rates of SARS-CoV-2 infection and hospitalizations related to it,[6] but this association has not been as strong as that seen in civilian populations.[7,8]

The military has a long history of mandating vaccination, starting with compulsory smallpox inoculation during the American Revolution.[9] All US military service members are required to receive routine childhood immunizations (e.g., hepatitis A, hepatitis B, seasonal influenza, tetanus, measles, mumps, rubella) at the time of entry into service unless they have evidence of immunity.[10] Additional vaccinations are required for overseas service members.[11] However, unless waived by the president for reasons of national security, the US military is prohibited by law from mandating the receipt of emergency-use vaccines.[12] After the US Food and Drug Administration fully approved the Pfizer vaccine in August 2021, the Secretary of Defense directed that all military service branches implement compulsory vaccination policies requiring active-duty service members to receive the vaccination by December 31, 2021, or potentially face military separation.[13,14] Service members had the ability to apply for administrative, medical, and religious exemptions for vaccination. Administrative exemptions were offered if the service member was pending military separation or retirement within 180 days. Permanent and temporary (< 365 day) medical exemptions were offered based on the underlying health condition of the recipient, such as cardiomyopathy, immunodeficiency, pharmacologic or radiation therapy, pregnancy, or previous adverse response to immunization. Religious exemptions were evaluated in accordance with service-specific policies, requiring the input of the services' members command, medical provider, judge advocate, and chaplain.[13] The US military has historically rarely granted exemptions to most mandated vaccines, although vaccine refusals did occur previously with the anthrax vaccine mandate in the 1990s.[9]

Following the COVID-19 vaccination mandate, there was considerable vaccine hesitancy and refusal among military service members and the US population as a whole,[15–17] with 22% of the US population expressing that they were likely or definitely not getting the vaccine.[15] Despite the long legal and historical precedent supporting its use,[9] and over the Defense Department's objection that this move would harm military readiness,[18] the US military's COVID-19 vaccine mandate was overturned by Congress in January 2023 through the 2023 National Defense Authorization Act.[19]

Data supporting the effect of vaccine mandates is often not formally analyzed or publicly available in civilian or military populations. In addition, while the military rapidly achieved near-complete vaccination coverage following the introduction of the mandate, thousands of service members remained unvaccinated because of residual vaccine hesitancy.[20] Of the 22 560 COVID-19 vaccine waivers requested, only 745 (3.3%) were for permanent medical exemptions and 1655 (7.3%) for temporary ones, while the vast majority were for administrative or religious accommodations.[21] Understanding the factors that are associated with this group of remaining unvaccinated service members is of substantial interest to the US military in promoting vaccination, force health protection, and military readiness. Given these gaps in the literature, the objective of this study was to assess (1) how the overall COVID-19 vaccination rate in the active component US military changed over time, with a specific interest in the association with the vaccine mandate, and (2) factors associated with postmandate vaccination in the US military.

## METHODS

In this retrospective cohort study, all active component service members were assessed for COVID-19 vaccination status from December 11, 2020, to January 1, 2022, by which time all nonexempted service members were required to be vaccinated or have officially requested a waiver. Vaccine status was defined as the completion of primary COVID-19 vaccine series—Moderna (vaccine administered [CVX] code = 207), Pfizer (CVX code = 208 217), Janssen (CVX code = 212), and Novavax (CVX code = 211)—over that period. Service members were considered fully vaccinated 2 weeks after the first dose of the Janssen vaccine or the second dose of the others. Data were collected from the Armed Forces Health Surveillance Division's Defense Medical Surveillance System. Individuals were included in the study if they were members of the active component of the US military during the surveillance period and had served at least 1 full month on active duty. Participants were excluded from the study if they were a member of the Reserves or National Guard components, or if discharge from military service occurred during the surveillance period or before January 1, 2022. Covariates of interest included age, sex, race and ethnicity, service branch, rank (officer or enlisted), education level, geographic region of current residence, military occupational group, years of military service, and history of SARS-CoV-2 infection. We defined geographic region (Northeast, Midwest, South, West, overseas, or unknown) as the location of participants in January 2022. We defined previous SARS-CoV-2 infection by positive reverse transcription polymerase chain reaction and antigen test laboratory-confirmed SARS-CoV-2 infection. The Armed Forces Health Surveillance Division maintained a complete list of all positive COVID-19 tests among military health system beneficiaries, including active-component service members, that was updated daily.[6]

We first compared trends in vaccination before and after the vaccine mandate between the US general population and the US active component military population. We obtained general US vaccination data from the Centers for Disease Control and Prevention's (CDC's) Overall Trends in number of COVID-19 vaccinations in the US data set, which includes COVID-19 vaccination data from all jurisdictional partner clinics, retail pharmacies, long-term care facilities, dialysis centers, Federal Emergency Management Agency,

Health Resources and Services Administration partner sites, and federal entity facilities in the United States.[22] We used the active component population found in the Defense Medical Surveillance System on January 1, 2022, who were also on active duty on December 1, 2021, as the denominator for the US military population. Because the Pfizer vaccine approval was expanded to individuals aged 12 to 15 years on May 10, 2021,[23] we used the US 12 years and older population estimates for 2019 (283 520 141 people) as the denominator for the vaccine-eligible US population (CDC Informatics and Data Analytics Branch, e-mail communication, July 10, 2024). When calculating weekly incidence rates, we removed all those who previously completed the vaccine from the denominator (i.e., using only the remaining population eligible to complete the series).

We performed both visual inspection and statistical analysis of the trend in vaccination over time. For the statistical analysis, cumulative proportions of vaccinated individuals among both US military and US general populations were logit-transformed for normality and analyzed using linear regression models for comparative interrupted time series analysis. We empirically divided the data into 3 time periods for this analysis: premandate; initial postmandate period from August 24 to November 6, 2021; and the postmandate period from November 6, 2021, to January 1, 2022. Models accounted for autocorrelation using Newey–West standard errors with a 2-period lag. We analyzed data for trends using the interrupted time series analysis procedure in Intercooled Stata version 18 (StataCorp LP, College Station, TX).

We performed all other analyses with SAS software, version 9.4 (SAS Institute, Cary, NC). We present the cumulative incidence of vaccination stratified by these time periods: (1) premandate—vaccination up to the time of the mandate on August 23, 2021; (2) postmandate—vaccination from August 24, 2021, to January 1, 2022, among those not already vaccinated before the mandate, and (3) overall cumulative incidence of vaccination on January 1, 2022—which includes vaccination from either period. We stratified by time period to assess heterogeneity in factors associated with vaccination between these time periods. We obtained unadjusted and adjusted odds ratios using logistic regression of the overall cumulative incidence of postmandate vaccination. We used these effect estimates to assess the associations between vaccination and the covariates of interest, and adjusted models included all the available covariates of interest.

## RESULTS

There were 1 317 792 military service members in the active component on January 1, 2022, of whom 1 305 159 (99.0%) were also in the active component on December 1, 2021. Figure 1 shows the large spike in primary COVID-19 vaccination among active component service members immediately following the vaccine mandate. As shown in Figure 2, 62.5% of the US population aged 12 years and older and 70.5% of active component service members had completed the primary COVID-19 vaccination series by August 21, 2021. By January 1, 2022, 1 242 364 (95.2%) of the eligible service members had completed the primary COVID-19 vaccination series, as compared with 74.7% of the US population aged 12 years and older.

There was no significant difference in the cumulative percentage vaccinated between active component service members and the US population initially in May 2021 ($P = .823$). However, the rate of increase was slightly higher among active component service members ($P = .012$) compared with the general US population during the 4 months before the Department of Defense vaccine mandate, as demonstrated by the difference between the premandate slopes shown in Figure A (available as a supplement to the online version of this article at https://ajph.org). During the initial 2 months after the Department of Defense mandate (August 28–November 6), vaccination increased at a significantly higher rate in the active component population ($P < .001$) compared with the earlier period, whereas vaccination in the US population increased at a significantly lower ($P = .018$) rate compared with the earlier period. Furthermore, the change in slope was significantly greater in the military population than in the US population ($P < .001$). Following that initial implementation period, cumulative vaccination rates demonstrated a significant leveling off in the military population ($P < .001$) but remained stable in the US population ($P = .087$).

As seen in Table 1, 70.5% of the US military received the vaccine before the mandate, and premandate vaccination was associated with increasing age, education levels, and time in service; officer ranks; overseas location; service in the Navy; and certain occupations such as health care workers and pilots. Previous documented infection with SARS-CoV-2 and non-Hispanic Black race were both associated with lower premandate vaccination. Of the remaining 29.5% of the population who did not receive premandate

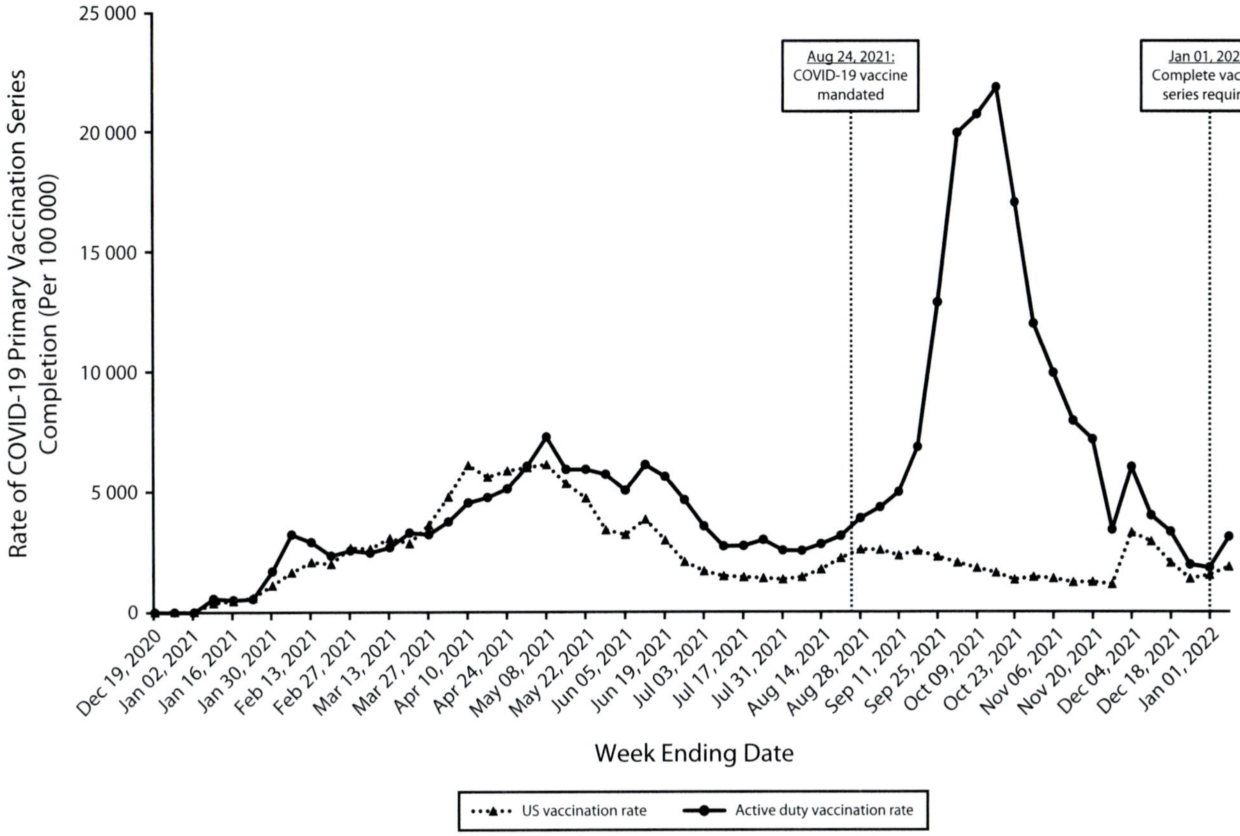


**FIGURE 1—** **Weekly Incidence Rates of Completion of the Primary COVID-19 Vaccination Series in the General US Population Aged 12 Years and Older Compared With the Rate Among US Active Duty Service Members: December 11, 2020, to January 1, 2022**

vaccination, 83.7% received the vaccination in the 3 months following the mandate. Previous SARS-CoV-2 infection was again associated with a lower incidence of postmandate vaccination. However, in contrast with the premandate associations, those who had younger ages, lower education levels, and lesser times in service were all associated with a higher incidence of postmandate vaccination, as were lower (enlisted) ranks. This is in contrast to the lower vaccine incidence seen in these groups in the premandate period. Also notable was the higher incidence of postmandate vaccination among non-Hispanic Blacks in contrast to the lower premandate incidence. Female sex was associated with a slightly lower incidence of vaccination in both periods.

As seen in Table 2, the strongest factor associated with overall postmandate vaccination status (including both the pre- and postmandate vaccination periods) was previous SARS-CoV-2 infection—those who had been infected previously had much lower odds of vaccination compared with those who had not (adjusted odds ratio [AOR] = 0.35; 95% confidence interval [CI] = 0.34, 0.35) after adjusting for other vaccine-related factors. Also of note, the adjusted odds of vaccination were significantly higher among Black, Hispanic, and those of other races and ethnicities compared with non-Hispanic White service members. Female (AOR = 0.86) service members had significantly lower and officers had significantly higher (AOR = 1.33) adjusted odds of vaccination compared with their male and enlisted counterparts, respectively. Health care workers (AOR = 1.21) and those stationed overseas (AOR = 1.87) had higher adjusted odds of vaccination compared with those in other professions and duty locations.

## DISCUSSION

The military's COVID-19 mandate was associated with both increasing the rate of vaccination and achieving high vaccination levels in the active component US military. The rate of vaccination

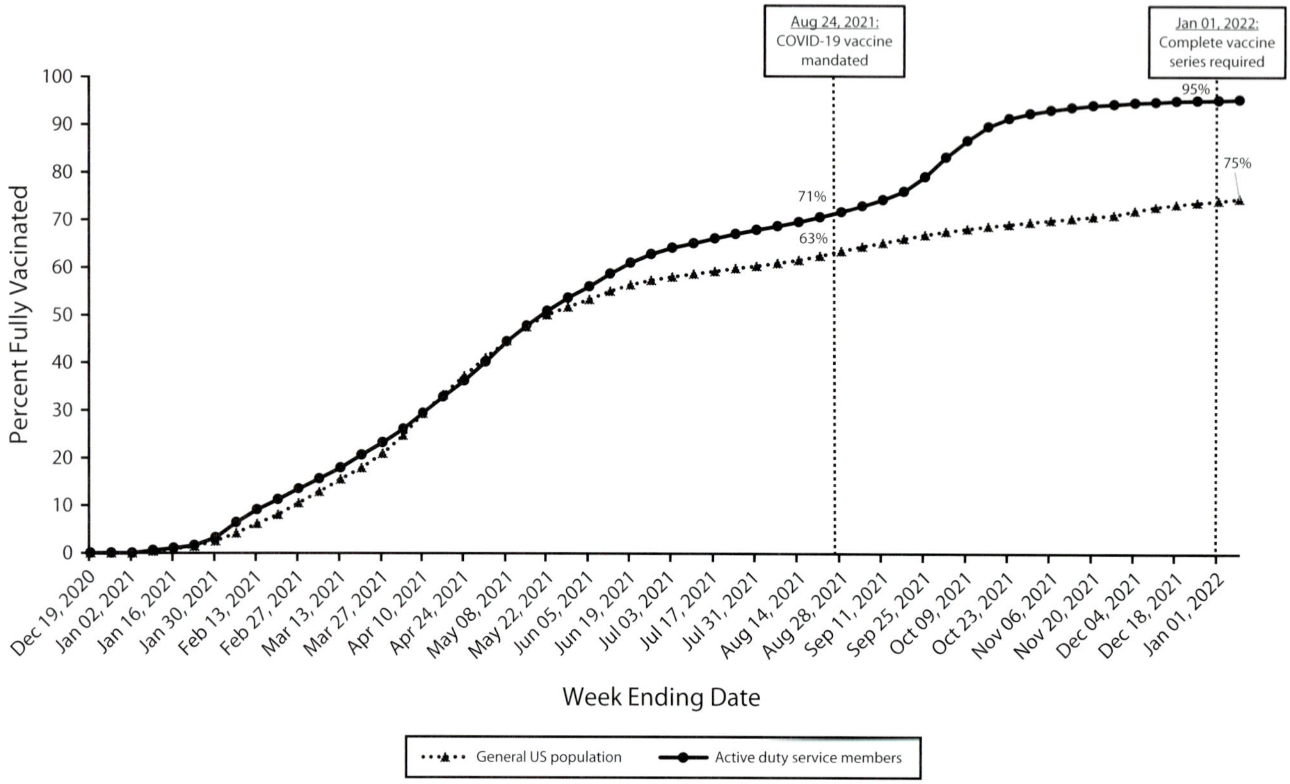


**FIGURE 2—** **Cumulative Incidence of Completion of the Primary COVID-19 Vaccination Series in the General US Population Aged 12 Years and Older Compared With the Incidence Among US Active Duty Service Members: December 11, 2020, to January 1, 2022**

immediately following the mandate was significantly greater than the rate seen in the general US population at the same time. Lower age, rank, and education level were associated with lower vaccination rates before the mandate but higher rates after the mandate. Similarly, while premandate vaccination was lower among Black service members, postmandate vaccination was higher among Black, Hispanic, and other races compared with White individuals. Other studies have shown lower vaccination coverage among racial and ethnic minorities in both military and civilian populations.[16,24] These results suggest that the US military COVID-19 vaccination mandate was effective not only at increasing overall vaccination rates but also in reducing disparities according to rank, education, and race and ethnicity. Similarly, mandates among municipal workers in New York City were also associated with reduced racial disparities in vaccination.[25]

Nevertheless, 4.8% of the active component population had not completed the primary COVID-19 vaccine series by January 2022. Some of these were individuals who waited until December to initiate the vaccine series, so they may have received the first dose only, and others had applied for waivers and had not received any vaccine doses. Consistent with previous research on military and civilian populations,[16,26] those servicemembers with a history of SARS-CoV-2 infection were less likely to be vaccinated (AOR = 0.35). A history of SARS-CoV-2 infection was not a qualification for medical exemption from vaccination, and vaccination was recommended 90 days after acute SARS-CoV-2 infection.[13] These results suggest that there are unmeasured (confounding) health beliefs that may be associated with both infection and vaccination.

Furthermore, unvaccinated service members after the mandate were more likely to be female, enlisted, stationed in the United States, serving in the Army or Air Force, and to have 12 or fewer years of formal education. Previous research has similarly shown increased primary and booster COVID-19 vaccination rates among service members with increasing rank, age, and education level and those

**TABLE 1— Active Component Service Members Who Received a Full Series of COVID-19 Vaccines Before and After the August 23, 2021, Mandate: United States, December 11, 2020, to January 1, 2022**

| | Total Population, No. | Completed the Full Vaccine Series Premandate (on or Before Aug 23, 2021), No. (%) | Population Who Did Not Complete the Full Vaccine Series Premandate (Aug 23, 2021), No. | Completed the Full Vaccine Series After Aug 23, 2021, but Before Jan 1, 2022, No. (%) | Total Postmandate Population Who Did Not Complete the Full Vaccine Series by Jan 1, 2022, No. (%) |
|---|---|---|---|---|---|
| Total | 1 305 159 | 919 606 (70.5) | 385 553 | 322 758 (83.7) | 62 795 (4.8) |
| Sex | | | | | |
| Male | 1 078 455 | 760 448 (70.5) | 318 007 | 266 818 (83.9) | 51 189 (4.7) |
| Female | 226 704 | 159 158 (70.2) | 67 546 | 55 940 (82.8) | 11 606 (5.1) |
| Age, y | | | | | |
| < 20 | 86 525 | 47 149 (54.5) | 39 376 | 34 230 (86.9) | 5 146 (5.9) |
| 20–24 | 416 537 | 268 325 (64.4) | 148 212 | 127 201 (85.8) | 21 011 (5.0) |
| 25–29 | 305 785 | 214 060 (70.0) | 91 725 | 78 427 (85.5) | 13 298 (4.3) |
| 30–34 | 210 385 | 156 043 (74.2) | 54 342 | 44 082 (81.1) | 10 260 (4.9) |
| 35–39 | 159 080 | 125 316 (78.8) | 33 764 | 26 221 (77.7) | 7 543 (4.7) |
| 40–44 | 80 698 | 67 627 (83.8) | 13 071 | 9 369 (71.7) | 3 702 (4.6) |
| ≥ 45 | 46 149 | 41 086 (89.0) | 5 063 | 3 228 (63.8) | 1 835 (4.0) |
| Race/ethnicity | | | | | |
| Non-Hispanic White | 704 255 | 501 097 (71.2) | 203 158 | 167 097 (82.2) | 36 061 (5.1) |
| Non-Hispanic Black | 208 572 | 131 391 (63.0) | 77 181 | 66 688 (86.4) | 10 493 (5.0) |
| Hispanic | 236 568 | 166 321 (70.3) | 70 247 | 60 256 (85.8) | 9 991 (4.2) |
| Other or unknown | 155 764 | 120 797 (77.6) | 34 967 | 28 717 (82.1) | 6 250 (4.0) |
| Service | | | | | |
| Army | 468 666 | 336 723 (71.8) | 131 943 | 107 179 (81.2) | 24 764 (5.3) |
| Navy | 339 278 | 269 239 (79.4) | 70 039 | 58 505 (83.5) | 11 534 (3.4) |
| Air Force | 321 549 | 207 847 (64.6) | 113 702 | 95 579 (84.1) | 18 123 (5.6) |
| Marines | 175 666 | 105 797 (60.2) | 69 869 | 61 495 (88.0) | 8 374 (4.8) |
| Rank | | | | | |
| Enlisted | 1 073 607 | 715 403 (66.6) | 358 204 | 303 609 (84.8) | 54 595 (5.1) |
| Officer | 231 552 | 204 203 (88.2) | 27 349 | 19 149 (70.0) | 8 200 (3.5) |
| Education level | | | | | |
| High school or less | 823 757 | 527 563 (64.0) | 296 194 | 254 038 (85.8) | 42 156 (5.1) |
| Some college | 154 279 | 113 061 (73.3) | 41 218 | 33 249 (80.7) | 7 969 (5.2) |
| Bachelor's or higher | 300 423 | 256 748 (85.5) | 43 675 | 32 041 (73.4) | 11 634 (3.9) |
| Other or unknown | 26 700 | 22 234 (83.3) | 4 466 | 3 430 (76.8) | 1 036 (3.9) |
| Geographic region | | | | | |
| Northeast | 37 442 | 28 844 (77.0) | 8 598 | 6 951 (80.8) | 1 647 (4.4) |
| Midwest | 79 100 | 50 192 (63.5) | 28 908 | 23 583 (81.6) | 5 325 (6.7) |
| South | 594 816 | 397 693 (66.9) | 197 123 | 169 467 (86.0) | 27 656 (4.6) |
| West | 339 038 | 233 237 (68.8) | 105 801 | 84 252 (79.6) | 21 549 (6.4) |
| Overseas | 148 556 | 121 179 (81.6) | 27 377 | 23 869 (87.2) | 3 508 (2.4) |
| Other or unknown | 106 207 | 88 461 (83.3) | 17 746 | 14 636 (82.5) | 3 110 (2.9) |
| DOD occupation | | | | | |
| Combat arms | 181 249 | 131 185 (72.4) | 50 064 | 40 859 (81.6) | 9 205 (5.1) |
| Motor transport | 39 412 | 24 913 (63.2) | 14 499 | 12 424 (85.7) | 2 075 (5.3) |

*Continued*

**TABLE 1— Continued**

| | Total Population, No. | Completed the Full Vaccine Series Premandate (on or Before Aug 23, 2021), No. (%) | Population Who Did Not Complete the Full Vaccine Series Premandate (Aug 23, 2021), No. | Completed the Full Vaccine Series After Aug 23, 2021, but Before Jan 1, 2022, No. (%) | Total Postmandate Population Who Did Not Complete the Full Vaccine Series by Jan 1, 2022, No. (%) |
|---|---|---|---|---|---|
| Pilot or aircrew | 46 848 | 38 811 (82.8) | 8 037 | 6 060 (75.4) | 1 977 (4.2) |
| Repair or engineering | 381 468 | 261 240 (68.5) | 120 228 | 102 373 (85.1) | 17 855 (4.7) |
| Communications or intelligence | 277 885 | 198 681 (71.5) | 79 204 | 65 789 (83.1) | 13 415 (4.8) |
| Health care | 108 935 | 87 717 (80.5) | 21 218 | 17 137 (80.8) | 4 081 (3.7) |
| Other or unknown | 269 362 | 177 059 (65.7) | 92 303 | 78 116 (84.6) | 14 187 (5.3) |
| Time in service, y | | | | | |
| < 1 | 124 508 | 68 196 (54.8) | 56 312 | 48 541 (86.2) | 7 771 (6.2) |
| 1–4 | 502 252 | 340 645 (67.8) | 161 607 | 137 412 (85.0) | 24 195 (4.8) |
| 5–10 | 285 982 | 200 989 (70.3) | 84 993 | 73 142 (86.1) | 11 851 (4.1) |
| > 10 | 392 417 | 309 776 (78.9) | 82 641 | 63 663 (77.0) | 18 978 (4.8) |
| Previous SARS-CoV-2 infection | | | | | |
| Yes | 125 640 | 74 476 (59.3) | 51 164 | 35 539 (69.5) | 15 625 (11.0) |
| No | 1 179 519 | 845 130 (71.7) | 334 389 | 287 219 (85.9) | 47 170 (4.1) |
| Vaccine type | | | | | |
| Moderna (CVX: 207) | | 330 983 (36.0) | | 43 762 (13.6) | |
| Pfizer (CVX: 208, 217) | | 484 478 (52.7) | | 261 197 (80.9) | |
| Janssen (CVX: 212) | | 104 112 (11.3) | | 17 797 (5.5) | |
| Novavax (CVX: 211) | | 33 (0.0) | | 2 (0.0) | |

*Note.* CVX = vaccine administered; DOD = US Department of Defense.

stationed overseas.[16,26] In contrast with the finding of lower incidence of vaccination among women in this study, Lang et al.[16] showed no association with COVID-19 vaccination, and Winkler et al.[26] showed increased acceptance of booster doses among female service members who had already received the primary vaccine series. Female service members who were pregnant could apply for a temporary (< 365 days) medical exemption to COVID-19 vaccination, and an estimated 16% of active-duty servicewomen are pregnant annually.[27] This may help explain why some female service members were less likely to get vaccinated compared with their male counterparts. The dynamic nature of the pandemic and attitudes about vaccination may also partially explain the small differences seen between this and previous studies. Awareness of these health disparities among women and enlisted service members may inform the US military's educational, policy, and research efforts at promoting vaccination.

Strengths of this study include a robust electronic vaccination registry that was required to be used and tracked by military regulation[10] and a large sample size. The most important limitation of this study is unmeasured confounding, in that we did not assess attitudes or beliefs such as trust in the vaccine, health care system, or government; political affiliation; or other potential underlying causal determinants of vaccination.[28] Lack of COVID-19 vaccination following the mandate does not necessarily imply vaccine hesitancy, as about 10.6% of service members had medical exceptions. The differences in demographics and cultures of vaccine acceptance between the US military and civilian populations may explain some of the differences in vaccination, as may the heterogeneity in vaccine mandates across federal and state jurisdictions. For this reason, the results of this research may not be generalizable to the general civilian population or other militaries around the world. In addition, the results

**TABLE 2— Overall Postmandate Adjusted Odds Ratios of Completing a COVID-19 Primary Vaccination Series Among Active Component Service Members: United States, January 2022**

| | Crude OR (95% CI) | Adjusted OR (95% CI) |
|---|---|---|
| Sex | | |
| Male (Ref) | 1 | 1 |
| Female | 0.92 (0.90, 0.94) | 0.86 (0.84, 0.88) |
| Age, y | | |
| < 20 (Ref) | 1 | 1 |
| 20–24 | 1.19 (1.15, 1.23) | 1.02 (0.99, 1.06) |
| 25–29 | 1.39 (1.35, 1.44) | 1.05 (1.00, 1.09) |
| 30–34 | 1.23 (1.19, 1.28) | 0.93 (0.88, 0.97) |
| 35–39 | 1.27 (1.22, 1.32) | 0.96 (0.91, 1.01) |
| 40–44 | 1.32 (1.26, 1.37) | 0.92 (0.87, 0.98) |
| ≥ 45 | 1.53 (1.45, 1.61) | 0.95 (0.88, 1.01) |
| Race/ethnicity | | |
| Non-Hispanic White (Ref) | 1 | 1 |
| Non-Hispanic Black | 1.02 (1.00, 1.04) | 1.08 (1.06, 1.11) |
| Hispanic | 1.22 (1.20, 1.25) | 1.32 (1.29, 1.35) |
| Other or unknown | 1.29 (1.26, 1.33) | 1.21 (1.18, 1.24) |
| Service | | |
| Army (Ref) | 1 | 1 |
| Navy | 1.59 (1.55, 1.62) | 1.49 (1.45, 1.53) |
| Air Force | 0.93 (0.92, 0.95) | 0.96 (0.94, 0.98) |
| Marines | 1.11 (1.09, 1.14) | 1.19 (1.16, 1.22) |
| Rank | | |
| Enlisted (Ref) | 1 | 1 |
| Officer | 1.46 (1.43, 1.49) | 1.33 (1.28, 1.38) |
| Education level | | |
| High school or less (Ref) | 1 | 1 |
| Some college | 0.99 (0.97, 1.01) | 1.06 (1.03, 1.09) |
| Bachelor's or advanced degree | 1.34 (1.31, 1.37) | 1.2 (1.16, 1.23) |
| Other or unknown | 1.34 (1.25, 1.42) | 1.01 (0.95, 1.08) |
| Geographic region | | |
| Northeast | 1.06 (1.01, 1.12) | 0.98 (0.93, 1.03) |
| Midwest | 0.68 (0.66, 0.70) | 0.7 (0.68, 0.72) |
| South (Ref) | 1 | 1 |
| West | 0.72 (0.71, 0.73) | 0.67 (0.66, 0.68) |
| Overseas | 2.02 (1.95, 2.09) | 1.87 (1.80, 1.94) |
| Other or unknown | 1.62 (1.56, 1.68) | 1.17 (1.12, 1.22) |
| DOD occupation | | |
| Infantry, artillery, armor, or combat engineer (Ref) | 1 | 1 |
| Motor transport | 0.96 (0.92, 1.01) | 0.89 (0.85, 0.94) |
| Pilot or aircrew | 1.21 (1.16, 1.28) | 0.91 (0.86, 0.96) |
| Repair or engineering | 1.09 (1.06, 1.12) | 0.97 (0.94, 1.00) |
| Communications or intelligence | 1.05 (1.03, 1.08) | 1 (0.97, 1.03) |
| Health care | 1.37 (1.32, 1.43) | 1.21 (1.16, 1.26) |
| Other or unknown | 0.96 (0.94, 0.99) | 0.9 (0.88, 0.93) |

*Continued*

## TABLE 2— Continued

| | Crude OR (95% CI) | Adjusted OR (95% CI) |
|---|---|---|
| Time in service, y | | |
| <1 (Ref) | 1 | 1 |
| 1–4 | 1.32 (1.28, 1.35) | 1.41 (1.36, 1.45) |
| 5–10 | 1.54 (1.50, 1.59) | 1.57 (1.51, 1.63) |
| >10 | 1.31 (1.27, 1.35) | 1.27 (1.21, 1.33) |
| Previous SARS-CoV-2 infection | | |
| Yes | 0.34 (0.33, 0.35) | 0.35 (0.34, 0.35) |
| No (Ref) | 1 | 1 |

*Note.* CI = confidence interval; CVX = vaccine administered; DOD = Department of Defense; OR = odds ratio.

of this study may not apply to the implementation of other vaccination and military vaccine mandates, as the acceptance of the COVID-19 vaccine was unusually and uniquely influenced by political affinity and polarization, as well as vaccine mis- and disinformation in the United States.[29]

Vaccine mandates have been demonstrated to be effective at increasing vaccine coverage. For example, COVID-19 vaccine mandates in 12 US states were followed by an 11.5% increase in vaccination compared with nonmandate states after 8 weeks[30]; mandates in Canada and New York City were associated with similar increases.[25,31] Routine childhood vaccines are also mandated for children to enter public schools in all 50 states because of their effectiveness in preventing illness and death. Vaccine mandates result in economic and social benefits by reducing lost productivity from illness, as well as from potentially accelerating transitions to normal activities during epidemics.[32] These benefits must be balanced against the risks of infringing upon personal autonomy, erosion of public trust if the vaccine fails to produce the anticipated benefits, or from mistrust because of politicization of the vaccine. The World Health Organization has recommended ethical principles to be used when considering vaccine mandates, along with other important scientific, legal, and practical issues.[33] While these recommendations included some unique settings for consideration, such as schools and health care settings, they did not address the unique military considerations, such as military readiness and its effect on national security.

The US military is at risk for SARS-CoV-2 infections and for hospitalizations and death from COVID-19,[4,5] and COVID-19 vaccines have been shown to effectively reduce these risks.[34] Vaccine mandates are an important intervention associated with dramatic increases in overall vaccination and rate of vaccination, and with reduced vaccination disparities. Without effective mandates, fewer service members may get vaccinated, and many of those who do get vaccinated may have their vaccination delayed. This may lead to decreased military readiness and increased rates of preventable disease and deaths, as has occurred in the past with this and other vaccine-preventable diseases.[4,35] The US military must retain the authority to mandate safe and effective vaccines as an important tool to promote health, readiness, and national security—particularly during health emergencies. The repeal of the COVID-19 vaccine mandate and politicization of the military's COVID-19 vaccine policy could pave the way for future resistance to other vaccines and other effective force health protection countermeasures. Nevertheless, each outbreak and public health event has unique circumstances, and the context of COVID-19 (e.g., in which a safe and effective vaccine was developed extremely rapidly) may not apply equally in all of these. The US military must continue to carefully assess the risks and benefits of each vaccine mandate—as well as all other force health protection countermeasures—and it must continue to defend the use of vaccine mandates when necessary to promote the health and readiness of the force. AJPH

## ABOUT THE AUTHORS

Elizabeth Dullea is with the Office of Student Affairs, School of Medicine, Uniformed Services University of the Health Sciences, Bethesda, MD. Angelia Cost is with the Armed Forces Health Surveillance Division, Public Health Directorate, Defense Health Agency, Silver Spring, MD. Cara Olsen and James Mancuso are with the Department of Preventive Medicine and Biostatistics, School of Medicine, Uniformed Services University of the Health Sciences, Bethesda.

**Note.** The contents of this publication are the sole responsibility of the authors and do not necessarily reflect the views, assertions, opinions, or policies of the Uniformed Services University of the Health Sciences, the Department of Defense, or the US government.

## CORRESPONDENCE

Correspondence should be sent to James Mancuso, USUHS Dept of PMB, 4301 Jones Bridge Road, Bethesda, MD 20814 (e-mail: james.mancuso@usuhs.edu). Reprints can be ordered at https://www.ajph.org by clicking the "Reprints" link.

## PUBLICATION INFORMATION

Full Citation: Dullea EJ, Eick-Cost AA, Olsen CH, Mancuso JD. COVID-19 vaccine mandate and vaccination rates in the US military, 2020–2022. *Am J Public Health*. 2025;115(7):1146–1156.

Acceptance Date: March 12, 2025.

DOI: https://doi.org/10.2105/AJPH.2025.308120

ORCID iDs:
Elizabeth J. Dullea https://orcid.org/0000-0003-4347-7864

James D. Mancuso https://orcid.org/0000-0002-0717-8202

## CONTRIBUTORS

E. Dullea, A. Cost, C. Olsen, and J. Mancuso all performed substantial contributions to the conceptualization or design of the work; or the acquisition, analysis, or interpretation of data for the work; drafted the work or revised it critically for important intellectual content; and gave final approval of the version to be published.

## CONFLICTS OF INTEREST

The authors report that they have no conflicts of interest.

## HUMAN PARTICIPANT PROTECTION

This study was approved by the Uniformed Services University institutional review board.

## REFERENCES

1. Centers for Disease Control and Prevention. COVID data tracker. Available at: https://covid.cdc.gov/covid-data-tracker/#deaths-landing. Accessed February 2, 2025.
2. National Center for Immunization and Respiratory Diseases. CDC releases new in-season estimates for COVID-19 and RSV. Available at: https://www.cdc.gov/ncird/whats-new/cdc-releases-new-in-season-estimates-for-covid-19-and-rsv.html. Accessed February 2, 2025.
3. US Department of Defense. Coronavirus: DOD response. 2022. Available at: https://www.defense.gov/Spotlights/Coronavirus-DOD-Response. Accessed March 20, 2024.
4. Kasper MR, Geibe JR, Sears CL, et al. An outbreak of Covid-19 on an aircraft carrier. *N Engl J Med*. 2020;383(25):2417–2426. https://doi.org/10.1056/NEJMoa2019375
5. Letizia AG, Ramos I, Obla A, et al. SARS-CoV-2 transmission among Marine recruits during quarantine. *N Engl J Med*. 2020;383(25):2407–2416. https://doi.org/10.1056/NEJMoa2029717
6. Young JM, Stahlman SL, Clausen SS, Bova ML, Mancuso JD. Racial and ethnic disparities in COVID-19 infection and hospitalization in the active component US military. *Am J Public Health*. 2021;111(12):2194–2201. https://doi.org/10.2105/AJPH.2021.306527
7. Gawthrop E. The color of coronavirus: COVID-19 deaths by race and ethnicity in the US. 2023. Available at: https://www.apmresearchlab.org/covid/deaths-by-race. Accessed March 20, 2023.
8. Shah M, Sachdeva M, Dodiuk-Gad RP. COVID-19 and racial disparities. *J Am Acad Dermatol*. 2020;83(1):e35. https://doi.org/10.1016/j.jaad.2020.04.046
9. Elliott CB, Chambers CS. A historical analysis of vaccine mandates in the United States military and its application to the COVID-19 vaccine mandate. *Vaccine*. 2022;40(51):7500–7504. https://doi.org/10.1016/j.vaccine.2022.08.017
10. US Department of Defense. Army Regulation 40–562/BUMEDINST 6230.15B/AFI 48–110_IP/CG COMDTINST M6230.4G: Immunizations and chemoprophylaxis for the prevention of infectious diseases. Available at: https://armypubs.army.mil/epubs/DR_pubs/DR_a/pdf/web/r40_562.pdf. Accessed April 24, 2025.
11. Defense Health Agency. Vaccine recommendations by AOR. 2023. Available at: https://www.health.mil/Military-Health-Topics/Health-Readiness/Immunization-Healthcare/Vaccine-Recommendations/Vaccine-Recommendations-by-AOR. Accessed March 20, 2024.
12. Emergency use products. 10 USC §1107a (2017). Available at: https://uscode.house.gov/view.xhtml?req=granuleid:USC-prelim-title10-section1107a&num=0&edition=prelim. Accessed April 24, 2025.
13. Immunizations and Chemoprophylaxis for the Prevention of Infectious Diseases. In: Regulation USA, Vol 40–562. BUMEDINST 6230.15B: Departments of the Army, Navy, Air Force, and Coast Guard; 2013:110.
14. Austin L. Memorandum for senior Pentagon leadership commanders of the Combatant Commands Defense Agency and DOD field activity directors. Subject: Mandatory coronavirus disease 2019 vaccination of Department of Defense service members. US Department of Defense. August 24, 2021. Available at: https://media.defense.gov/2021/Aug/25/2002838826/-1/-1/0/MEMORANDUM-FOR-MANDATORY-CORONAVIRUS-DISEASE-2019-VACCINATION-OF-DEPARTMENT-OF-DEFENSE-SERVICE-MEMBERS.PDF. Accessed April 24, 2025.
15. Khubchandani J, Sharma S, Price JH, Wiblishauser MJ, Sharma M, Webb FJ. COVID-19 vaccination hesitancy in the United States: a rapid national assessment. *J Community Health*. 2021;46(2):270–277. https://doi.org/10.1007/s10900-020-00958-x
16. Lang MA, Stahlman S, Wells NY, et al. Disparities in COVID-19 vaccine initiation and completion among active component service members and health care personnel, 11 December 2020–12 March 2021. *MSMR*. 2021;28(4):2–9.
17. Theis SR, Li PC, Kelly D, et al. Perceptions and concerns regarding COVID-19 vaccination in a military base population. *Mil Med*. 2022;187(11-12):e1255–e1260. https://doi.org/10.1093/milmed/usab230
18. Myers M. The fallout of the military's COVID-19 vaccine mandate. *Military Times*. March 27, 2023. Available at: https://www.militarytimes.com/news/your-military/2023/03/27/the-fallout-of-the-militarys-covid-19-vaccine-mandate. Accessed March 20, 2024.
19. US Congress. H.R.7776 - James M. Inhofe National Defense Authorization Act for Fiscal Year 2023. Pub L No: 117-263. Available at: https://www.congress.gov/bill/117th-congress/house-bill/7776. Accessed April 24, 2025.
20. Garamone J. Almost all active duty service members receive vaccines. *DOD News*. December 16, 2021. Available at: https://www.defense.gov/News/News-Stories/Article/Article/2877173/almost-all-active-duty-service-members-receive-vaccines. Accessed March 20, 2024.
21. Department of Defense Inspector General. Report no. DODIG-2024-061: Audit of military services' processing of coronavirus disease—2019 vaccination exemptions and discharges for active duty service members. March 12, 2024. Available at: https://media.defense.gov/2024/Mar/14/2003413066/-1/-1/1/DODIG-2024-061_AUDIT_VACCINEEXEMPT_REDACTED_SECURED.PDF. Accessed February 2, 2025.
22. National Center for Immunization and Respiratory Diseases. COVID-19 vaccination trends in the United States, national and jurisdictional. Atlanta, GA: Centers for Disease Control and Prevention; 2021.
23. Assistant Secretary for Public Affairs. COVID-19 vaccines. 2024. Available at: https://www.hhs.gov/coronavirus/covid-19-vaccines/index.html. Accessed July 7, 2024.
24. Gertz A, Rader B, Sewalk K, Brownstein JS. Emerging socioeconomic disparities in COVID-19 vaccine second-dose completion rates in the United States. *Vaccines (Basel)*. 2022;10(1):121. https://doi.org/10.3390/vaccines10010121
25. Rubenstein BL, Amiel PJ, Ternier A, et al. Increases in COVID-19 vaccination among NYC municipal employees after implementation of vaccination requirements. *Health Aff (Millwood)*. 2023;42(3):357–365. https://doi.org/10.1377/hlthaff.2022.00809
26. Winkler EL, Stahlman SL, Wells NY, et al. COVID-19 booster vaccination in the US Military, August 2021–January 2022. *Am J Prev Med* 2023;64(2):270–274. https://doi.org/10.1016/j.amepre.2022.07.017
27. Meadows SO, Collins RL, Schuler MS, Beckman RL, Cefalu M. The Women's Reproductive Health Survey (WRHS) of active-duty service members. *Rand Health Q*. 2023;10(2):11.
28. Sapienza A, Falcone R. The role of trust in COVID-19 vaccine acceptance: considerations from a systematic review. *Int J Environ Res Public Health*. 2022;20(1):665. https://doi.org/10.3390/ijerph20010665
29. Bolsen T, Palm R. Politicization and COVID-19 vaccine resistance in the US. *Prog Mol Biol Transl Sci*. 2022;188(1):81–100. https://doi.org/10.1016/bs.pmbts.2021.10.002

30. Howard-Williams M, Soelaeman RH, Fischer LS, McCord R, Davison R, Dunphy C. Association between state-issued COVID-19 vaccine mandates and vaccine administration rates in 12 US states and the District of Columbia. *JAMA Health Forum*. 2022;3(10):e223810. https://doi.org/10.1001/jamahealthforum.2022.3810
31. Maquiling A, Jeevakanthan A, Fane BHM. The effect of vaccine mandate announcements on vaccine uptake in Canada: an interrupted time series analysis. *Vaccine*. 2023;41(18):2932–2940. https://doi.org/10.1016/j.vaccine.2023.03.040
32. Canning AG, Watson KE, McCreedy KE, Olawepo JO. Ethics and effectiveness of US COVID-19 vaccine mandates and vaccination passports: a review. *J Res Health Sci*. 2022;22(2):e00546. https://doi.org/10.34172/jrhs.2022.81
33. *COVID-19 and Mandatory Vaccination: Ethical Considerations: Policy Brief*. Geneva, Switzerland: World Health Organization; 2022.
34. Lin DY, Gu Y, Wheeler B, et al. Effectiveness of Covid-19 vaccines over a 9-month period in North Carolina. *N Engl J Med*. 2022;386(10):933–941. https://doi.org/10.1056/NEJMoa2117128
35. Radin JM, Hawksworth AW, Blair PJ, et al. Dramatic decline of respiratory illness among US military recruits after the renewed use of adenovirus vaccines. *Clin Infect Dis*. 2014;59(7):962–968. https://doi.org/10.1093/cid/ciu507

# A Decarceral Response to HIV Criminalization in the Black LGBTQIA+ Community

Louis Listerud, BA, Steven Meanley, PhD, MPH, Alana Richards, MA, Blake Kosciow, BA, and Stephen Bonett, RN, MA, PhD

See also Csete, p. 988.

HIV criminalization statutes continue to disproportionately impact Black queer and trans individuals, particularly Black transgender and gender-expansive people and sex workers, and have historically served as a way to inequitably punish communities for a disease that affects them because of inequitable systems rooted in the legacy of slavery.

To achieve the Centers for Disease Control and Prevention's 2030 goals for Ending the HIV Epidemic in the US, it is essential to take bold steps to decriminalize HIV and interrogate the role of criminalization in reinforcing stigma, exacerbating the social determinants of health, and further disenfranchising marginalized communities. Through the analysis of the theory of racial capitalism, we aim to make the argument for complete decriminalization of HIV as a small step in the ultimate goal of prison abolition and decarceration of all peoples.

We advocate rejecting efforts aiming to modernize statutes that further concretize the punitive role prisons play in a capitalist society and systematically revoke HIV-affected communities' right to freedom. Multilevel policies must address the racialized nature of HIV criminalization. (*Am J Public Health*. 2025;115(7):1157–1165. https://doi.org/10.2105/AJPH.2025.308110)

AJPH July 2025, Vol. 115, No. 7

The public health issue of HIV disparities between Black queer and trans communities and their White counterparts has been well documented.[1] While Black people make up around 12% of the population, they constitute 40% of all HIV infections.[2] This inequity, rooted in historical, racial, and structural violence, is further exacerbated by the criminalization of HIV, which disproportionately impacts Black queer and trans individuals and sex workers, specifically Black women, queer men, and transgender and gender-expansive people. This analytic essay explores (1) how the United States has instituted HIV criminalization as a public health measure that inherently criminalizes the conditions of poverty and Black people in the process, (2) how the theory of racial capitalism can be utilized as a tool to understand the root of this country's history of criminalizing HIV, (3) how reforming and modernizing HIV criminalization statutes divert us away from the path to full prison abolition, and (4) recommendations for more equitable interventions that address racism in carceral practices. By examining the history of HIV-based stigma and interconnected racial discrimination, we can more effectively pave a way toward justice-informed decarceral solutions.

## HIV/AIDS CRIMINALIZATION HISTORY

When HIV began to spread in the United States, it was immediately associated with queerness. Originally referred to as the gay-related immunodeficiency disease, HIV was both perceived as a disease of "choice" and attached to a sense of "morality," making it easier to criminalize when HIV inevitably spread from queer communities to heterosexual populations.[3] Ronald Reagan and his administration codified these policies with his stance on criminal policies and the 1987 Reagan Commission on the HIV Epidemic.[4] The report explicitly proposed that states enact laws around "affirmative personal responsibility" for people with HIV (PWH) to disclose their HIV status to sexual partners and intravenous drug use partners before participating in activities associated with chances of transmission. This theory failed to consider that many were not aware of their HIV status, as acute HIV infection has ambiguous symptoms.[5] Testing was not universally available, diminishing one's ability to take "affirmative personal responsibility."[6] The Reagan administration relied on this individualization rhetoric to place blame onto marginalized individuals instead of the social issues they were exacerbating and actively promoting through policy.[7]

The first HIV criminalization statutes were established in 1986 in Tennessee (Tenn Code Ann §68-32-104 for donation of tissue, blood, and fluids), Washington (Wash Rev Code Ann §9A.36.011 for knowing exposure), and Florida (Fla Stat Ann §384.24[2] for sexual exposure and Fla Stat Ann §796.08[5] for sex work).[8] In the following year, the same year as the Commission's creation, Representative Kernan "Skip" Hand of Jefferson Parish, Louisiana, introduced House Bill 1728 to criminalize intentional exposure to HIV to "deter those who are infected with the AIDS virus from remaining sexually active in the community" mirroring the language around blame the Reagan administration propagated.[9(p109)] Similar to several other states, this law was updated to include additional infractions for exposing a police officer, including "spitting, biting, stabbing with an AIDS-contaminated object, or throwing of blood or other bodily substances."[9(p110)]

In 1990, under George H. W. Bush, the Ryan White Comprehensive AIDS Resources Emergency (CARE) Act was passed, giving PWH access to education and medication through federal grants to states. However, Ryan White funds were predicated on the "affirmative responsibility" clause, also known as "duty to warn," in state law.[3] Some states created HIV-specific statutes for criminalization, while others elected for "sentence enhancements under traditional criminal codes," like aggravated assault. Although public health recommendations for reducing HIV transmission were being developed and distributed at this time, these laws did not have exceptions for cases where transmission risk was low.

Depending on the state, PWH may be charged with bioterrorism, attempted murder, aggravated assault, and other violent infractions, even in cases of nontransmission or where transmission was not willful.[3] However, bioterrorism laws (specific to Michigan), for example, are rarer and less easily prosecuted. Two specific notable cases occurred in *People v Odem* in which a person with HIV allegedly spat on a correctional officer. Because this man was bleeding from his mouth at the time, his saliva was characterized as a "harmful biological substance," and he received an enhanced sentence of 5 to 15 years.[10] In another case, a person with HIV was charged under this statute for allegedly biting his neighbor in an altercation; however, the charge was dismissed because there was no evidence that his mouth was bleeding during the interaction. Given Centers for Disease Control and Prevention (CDC) guidelines around nonexistent transmission rates for saliva, the specific bioterrorism charge was dropped. This case still affirmed the *Odem* decision, arguing that blood from PWH continues to be considered a "harmful biological substance."[10] It also further emphasizes how minimally modernized statutes are still insufficient.[10]

## HIV DISPARITIES (IN CRIMINALIZATION)

Roughly 1 decade after the start of the epidemic in the United States, the public faces of HIV shifted from White gay men (i.e., "regime of Black American exclusion," 1981–1992) to Black people ("regime of Black American inclusion," 1993–present), even though this phenomenon was not based in evidence.[11] Evidence of disproportionate conviction rates by race emerged soon after in the 1990s when state-level criminalization statutes were implemented.[12] Experts and community advocates described this criminalization as a form of racial–sexual terror given that "HIV status is most often a function of poverty and not sexual promiscuity."[3(p140)] HIV had become racialized, leading to structural determinants of HIV. For Black queer and trans people, in particular, there are numerous barriers and disparities along the entire HIV continuum, including prevention and preexposure prophylaxis (PrEP) use, testing and awareness, treatment and viral suppression, and mortality.[13–15] For example, up to 60 000 PWH live in states that have failed to expand Medicaid coverage, actively harming Black PWH who are more likely to be insured by Medicaid compared with their White counterparts. In addition, previous studies have found Medicaid expansion to be associated with greater uptake of PrEP, increased viral suppression, and reduced HIV incidence.[16] Thus, HIV becomes underprioritized and criminalized for predominately Black queer and trans communities, particularly in the US South, because of pervasive racial segregation and subsequent lack of resources, rather than treated as a public health priority rooted in systemic racism and the legacy of slavery.[17]

Recent estimates indicate that the US South accounted for 52% of new HIV diagnoses in 2022.[18,19] Racial disparities in HIV prevalence and HIV criminalization are clear. In Florida, for example, Black people constitute only 16% of the population but represent 45% of PWH. Yet, they further represent 56% of those convicted of an HIV-related "crime."[20] Black people in the South are also more likely to be convicted after being arrested for HIV-related offenses compared with other racial groups, as well as to be overrepresented on sex-offender registries and to receive longer prison sentences for the same conviction.[20] The Movement Advancement Project supports the claim that these criminalization laws are disproportionately pushing queer and trans people of color into the carceral system.[21] While Black transgender women who engage in sex work are particularly vulnerable, Black cisgender women in sex work are also often charged, in addition to Black men (often straight) who have had interactions with law enforcement.[22,23] Though racism and transphobia and homophobia absolutely exacerbate each other, this demonstrates that racism can at times be a more salient factor than homophobia and transphobia in conviction. This is a specific area that requires more intersectional research to clarify these disparities. Currently, 35 states in the United States hold HIV criminalization statutes.[24]

## SOCIAL AND HEALTH OUTCOMES RELATED TO HIV

While disparities in the prevalence of and mortality attributable to HIV are clearly linked to health and health outcomes, the additional social effects of HIV status are significant. Living with HIV is linked to increased external and internalized stigma (resulting in repressed sexuality and gender expression and worse health outcomes), discrimination, and violence.[1,25,26] In this way, the social elements of HIV (e.g., stigma) can be just as damaging as the physical health impacts, and HIV criminalization reinforces the negative social outcomes, all while not promoting positive physical health outcomes. In addition, while the presumed purpose of HIV criminalization laws was to dissuade and reduce transmission, some research has found HIV to have been transmitted in prisons through condomless sex and injection drug use.[27,28] The abject neglect of this hypermarginalized community in need of care, treatment, and prevention is also its own form of structural violence.

## THEORY

The disproportionate impact of HIV criminalization on Black queer and trans communities highlights how systemic racism continues to shape health and social outcomes in the United States. To better understand the roots of this discriminatory approach to public health, it is essential to examine the issue through the lens of critical theory.

Racial capitalism asserts that racialized exploitation and capital accumulation are mutually reinforcing.[29] While the "queerification" of HIV laid the groundwork for the subsequent criminalization of HIV, the shifting face of HIV later drastically racialized this issue and even included cisgender and heterosexual Black men and women. This suggests that while these laws were enacted to punish White cis gay men, punishments disproportionately affected Black communities.[22] This process allows a capitalist system to "dispose" of surplus populations through incarceration and neglect their health needs, reducing the monetary "drain" of health care provision.[27] Surplus populations are "working-age population[s], who are surplus to the immediate needs of capital for waged labor at any given place and time"[30(p412)] characterized by un- or underemployment, absence of a living wage, inability to meet basic needs, and "hyper-exploitative" work.[30]

In the prison industrial complex, especially in the cases of privatized prisons, surplus populations are exploited for labor, enriching stakeholders. These disparities are deeply racialized. In 2015, more than 17 150 of incarcerated people in the United States were PWH, the vast majority attributable to contraction outside of the prison system.[31] HIV researchers argue that health care in prison is an opportunity to engage incarcerated PWH in HIV treatment (as part of an HIV-prevention strategy).[32] They also cite that PWH from multiple marginalized backgrounds lack consistent access to HIV care outside of prisons.[32] Realistically, efforts outside incarceration are insufficiently addressing social determinants of health and the role of racism, homophobia, and transphobia in their HIV treatment and prevention strategies. Racist incarceration practices should not have to be a way to gain access to consistent HIV-related care.

AJPH July 2025, Vol. 115, No. 7

Estimates for those charged under HIV statutes vary and are often underreported because of a reliance on media or recorded court reports. Some of these estimates rely on HIV-specific statute indictments but neglect those prosecuted under general statutes. One study identified 310 cases between 1986 and 2001 and 350 between 2008 and 2011.[33] Other sources, such as the HIV Justice Network, which include cases between 2008 and 2024, cite 2574 cases.[34] Thus, there is less consistency in reporting whether individuals were just arrested versus charged or convicted, as most cases are based on media coverage after police involvement. For example, the HIV Justice Network found 629 cases in Florida, but the Williams Institute cites that only 35% of arrests end in conviction.[34,35] The intersections of race, gender, sexual orientation, and socioeconomic status add complexity to this issue, underscoring the way that these coalescing oppressions serve to exacerbate one another.

While racial capitalism and intersectionality are essential lenses from which to view these inequities, additional theories, like the social determinants of health and neighborhood effects framework, add nuance to racial HIV disparities and criminalization. A social determinants of health lens sheds light on how disparities in access to basic needs and resources (e.g., income, housing, freedom from incarceration) drive the HIV epidemic. These poverty-related factors, particularly housing, employment, income, insurance, and health care access, present barriers to HIV resources.[1,16] Of note, these frameworks overlap in violent and racialized ways that form a vicious cycle of disenfranchisement for marginalized communities, like Black queer and trans people. It is essential to acknowledge the role that racism and racial capitalism play in shaping social determinants and reinforcing disparities in these communities.

Relatedly, the neighborhood effects framework highlights how structural environments shape neighborhood conditions that influence health, particularly for racially marginalized communities.[36] For example, a Chicago study found that an additional HIV-positive individual in one's sexual network increased seroconversion risk 13-fold.[37] Segregated residential patterns concentrate high rates of HIV and unsuppressed viral loads within small geographic areas, increasing the likelihood of exposure to an HIV-positive partner.[38] Not only does this unsurprisingly map onto some of the CDC's Ending the HIV Epidemic districts, but the enforcement of HIV criminalization statutes against (Black) PWH is also harsher, with increased rates of conviction. In Missouri, for instance, Black residents make up only 12% of the population but account for 45% of PWH and 61% of HIV-related convictions, reflecting entrenched segregation and inequities like St. Louis's "Delmar Divide."[20,33,39]

Overall, HIV criminalization is a symptom of a larger violent system purposefully built to further entrench racial injustice, including what is essentially slave prison labor, in our society. While, numerically, the impact of HIV decriminalization is small compared with the vast number of those incarcerated on other charges, efforts to decarcerate have a drastic impact on individuals' lives. Michael Johnson, sentenced to 30 years in prison in Missouri on a felony charge for allegedly "knowingly" transmitting HIV to a (White) man and 4 charges for potentially exposing 4 other men who did not contract HIV, was freed after 5 years on appeal. In prison, he was placed in solitary confinement for 23 hours a day, saying, "I'm HIV-positive and they feel like I could harm someone, or they feel like because people don't want to be around me, they have to isolate me," and that, "certain people feel like they can mistreat me just because I'm a little different."[40] Solitary confinement is a particularly brutal practice with devastating impacts on individuals' health. Even after release, these individuals face higher rates of premature death from opioid overdose, homicide, and suicide, which further underscores the potential significance and impact that HIV decriminalization and decarceration may have on other priority public health issues.[41]

## DECRIMINALIZATION AND DECARCERATION VS MODERNIZATION

The debate over modernizing or reforming HIV criminalization statutes versus abolishing them entirely remains contentious. In this policy insight, the language used to describe these approaches is drawn from abolitionist activists: "reformist reforms" and "abolitionist steps." Abolitionist steps steadily deconstruct and reduce the overall impact of violent institutions like prisons, while reformist reforms continue to promote or expand the reach of these institutions' power.[42] Reformist reforms take the shape of HIV modernization that may decrease sentence severity, place stricter criteria for criminalization, or combine HIV criminalization under general codes or other contagious disease criminalization statutes.[43] These "reformist" reforms make it more difficult to charge people with a crime or may decrease sentence length but further serve to concretize criminalization. These reforms may still be inequitably applied by race, implicitly dictating who society believes still deserves to have their freedom revoked. They remain HIV criminalization statutes rebranded under a new name, effectively maintaining the status quo of criminalization, and may eventually be more difficult to abolish. Generally, reforms proposed by institutions that benefit from the exploitation of those demanding racial justice are insufficient. These reforms attempt to placate dissenters while upholding White supremacy to maintain power and control. Abolition requires individuals to work and deconstruct reforms outside of oppressive systems to bring about genuine change, as oppressive systems will not plot their own demise.

Reformist reforms may reduce incarceration, but may do little to address HIV stigma, with devastating consequences.[44] A key example of a reformist reform is the institution of general communicable disease statutes, such as Iowa's criminalization law (2014 Iowa Legis Serv Ch 1119 [SF 2297] [West]).[45] Despite repealing its HIV-specific criminalization statutes, Iowa legislators adopted a broad contagious disease transmission law that criminalizes people with hepatitis, meningococcal disease, and tuberculosis, in addition to HIV.[45]

Bolder initiatives are needed to intervene at the root of the racial capitalist criminal justice system that is the prison industrial complex. The American Public Health Association outlines concrete evidence-based steps in its 2021 policy statement on prison abolition, arguing that "an abolitionist public health approach advocates primary prevention by disrupting the ideologies and structural determinants that shape incarceration prevalence, target marginalized populations, and increase the risk of adverse health outcomes."[46] Abolitionist steps, in contrast to reformist reforms, work to steadily reduce the power, money, or influence of oppressive institutions as part of the long process toward an end goal of true abolition. The current status quo of stagnancy is moving away from the CDC's 2025 Ending the HIV Epidemic goals.[47]

It is important to acknowledge that abolitionist changes are often incremental and to prioritize addressing aspects of decriminalization and decarceration iteratively. Abolitionist approaches

1. effectively decrease the number of people who are incarcerated by removing the statutes completely,
2. make an explicit statement that under no conditions is a person to be incarcerated as a public health intervention for a disease often rooted in poverty (noting that poverty and social and racial inequities are the root of many charges),
3. limit this oppressive institution's power and monetary income (funds that can then be utilized in health-promoting ways instead of punitively), and
4. are a small step in the full decarceration of all peoples.

Supposed crimes against law enforcement officers should also be stricken from the law.

Abolitionist efforts must confront common assumptions and missteps. Some suggest creating "evidence-based" policies to replace unsupported criminalization practices, but no evidence supports criminalization as a public health, rehabilitative, or accountability measure.[12] Another harmful assumption is the belief that abolishing only some statutes implies that those incarcerated for other reasons are more "deserving" of imprisonment, reinforcing narratives of "nonviolent exceptions." True abolition requires addressing these issues alongside mass decarceration, closing prisons without replacement, eliminating funding for jails and prisons, reducing policing and community contact with police, and establishing accessible community-led services that address the root of harm.

Full decarceration does not equate to a lack of accountability but, instead, opens the door for new forms of accountability, such as models of transformative justice, which center healing and humanity for both survivors and perpetrators of harm. Transformative justice is a political framework that responds to violence without relying on the state, avoiding reinforcement of systemic violence. It emphasizes prevention measures through "healing, accountability, resilience, and safety for all."[48] Beyond interpersonal accountability, transformative justice seeks to restructure society to prioritize the flourishing and healing of all, particularly those harmed by racist oppressive systems, offering a pathway to address harm without perpetuating cycles of violence and dehumanization.

## SOLUTION BUILDING

The complex, piecework system of HIV criminalization requires multifaceted solutions that address HIV as a public health issue and deconstruct the longstanding harms of criminalization by using transformative justice tenets as a framework to repair and prevent harm on a structural level.

AJPH July 2025, Vol. 115, No. 7

## REDISTRIBUTING FUNDS

Criminalizing HIV is, in and of itself, a policy supposedly instituted to reduce the transmission of HIV; yet, HIV continues to spread among incarcerated people in the prison system.[27] Incarceration serves as a punishment for a disease, not treatment or prevention. Not only are these statutes ineffective, but they are also incredibly costly. Florida diverted an estimated $15.2 million to incarceration costs for HIV-related convictions between 1997 and 2020, while Georgia spent $9 million between 2000 and 2020.[49,50] Criminalization policies disproportionately affect Black people, as reflected in Nevada, where Black individuals constitute 40% of those convicted under HIV statutes despite representing only 10% of the state's population.[51]

Funds dedicated to incarceration can be redistributed to provide treatment services for PWH (e.g., antiretroviral treatment access) and prevention efforts (e.g., access to testing, PrEP, condoms, substance use treatment, and education). This is essential, as the United States is far behind in meeting its Ending the HIV Epidemic benchmark of reducing new HIV infections by 75% by 2025, decreasing only 12% between 2017 and 2021.[47] These funds can also be directed toward advocacy organizations that are leveraging antiracist approaches to policy change.

## STIGMA AND PREVENTION

The coalescence of racism, HIV stigma, homophobia, and linked socioeconomic factors creates significant barriers to health and positive health outcomes for treatment and prevention. While evidence is mixed, some studies suggest that states with enacted HIV criminalization laws report higher levels of HIV stigma and discrimination, which may discourage testing, prevention measures, and disclosure.[12,26] This relationship may be mediated by mass-media portrayals of criminalized cases, which amplify stigma by framing PWH as dangerous or deviant.[52] Such stigma, however, is not independent of racial discrimination; rather, it intersects with and exacerbates racial inequities, as Black and other marginalized communities bear the brunt of both criminalization and systemic oppression. Confronting these structural and social barriers, along with improving access to high-quality care, housing, and HIV prevention, can improve these health outcomes, including linkage to HIV medical care and increased viral suppression, ultimately reducing transmissibility.[53]

Decreasing criminalization can be advanced by promoting accessible and equitable prevention strategies, particularly those that address racial inequities.[54] Current prevention methods, like PrEP, must reach the most vulnerable populations, including Black transgender women, especially those engaged in sex work (which is 27% of Black trans women).[55] Nearly half (47%) of Black transgender individuals have been incarcerated at some point in their lives, where they experience disproportionate rates of sexual violence, a result of poverty, houselessness, discrimination, criminalization of sex work, and law enforcement bias.[56] These women are 13 times more likely to live with HIV, and sex work criminalization amplifies stigma and violence.[23] Incarceration is particularly dehumanizing for Black trans women, who are often placed in male prisons, denied gender-affirming care, subjected to violence, and confined in solitary under the guise of "protection."[57] Addressing these injustices requires accessible prevention, harm reduction (e.g., clean needle programs), antistigma campaigns, and policies targeting violence against transgender people. Funding should prioritize trusted, local, antiracist community-based organizations and governmental initiatives that advocate for decriminalization, provide services, and combat stigma to effectively support prevention and empowerment.

## ONGOING AND ANTICIPATED CHALLENGES

Abolition initiatives face several barriers, particularly from powerful stakeholders who profit from carceral practices, including private prison owners, law enforcement, politicians, and the justice system. Privatized prisons generate $374 million annually, incentivizing law enforcement to increase low-level arrests and incarcerate "surplus" populations deemed unfit for society but exploitable for labor.[58] According to 2017 data, the justice system benefits directly, with the government paying approximately $3.9 billion annually to companies managing private prisons, which also profit from supplying commissary goods and telephone services.[59] Penal labor further enriches both public and private prisons, generating $9 billion in prison maintenance services and $2 billion in goods annually, while incarcerated individuals earn pennies.[60] For example, Dominique Morgan cited being paid $2.25 a day as a chef working from 4 AM through dinner despite his HIV diagnosis.[58] Notably, there has been a recent shift in for-profit prisons with an increasing amount being converted into US Immigration and Customs Enforcement facilities.[61] Nevertheless, there have been reported abuses within these facilities against persons who are queer, trans, and living with HIV, including sexual abuse and being denied adequate health care, dehumanizing and violating these communities.[62]

The historical devaluation of Black queer and trans lives poses another barrier to implementing meaningful, multipronged interventions. This systemic degradation and subjugation have created a chronic undervaluation of these communities, underscoring the need for a collective movement to extend care and support. Antistigma campaigns are critical to raising awareness, disseminating evidence-based knowledge, and humanizing the deleterious effects of criminalization on marginalized and often neglected communities. Despite substantial opposition and extensive challenges, forward momentum must be maintained. Small legislative changes in reforming HIV criminalization across the United States, while insufficient, signal a growing willingness to address these injustices and advance a more equitable and just society.

## CONCLUSION

To address racial, sexual orientation–, and gender-based disparities in HIV prevalence in the United States, it is essential to confront the racialized root causes of these inequities. This requires immediate decarceration of individuals imprisoned under HIV criminalization statutes, the eradication of these statutes, and comprehensive prevention and treatment efforts. By redistributing resources and wealth and intentionally valuing marginalized communities, particularly Black queer and trans communities, we can prioritize their health and well-being. Decriminalizing HIV is a small step toward full prison abolition, affirming that no one deserves to lose their freedom. This path reflects a commitment to honoring the humanity of all, especially those historically oppressed by exploitative systems. AJPH

## ABOUT THE AUTHORS

Louis Listerud, Steven Meanley, Alana Richards, Black Kosciow, and Stephen Bonett are with the Department of Family and Community Health, University of Pennsylvania School of Nursing, Philadelphia, PA.

## CORRESPONDENCE

Correspondence should be sent to Louis Listerud, 418 Curie Blvd, Rm: 2013C, Philadelphia, PA 19104 (e-mail: louis1@nursing.upenn.edu). Reprints can be ordered at https://www.ajph.org by clicking the "Reprints" link.

## PUBLICATION INFORMATION

Full Citation: Listerud L, Meanley S, Richards A, Kosciow B, Bonett S. A decarceral response to HIV criminalization in the Black LGBTQIA+ community. *Am J Public Health*. 2025;115(7):1157–1165.

Acceptance Date: March 5, 2025.

DOI: https://doi.org/10.2105/AJPH.2025.308110

ORCID iDs:

Louis Listerud https://orcid.org/0000-0001-5337-0265

Steven Meanley https://orcid.org/0000-0002-6098-9733

Alana Richards https://orcid.org/0009-0001-7602-5488

Blake Kosciow https://orcid.org/0009-0006-8912-8773

Stephen Bonett https://orcid.org/0000-0002-7608-3741

## CONTRIBUTORS

L. Listerud made substantial contributions to the conceptualization, drafting, and revising of the work. S. Meanley, A. Richards, B. Kosciow, and S. Bonnet revised the work critically for important intellectual content and approved the final version to be published.

## ACKNOWLEDGMENTS

We would like to extend our deepest gratitude to Seleeke Flingai for his encouragement, instruction, and guidance.

## CONFLICTS OF INTEREST

The authors have no potential or actual conflicts of interest from funding or affiliation-related activities to report.

## HUMAN PARTICIPANT PROTECTION

This analytic essay did not include any human participants.

## REFERENCES

1. Burns PA. Perspective chapter: Centering race, stigma and discrimination—structural racism and disparities in HIV among Black sexual minority men. In: Guerrero E. *Effective Elimination of Structural Racism*. London, England: IntechOpen; 2022. https://doi.org/10.5772/intechopen.101528
2. Centers for Disease Control and Prevention. Fast facts: HIV in the US by race and ethnicity. HIV. June 27, 2024. Available at: https://www.cdc.gov/hiv/data-research/facts-stats/race-ethnicity.html. Accessed August 26, 2024.
3. Wilson TA. HIV criminalization: a continuation of racial–sexual terror exacted on the bodies of Black MSM. In: Brock R, Nix-Stevenson D, Miller PC. *Critical Black Studies Reader*. New York, NY: Peter Lang Group; 2017. https://doi.org/10.3726/978-1-4539-1896-8
4. Ronald Reagan. Executive Order 12601—Presidential Commission on the Human Immunodeficiency Virus Epidemic. June 24, 1987. Available at: https://www.reaganlibrary.gov/archives/speech/executive-order-12601-presidential-commission-human-immunodeficiency-virus-epidemic. Accessed August 26, 2024.
5. National Institutes of Health. Guidelines for the Use of Antiretroviral Agents in Adults and Adolescents With HIV. 2023. Available at: https://clinicalinfo.hiv.gov/en/guidelines/hiv-clinical-guidelines-adult-and-adolescent-arv/early-acute-and-recent-hiv-infection. Accessed August 26, 2024.
6. American Psychological Association. 1990s HIV/AIDS Timeline. Available at: https://www.apa.org/pi/aids/youth/nineties-timeline. Accessed August 26, 2024.
7. Pimm L. *The Reagan Administration and the AIDS Epidemic: The Relationship Between Rhetoric and Marginalization*. Honors Thesis. Hattiesburg, MS: University of Southern Mississippi; 2021. Available at: https://aquila.usm.edu/cgi/viewcontent.cgi?article=1778&context=honors_theses. Accessed October 7, 2024.
8. Lehman JS, Carr MH, Nichol AJ, et al. Prevalence and public health implications of state laws that criminalize potential HIV exposure in the United States. *AIDS Behav*. 2014;18(6):997–1006. https://doi.org/10.1007/s10461-014-0724-0
9. Brown R. When the body is a weapon: an intersectional feminist analysis of HIV criminalization in Louisiana. *Berkeley J Gend Law Justice*. 2020;35(1):91–136. https://doi.org/10.15779/Z38NS0KZ4H
10. The Center for HIV Law and Policy. *HIV Criminalization in the United States. A Sourcebook on State and Federal HIV Criminal Law and Practice*. Available at: https://www.hivlawandpolicy.org/sites/default/files/HIV%20Criminalization%20in%20the%20U.S.%20A%20Sourcebook%20on%20State%20Fed%20HIV%20Criminal%20Law%20and%20Practice%20022722.pdf. Accessed October 6, 2024.
11. Moseby KM. Two regimes of HIV/AIDS: the *MMWR* and the socio-political construction of

HIV/AIDS as a 'Black disease.' *Sociol Health Illn.* 2017;39(7):1068–1082. https://doi.org/10.1111/1467-9566.12552

12. Cann D, Harrison SE, Qiao S. Historical and current trends in HIV criminalization in South Carolina: implications for the Southern HIV epidemic. *AIDS Behav.* 2019;23(suppl 3):233–241. https://doi.org/10.1007/s10461-019-02599-1
13. Hawkins DS. "What if I aint ate in 2 days, why the hell would I want you to poke into my arm": a critical cultural analysis of Testing Makes Us Stronger. *Front Commun (Lausanne).* 2020;5:26. https://doi.org/10.3389/fcomm.2020.00026
14. Centers for Disease Control and Prevention. HIV and gay and bisexual men. November 30, 2021. Available at: https://www.cdc.gov/vitalsigns/hivgaybimen/index.html. Accessed January 13, 2025.
15. Centers for Disease Control and Prevention. Health disparities in Black or African American people. November 21, 2024. Available at: https://www.cdc.gov/health-disparities-hiv-std-tb-hepatitis/populations/black-african-american.html. Accessed January 13, 2025.
16. Millett GA. New pathogen, same disparities: why COVID-19 and HIV remain prevalent in US communities of colour and implications for ending the HIV epidemic. *J Int AIDS Soc.* 2020;23(11):e25639. https://doi.org/10.1002/jia2.25639
17. KFF. The Impact of HIV on Black People in the United States. September 9, 2024. Available at: https://www.kff.org/hivaids/fact-sheet/black-americans-and-hivaids-the-basics. Accessed October 17, 2022.
18. Marano M, Stein R, Song W, et al. HIV testing, linkage to HIV medical care, and interviews for partner services among Black men who have sex with men—non–health care facilities, 20 southern US jurisdictions, 2016. *MMWR Morb Mortal Wkly Rep.* 2018;67(28):778–781. https://doi.org/10.15585/mmwr.mm6728a3
19. Centers for Disease Control and Prevention. CDC publishes new HIV surveillance reports. National Center for HIV, Viral Hepatitis, STD, and Tuberculosis Prevention. May 21, 2024. Available at: https://www.cdc.gov/nchhstp/director-letters/cdc-publishes-new-hiv-surveillance-reports.html. Accessed January 13, 2025.
20. UCLA School of Law Williams Institute. HIV criminalization in the United States. Available at: https://williamsinstitute.law.ucla.edu/visualization/hiv-criminalization. Accessed January 13, 2025.
21. Movement Advancement Project and Center for HIV Law & Policy. LGBT policy spotlight: HIV criminalization laws. December 2016. Available at: https://www.lgbtmap.org/policy-and-issue-analysis/policy-spotlight-HIV-criminalization. Accessed February 24, 2025.
22. Catherine Hanssens on HIV Criminalization in the US. AIDSVu. May 10, 2021. Available at: https://aidsvu.org/news-updates/catherine-hanssens-on-hiv-criminalization-in-the-u-s. Accessed February 24, 2025.
23. Holston-Zannell LB. Reducing HIV transmission requires decriminalizing sex work. News & Commentary. American Civil Liberties Union. December 2019. Available at: https://www.aclu.org/news/hiv/reducing-hiv-transmission-requires-decriminalizing-sex-work. Accessed December 19, 2022.
24. Centers for Disease Control and Prevention. HIV and STD criminalization laws. Available at: https://web.archive.org/web/20241201180756/https://www.cdc.gov/hiv/policies/law/states/exposure.html. Accessed October 17, 2022.
25. Chestnut S, Dixon E, Jindasurat C. Lesbian, gay, bisexual, transgender, queer and HIV-affected hate violence in 2012. National Coalition of Anti-Violence Programs. 2012. Available at: https://avp.org/reports. Accessed October 5, 2024.
26. Baugher AR, Whiteman A, Jeffries WL, Finlayson T, Lewis R, Wejnert C. Black men who have sex with men living in states with HIV criminalization laws report high stigma, 23 US cities, 2017. *AIDS.* 2021;35(10):1637–1645. https://doi.org/10.1097/QAD.0000000000002917
27. Horley J. Sexuality and sexual health in prisons. *Sex Cult.* 2019;23(4):1372–1386. https://doi.org/10.1007/s12119-019-09619-1
28. Valera P, Chang Y, Lian Z. HIV risk inside US prisons: a systematic review of risk reduction interventions conducted in US prisons. *AIDS Care.* 2017;29(8):943–952. https://doi.org/10.1080/09540121.2016.1271102
29. Robinson CJ. *Black Marxism: The Making of the Black Radical Tradition.* Chapel Hill, NC: University of North Carolina Press; 2000.
30. Bernards N, Soederberg S. Relative surplus populations and the crises of contemporary capitalism: reviving, revisiting, recasting. *Geoforum.* 2021;126:412–419. https://doi.org/10.1016/j.geoforum.2020.12.009
31. Parsons S. The "wear and tear" of African Americans in Louisiana with HIV/AIDS: more than HIV. *SunKrist Public Health Res J.* 2020;2(2):1–15.
32. Meyer JP, Chen NE, Springer SA. HIV treatment in the criminal justice system: critical knowledge and intervention gaps. *Aids Res Treat.* 2011; 2011(1):680617. https://doi.org/10.1155/2011/680617
33. Harsono D, Galletly CL, O'Keefe E, Lazzarini Z. Criminalization of HIV exposure: a review of empirical studies in the United States. *AIDS Behav.* 2017;21(1):27–50. https://doi.org/10.1007/s10461-016-1540-5
34. HIV Justice Network. USA. Available at: https://www.hivjustice.net/country/us. Accessed February 24, 2025.
35. Williams Institute. HIV criminalization in Florida. October 2018. Available at: https://williamsinstitute.law.ucla.edu/publications/hiv-criminalization-fl. Accessed January 13, 2025.
36. Diez Roux AV. Neighborhoods and health: where are we and where do we go from here? *Rev Epidemiol Sante Publique.* 2007;55(1):13–21. https://doi.org/10.1016/j.respe.2006.12.003
37. Morgan E, Skaathun B, Duvoisin R, Michaels S, Schneider J. Are HIV seroconversions among young men who have sex with men associated with social network proximity to recently or long-term HIV-infected individuals? *J Acquir Immune Defic Syndr.* 2018;77(2):128–134. https://doi.org/10.1097/QAI.0000000000001586
38. Akers AY, Muhammad MR, Corbie-Smith G. "When you got nothing to do, you do somebody": a community's perceptions of neighborhood effects on adolescent sexual behaviors. *Soc Sci Med.* 2011;72(1):91–99. https://doi.org/10.1016/j.socscimed.2010.09.035
39. For the Sake of All. A Report on the Health and Well-Being of African Americans in St. Louis and Why It Matters for Everyone. Washington University in St Louis, Saint Louis University. 2014. Available at: https://forthesakeofall.wordpress.com/wp-content/uploads/2014/05/for-the-sake-of-all-report.pdf. Accessed December 2, 2024.
40. HIV Justice Network. [Update] US: Michael Johnson set free after spending 5 years in prison. July 9, 2019. Available at: https://www.hivjustice.net/cases/us-missouri-supreme-court-upholds-reversal-of-michael-johnson-conviction. Accessed February 24, 2025.
41. Herring T. The research is clear: solitary confinement causes long-lasting harm. Prison Policy Initiative. December 8, 2020. Available at: https://www.prisonpolicy.org/blog/2020/12/08/solitary_symposium. Accessed February 24, 2025.
42. Community Resource Hub. Reformist reforms vs. abolitionist steps to end imprisonment. Available at: https://communityresourcehub.org/resources/reformist-reforms-vs-abolitionist-steps-in-policing. Accessed August 26, 2024.
43. Centers for Disease Control and Prevention. HIV criminalization and ending the HIV epidemic. January 30, 2024. Available at: https://web.archive.org/web/20240718225122/https://www.cdc.gov/hiv/policies/law/criminalization-ehe.html. Accessed August 26, 2024.
44. Turan B, Budhwani H, Fazeli PL, et al. How does stigma affect people living with HIV? The mediating roles of internalized and anticipated HIV stigma in the effects of perceived community stigma on health and psychosocial outcomes. *AIDS Behav.* 2017;21(1):283–291. https://doi.org/10.1007/s10461-016-1451-5
45. Iowa Legislature. Chapter 1119, Criminal Transmission of Contagious or Infectious Diseases, S.F. 2297. 2014. Available at: https://www.legis.iowa.gov/docs/publications/iactc/85.2/CH1119.pdf. Accessed December 6, 2024.
46. American Public Health Association. Advancing public health interventions to address the harms of the carceral system. October 25, 2021. Available at: https://www.apha.org/policies-and-advocacy/public-health-policy-statements/policy-database/2022/01/07/advancing-public-health-interventions-to-address-the-harms-of-the-carceral-system. Accessed August 26, 2024.
47. Centers for Disease Control and Prevention. Ending the HIV Epidemic in the US Goals. Ending the HIV Epidemic in the US. May 14, 2024. Available at: https://www.cdc.gov/ehe/php/about/goals.html. Accessed August 26, 2024.
48. Mingus M. Transformative justice: a brief description. TransformHarm. 2019. Available at: https://transformharm.org/tj_resource/transformative-justice-a-brief-description. Accessed January 13, 2025.
49. Williams Institute. HIV criminalization in Florida: length of incarceration and fiscal implications. July 2021. Available at: https://williamsinstitute.law.ucla.edu/publications/hiv-incarceration-fl. Accessed December 19, 2022.
50. Williams Institute. HIV criminalization in Georgia: length of incarceration and fiscal implications. June 2021. Available at: https://williamsinstitute.law.ucla.edu/publications/hiv-incarceration-ga. Accessed December 19, 2022.
51. Williams Institute. Enforcement of HIV criminalization in Nevada. May 2021. Available at: https://williamsinstitute.law.ucla.edu/publications/hiv-criminalization-nevada. Accessed December 19, 2022.
52. Conway P. Media-driven stigma continues with new HIV criminalization case. AIDS Foundation

Chicago. June 9, 2015. Available at: https://www.aidschicago.org/media-driven-stigma-continues-with-new-hiv-criminalization-case. Accessed January 14, 2025.

53. Centers for Disease Control and Prevention. HIV and African American gay and bisexual men: prevention challenges. September 14, 2022. Available at: https://web.archive.org/web/20240408233840/https://www.cdc.gov/hiv/group/bmsm/prevention-challenges.html. Accessed November 25, 2022.
54. Centers for Disease Control and Prevention. HIV and African American gay and bisexual men: HIV prevention. September 14, 2022. Available at: https://web.archive.org/web/20231206032946/https://www.cdc.gov/hiv/group/bmsm/hiv-prevention.html. Accessed November 25, 2022.
55. Greene J. The cost of crossing gender boundaries: trans women of color and the racialized workplace gender order. *Gend Work Organ.* 2024;31(6):2585–2600. https://doi.org/10.1111/gwao.13108
56. National Center for Transgender Equality. Prison and detention reform. Available at: https://transequality.org/sites/default/files/docs/resources/NCTE_Blueprint_for_Equality2012_Prison_Reform.pdf. Accessed October 3, 2024.
57. Coppola F. Gender identity in the era of mass incarceration: the cruel and unusual segregation of trans people in the United States. *Int J Const Law.* 2023;21(2):649–672. https://doi.org/10.1093/icon/moad046
58. Payne S. The economic impact of prison labor for incarcerated individuals and taxpayers. *Princeton Legal Journal.* 2023;2(1). Available at: https://legaljournal.princeton.edu/the-economic-impact-of-prison-labor-for-incarcerated-individuals-and-taxpayers. Accessed August 26, 2024.
59. Wagner P, Rabuy B. Following the money of mass incarceration. Prison Policy Initiative. 2017. Available at: https://www.prisonpolicy.org/reports/money.html. Accessed August 26, 2024.
60. US prison labor programs violate fundamental human rights, new report finds. *UChicago News.* June 16, 2022. Available at: https://news.uchicago.edu/story/us-prison-labor-programs-violate-fundamental-human-rights-new-report-finds. Accessed August 26, 2024.
61. American Civil Liberties Union. Privatized immigrant detention. Available at: https://www.aclu.org/issues/immigrants-rights/immigrants-rights-and-detention/privatized-immigration-detention. Accessed February 24, 2025.
62. Immigration Equality. New report finds widespread abuse of LGBTQ and HIV-positive people in ICE and CBP jails. June 18, 2024. Available at: https://immigrationequality.org/press/press-releases-2/new-report-finds-widespread-abuse-of-lgbtq-and-hiv-positive-people-in-ice-and-cbp-jails. Accessed February 24, 2025.

# Minimum Legal Age of Nonmedical Cannabis Purchase Laws and Cannabis-Related Hospitalizations in Canada, 2015 to 2022

Daniel T. Myran, MD, Robert Talarico, MSc, Rosalie Liccardo Pacula, PhD, Jennifer Xiao, MSc, Doug Manuel, MD, Erin Hobin, PhD, Lauren Konikoff, MA, Peter Tanuseputro, MD, and Monica Taljaard, PhD

See also Dilley and Hendrickson, p. 979.

AJPH July 2025, Vol. 115, No. 7

**Objectives.** To determine whether the minimum legal age (MLA) for cannabis purchases is associated with reductions in cannabis-related hospitalizations in youths.

**Methods.** We performed a population-based study examining all hospitalizations for cannabis use in Canada for individuals aged 15 to 44 years (n = 14.6 million in 2018) between January 1, 2015, and March 31, 2022. MLAs varied across Canada. We used a controlled interrupted time series design to compare changes in cannabis-related hospitalizations between individuals above and below the MLA.

**Results.** There were 137 901 cannabis-related hospitalizations during the study. Prelegalization rates of hospitalizations were increasing by 2% per quarter for individuals above and below the MLA. After legalization, hospitalizations began declining by 2% per quarter in individuals below the MLA (rate ratio [RR] quarterly slope change = 0.96; 95% confidence interval [CI] = 0.95, 0.98) with no slope change for individuals above the MLA. The total effect, 3.5 years after legalization, was a 34% reduction (relative difference = 0.66; 95% CI = 0.49, 0.91; *P* = .011) in hospitalizations for those below relative to those above the MLA.

**Conclusions.** Nonmedical cannabis legalization in Canada was associated with reductions in cannabis-related hospitalizations for youths below the MLA and with ongoing increases for individuals above the MLA.

**Public Health Implications.** The results suggest that cannabis legalization may increase cannabis-related hospitalizations in adults but that MLAs may prevent such increases for at-risk young people in regions pursuing cannabis legalization. (*Am J Public Health*. 2025;115(7):1166–1174. https://doi.org/10.2105/AJPH.2025.308090)

Many US states and countries around the world have legalized or are considering legalizing recreational, or nonmedical, cannabis for adult use. On October 17, 2018, Canada became the second country to legalize nonmedical cannabis for adults at the national level and the first to create a commercial cannabis market through the Cannabis Act.[1] The Cannabis Act allowed the personal possession of 30 grams of cannabis, limited home cultivation of cannabis, and the purchase of cannabis from regulated legal cannabis growers and sellers for adults. The Cannabis Act also decriminalized cannabis possession in youths of up to 5 grams for personal use.[1]

A major concern is that legalization may increase cannabis use in youths and young adults, a population that is particularly vulnerable to cannabis-related impacts on brain development and mental health harms.[2–6] Consequently, the Cannabis Act specifically sought to reduce cannabis use in youths through a variety of regulations, including setting a national minimum legal age (MLA) for cannabis purchase from legal sources (e.g., online or retail stores) of 18 years.[1] Evidence suggests that MLA restrictions are effective at reducing youth use and consequent harms of alcohol and tobacco.[7–9] Importantly, before cannabis legalization in Canada (and other countries that may pursue legalization), there was an established illicit cannabis market.[10] Critics of setting a higher MLA argue that youths will continue to access cannabis through the illicit market. In contrast, proponents of a higher MLA suggest that it will reduce youth cannabis use and associated harms by decreasing overall access to cannabis through a combination of a shrinking illicit market and excluding youths below the MLA from accessing the legal market. Importantly, the effect of cannabis MLAs on youth cannabis use and associated harms and whether higher age limits may be more protective remains uncertain.

The Cannabis Act required all provinces (n = 10) and territories (n = 3) to have an MLA of at least 18 years but permitted setting higher MLAs if desired. At the onset of legalization, 8 provinces and 3 territories set an MLA of 19 years, while Alberta (fourth-most-populous province) and Quebec (second-most-populous province) set an MLA of 18 years. In January 2020, Quebec increased the MLA from 18 to 21 years.[11] The different MLA policies across provinces and territories and the use of health administrative data capturing all hospitalizations in Canada provides a unique opportunity to examine the effect of MLA policies on cannabis-related hospitalizations in youths and young adults.

## METHODS

We completed a population-based interrupted time series study of hospitalizations in individuals aged 15 to 44 years for all provinces and territories in Canada (population of 14.6 million individuals in 2018) between January 1, 2015, and March 31, 2022. These data capture all hospitalizations for individuals eligible for a province or territory's universal health system. Canada's universal health system covers all hospital-based care and primary and specialty physician services for an estimated 97% of people living in Canada, including Canadian citizens, permanent residents, individuals with work permits, immigrants applying for permanent residence, and some refugees.[12] We used a controlled interrupted time series design to estimate the differential effects of MLA restrictions of nonmedical cannabis legalization on individuals above and below the MLA. We evaluated effects in Canada overall, across regions with different MLAs, and in Quebec, which changed its MLA in 2020.

### Data Sources

We obtained data from the Canadian Institutes for Health Information and ICES (formerly the Institute for Clinical Evaluative Sciences). We used 3 databases to capture all acute care and specialized mental health hospitalizations in Canada (see Appendix Methods 1, available as a supplement to the online version of this article at https://ajph.org, for details on databases). These data sets were linked using unique encoded identifiers and analyzed at ICES. We obtained aggregate counts of cannabis-related hospitalizations by age group each quarter for Ontario, Quebec, Alberta, and the rest of Canada. We generated age- and region-specific quarterly rates of cannabis-related hospitalizations using the estimated population obtained from Statistics Canada.[13]

### Minimum Legal Age

We considered age-specific quarterly rates to be above or below MLA at the time by using region-specific MLA policies. In Alberta (MLA = 18 years), individuals aged 15 to 17 years were below the MLA, and those who were aged 18 to 44 years were above the MLA. In Quebec (MLA = 18 years, then increased to 21 years in January 2020), individuals aged 15 to 17 years were below the MLA, individuals aged 18 to 20 years were above the MLA in period 1 and below the MLA in period 2, and individuals aged 21 to 44 years were always above the MLA. For the rest of Canada (MLA = 19 years), individuals aged 15 to 18 years were below the MLA, and those aged 19 to 44 years were above the MLA.

### Observation Period

We divided our study period into 2 policy periods: prelegalization (January 2015–September 2018) and postlegalization (October 2018–March 2022). Within the postlegalization period, we examined 2 periods: period 1 (October 2018 to December 2019) and period 2 (January 2020 to March 2022). These periods were selected based on increases in legal cannabis product and store availability and Quebec's MLA switch from 18 to 21 years in January 2020.[11,14,15] In period 1, provinces and territories were only allowed to sell dried cannabis flower, and there were restrictions on cannabis stores. In period 2, provinces and territories were also allowed to sell cannabis vapes, edibles, and concentrates, and per-capita stores increased 3.6-fold between April 2020 and April 2022 (2.6 vs 9.3 stores per 100 000 individuals).[15]

### Outcome

The outcome of interest was a cannabis-related hospitalization. In the Discharge Abstract Database and the Hospital Morbidity Database, we defined a cannabis-related hospitalization when 1 of the following *International Classification of Diseases, 10th Revision, Clinical Modification* (*ICD-10-CM*; https://secure.cihi.ca/free_products/canadian-coding-standards-2022-en.pdf) codes was listed as the main or contributing reason for hospitalization: T40.7 (poisonings by cannabis, including derivatives) and F12.X (mental and behavioral disorders due to use of cannabinoids including intoxication, harmful use, dependence, withdrawal, psychosis, and other). In the Ontario Mental Health Reporting System database, we defined a cannabis-related hospitalization when 1 of the following *International Classification of Diseases, 9th Revision, Clinical Modification* (*ICD-9-CM*, https://secure.cihi.ca/free_products/canadian-coding-standards-2022-en.pdf) codes was listed as a main or contributing reason for hospitalizations: 304.30 (cannabis dependence) or 305.20 (cannabis abuse), along with the same *ICD-10-CM* codes, T40.7 and F12.X. Previous work has found that the majority of cannabis-related hospitalizations in Canada are for cannabis use disorder (67.4%), with cannabis-induced psychosis (9.7%) and cannabis intoxication or poisoning (6.1%) being the second- and third-most-common reason for hospitalization.[16]

## Statistical Analyses

We presented the quarterly rates of cannabis-related hospitalizations per 100 000 individuals using time series plots and summarized the data across the different regulatory periods (prelegalization, overall postlegalization, and postlegalization period 1 and period 2) using annualized rates.

We used segmented linear regression analyses to examine immediate (intercept) and gradual (slope) changes in the quarterly rates of cannabis-related hospitalizations after legalization among those above versus below MLA. To account for nonlinearity in trends over time and improve normality, we conducted analyses on the log-transformed scale and estimated intercept and exponentiated slope changes in each series to provide rate ratios (RRs) with accompanying 95% confidence intervals (CIs). We estimated models by using restricted maximum likelihood and included a first-order autoregressive covariance structure as recommended for interrupted time series studies.[17] To obtain the total effect (combined intercept and slope changes), we compared the model-based estimate at the end of the study (i.e., in Q1 2022) to the counterfactual projected rate based on the trend from the preintervention period (e.g., the rate that would have been observed had legalization not occurred).[17] We used ratios of ratios to generate relative differences between groups, with individuals below the MLA considered as the reference group. All analyses were completed using SAS version 9.4 (SAS Institute, Cary, NC). See Appendix Methods 2 (available as a supplement to the online version of this article at https://ajph.org) for details on model specifications.

We completed 2 primary analyses. First, we completed a national analysis (excluding Quebec) of the quarterly rate for individuals above compared with those below the MLA, where age groups were assigned to the national aggregate rate based on region-specific MLA policies. The analysis contained 29 time points (15 quarters prelegalization, 14 quarters postlegalization) for 2 groups for a total of 58 data points. Second, we completed a Quebec-specific analysis leveraging the change from an MLA of 18 to 21 years in January 2020 to assess the robustness of our findings. We first examined changes for quarterly rates for ages 18 to 20 years and 21 years or older immediately after legalization when both groups were above the MLA. Next, we examined changes after January 2020 in rates for ages 18 to 20 years and 21 years or older when individuals aged 18 to 20 years switched to being below the MLA and those aged 21 years or older continued to be above the MLA.

We completed a series of prespecified sensitivity analyses using stratified models. We completed separate analyses for an MLA of 18 years (Alberta) and an MLA of 19 years (Canada excluding Alberta and Quebec) to examine for consistency in findings. We completed an analysis of just Ontario (MLA = 19 years) to independently assess influences of the transition of Ontario's OMHRS database from *ICD-9-CM* to *ICD-10-CM* coding in April 2019. To support the policy relevance of our findings (e.g., MLAs unlikely to be set above 25 years), we completed our primary national analysis, where we excluded rates for those aged 25 to 44 years.

# RESULTS

During the 7-year study period, there were 137 901 hospitalizations related to cannabis in Canada (130.4 hospitalizations per 100 000 person-years). For individuals above the MLA, the rate of cannabis-related hospitalizations per 100 000 person-years increased from 114.7 before to 139.4 after legalization (a 21.6% relative increase), and for individuals below the MLA, it increased

**TABLE 1— Hospitalizations for Cannabis Use by Region and Minimum Legal Age (MLA) of Cannabis Purchase: Canada, January 2015–March 2022**

| | No. or Annualized Rate Per 100 000 Individuals | | | | Crude Percent Change[a] | | |
|---|---|---|---|---|---|---|---|
| Region (Population Aged 15–44 y, 2018) | Prelegalization, January 2015–September 2018 | Postlegalization, October 2018–March 2022 | Period 1, October 2018–December 2019 | Period 2, January 2020–March 2022 | Postlegal vs Prelegal | Period 1 vs Prelegal | Period 2 vs Prelegal |
| Canada (14 570 157) | 63 817 | 74 084 | 24 518 | 49 566 | | | |
| Below MLA | 157.5 | 161.5 | 167.4 | 158.7 | 2.5 | 6.3 | 0.8 |
| Above MLA | 114.7 | 139.5 | 128.8 | 145.4 | 21.6 | 12.3 | 26.7 |
| Ontario (5 691 204) | 13 661 | 17 658 | 5 610 | 12 048 | | | |
| Below MLA | 130.4 | 116.9 | 120.9 | 114.7 | −10.3 | −7.3 | −12.1 |
| Above MLA | 57.2 | 81.9 | 71.8 | 87.4 | 43.4 | 25.7 | 53.0 |
| Alberta (1 848 997) | 7 894 | 8 862 | 2 929 | 5 933 | | | |
| Below MLA | 178.8 | 186.1 | 191.0 | 183.4 | 4.1 | 6.8 | 2.6 |
| Above MLA | 109.1 | 130.6 | 120.0 | 136.5 | 19.7 | 9.9 | 25.0 |
| Quebec (3 144 225) | 19 277 | 23 889 | 7 901 | 15 988 | | | |
| Age 15–17 y | 111.4 | 105.7 | 109.3 | 103.8 | −5.1 | −1.9 | −6.8 |
| Age 18–20 y | 215.6 | 238.4 | 246.5 | 233.9 | 10.6 | 14.4 | 8.5 |
| Age ≥ 21 y | 165.2 | 222.1 | 202.6 | 232.9 | 34.4 | 22.6 | 41.0 |
| Rest of Canada (3 885 731) | 22 985 | 23 675 | 8 078 | 15 597 | | | |
| Below MLA | 216.1 | 222.4 | 260.7 | 200.8 | 3.0 | 20.7 | −7.1 |
| Above MLA | 153.7 | 163.4 | 151.7 | 169.8 | 6.3 | −1.3 | 10.4 |

[a]Calculated as (postlegal rate–prelegal rate)/prelegal rate * 100.

from 157.5 before to 161.5 after legalization (a 2.5% relative increase; Table 1). Hospitalizations by age and province are available in Appendix Table A.

Figure 1a displays the results of the segmented linear regression analyses of quarterly rates of hospitalizations related to cannabis for Canada, excluding Quebec, with model results in Table 2. Prelegalization rates of hospitalizations were increasing at a similar rate of 2.0% per quarter for individuals below and above the MLA (relative difference = 1.00; 95% CI = 0.99, 1.01; $P$ = .866). After legalization, there were no immediate changes in either group and no slope change for individuals above the MLA (RR = 1.00; 95% CI = 0.98, 1.01) with rates of hospitalization continuing to increase by 2.0% per quarter. However, there was a slope change for individuals below the MLA (RR = 0.96; 95% CI = 0.95, 0.98), with rates of hospitalizations now declining by 2.0% per quarter. Overall, in Q1 2022 (3.5 years after legalization), rates of cannabis-related hospitalizations were 39.0% (RR = 0.61; 95% CI = 0.49, 0.76) lower than expected based on prelegalization trends in those below the MLA and not different than expected in those above the MLA (RR = 0.92; 95% CI = 0.73, 1.14). Overall, legalization was associated with a 34.0% (relative difference = 0.66; 95% CI = 0.49, 0.91; $P$ = .011) reduction in cannabis-related hospitalizations in those below the MLA relative to those above.

Figure 1b displays the results of the segmented linear regression analyses of quarterly rates of cannabis-related hospitalizations for Quebec with model results in Table 3. In Quebec, rates of hospitalizations were increasing before legalization in ages 18 to 20 years and 21 years or older. There were no immediate or gradual changes after legalization in October 2018 when the MLA was 18 years. Before the MLA change, hospitalizations were increasing by 2.0% per quarter in ages 18 to 20 years and 3.0% for ages 21 years or older with no difference in trends (RR = 0.99; 95% CI = 0.98, 1.00; $P$ = .068).

After the change in MLA from 18 years to 21 years in January 2020, there was a larger immediate decrease in hospitalizations (relative difference = 0.94; 95% CI = 0.76, 1.17) for ages 18 to 20 years relative to ages 21 years and

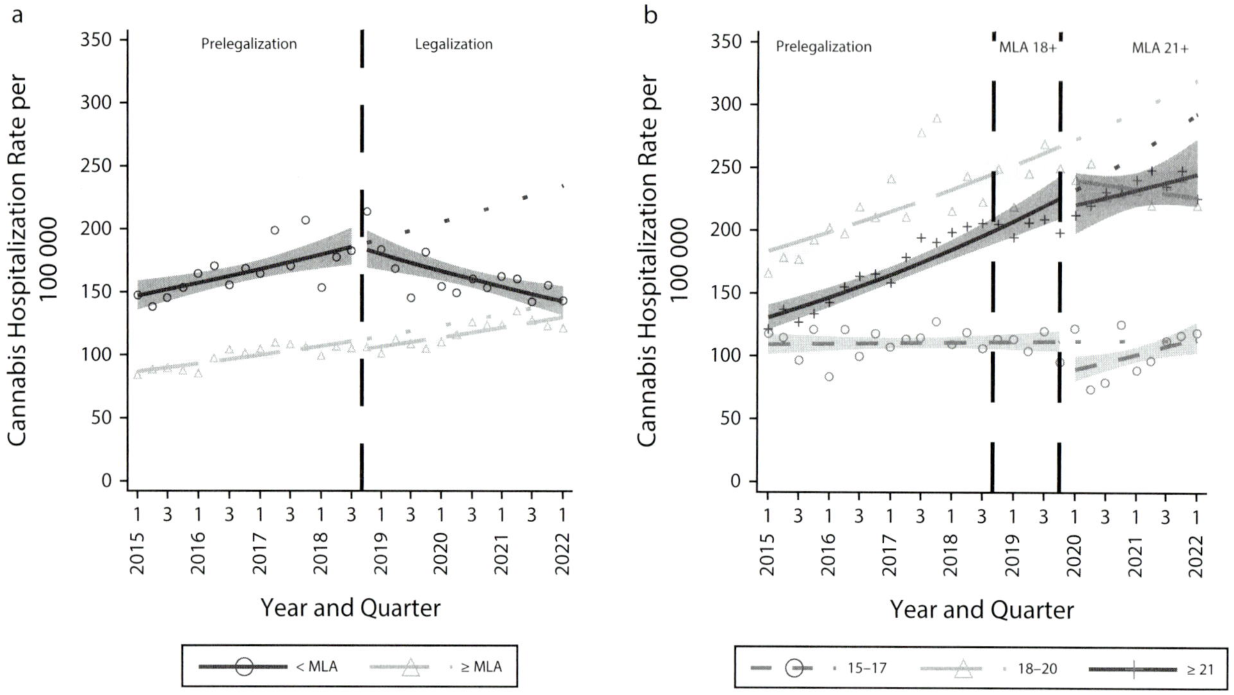


**FIGURE 1— Quarterly Rates of Cannabis-Related Hospitalizations in (a) Canada (except Quebec) for Individuals Above and Below the Minimum Legal Age (MLA) and (b) Quebec for Individuals Aged 15–17, 18–20, and 21–44 Years: January 2015–March 2022**

*Note.* The MLA in Quebec was initially 18 years, and it switched to 21 years in January 2020. Points show observed data, and solid lines show model fit with the shaded regions, indicating 95% confidence intervals. The colored dashed line represents the projected counterfactual (e.g., assuming continuation of trends from the prelegalization period) for individuals above and below the MLA.



older. Similarly, there was a greater slope change for ages 18 to 20 years than for those aged 21 years or older (relative difference = 0.99; 95% CI = 0.96, 1.02), and visits began declining by 1.0% a quarter in ages 18 to 20 years while continuing to increase by 1.0% a quarter for individuals aged 21 years or older. The combined effect 2.5 years (in Q1 2022) after the MLA change was a 29.0% reduction (RR = 0.71; 95% CI = 0.60, 0.84) in rates of hospitalizations in those aged 18 to 20 years compared with the counterfactual (had the pre-MLA change trend continued) and a

**TABLE 2— Segmented Regression Analyses of Cannabis-Related Hospitalizations After Legalization in October 2018 for Individuals Below the MLA Relative to Those Above the MLA for All of Canada Excluding Quebec: January 2015–March 2022**

| | RR (95% CI) | | |
|---|---|---|---|
| | Below MLA | Above MLA | Relative Difference Below vs Above MLA |
| Prelegalization quarterly slope | 1.02 (1.01, 1.03) | 1.02 (1.01, 1.03) | 1.00 (0.99, 1.01) |
| Immediate change (level change) | 1.01 (0.90, 1.13) | 0.93 (0.83, 1.05) | 1.08 (0.92, 1.28) |
| Gradual change (slope change per quarter) | 0.96 (0.95, 0.98) | 1.00 (0.98, 1.01) | 0.97 (0.95, 0.99) |
| Postlegalization quarterly slope | 0.98 (0.97, 0.99) | 1.02 (1.01, 1.03) | 0.96 (0.95, 0.98) |
| Total effect relative to counterfactual[a] | 0.61 (0.49, 0.76) | 0.92 (0.73, 1.14) | 0.66 (0.49, 0.91) |

*Note.* CI = confidence interval; MLA = minimum legal age of cannabis purchase; RR = rate ratio.
[a]Combined intercept and slope change relative to projected prelegalization trend at the end of the study period (March 2022).

**TABLE 3—** Segmented Regression Analyses of Cannabis-Related Hospitalizations After Change in MLA From 18 to 20 Years in January 2020 for Individuals Aged 15–17, 18–20 and 21 Years or Older in Quebec: January 2015–March 2022

| | RR (95% CI) | | | |
|---|---|---|---|---|
| | Age 15–17 y | Age 18–20 y | Age ≥ 21 y | Relative Difference (18–20 y vs ≥ 21 y) |
| Prechange quarterly slope | 1.00 (0.99, 1.01) | 1.02 (1.01, 1.03) | 1.03 (1.02, 1.04) | 0.99 (0.98, 1.00) |
| Immediate change (level change) | 0.78 (0.67, 0.90) | 0.91 (0.78, 1.05) | 0.96 (0.83, 1.12) | 0.94 (0.76, 1.17) |
| Gradual change (slope change per quarter) | 1.03 (1.01, 1.06) | 0.97 (0.95, 1.00) | 0.98 (0.96, 1.01) | 0.99 (0.96, 1.02) |
| Postchange quarterly slope | 1.03 (1.01, 1.06) | 0.99 (0.97, 1.02) | 1.01 (0.99, 1.04) | 0.98 (0.95, 1.01) |
| Total effect relative to counterfactual[a] | 1.01 (0.85, 1.20) | 0.71 (0.60, 0.84) | 0.84 (0.70, 0.99) | 0.85 (0.61, 1.18) |

*Note.* CI = confidence interval; MLA = minimum legal age of cannabis purchase; RR = rate ratio.
[a]Combined intercept and slope change relative to projected prelegalization trend at the end of the study period (March 2022).

16.0% reduction for ages 21 years or older (RR = 0.84; 95% CI = 0.70, 0.99). The relative difference estimate for the association between the MLA change was a 15.0% reduction (relative difference = 0.85; 95% CI = 0.61, 1.18; *P* = .322) in the rate of cannabis-related hospitalizations for ages 18 to 20 years relative to ages 21 years or older though the confidence intervals crossed 1.

## Sensitivity Analyses

The same pattern of increasing visits before legalization that began declining after legalization for those below but not above the MLA was consistent across regions. In regions of Canada with an MLA of 19 years (Canada excluding Quebec and Alberta), legalization was associated with 34% (relative difference = 0.66; 95% CI = 0.47, 0.94; *P* = .021) reduction (combined intercept and slope change) in rates of hospitalization rates for age groups below relative to above the MLA. In Alberta, with an MLA of 18 years, legalization was associated with a 24% reduction (relative difference = 0.76; 95% CI = 0.50, 1.18; *P* = .221) in rates of hospitalizations for age groups below relative to above the MLA. In models excluding the 25- to 44-year age group, legalization was associated with a 29.0% (relative difference = 0.71; 95% CI = 0.51, 1.00; *P* = .050) reduction in rates of hospitalizations for age groups below relative to above the MLA (see Appendix Figure A and Appendix Table B for regression coefficients).

## DISCUSSION

In this quasi-experimental study, we explored changes in cannabis-related hospitalizations after legalization for individuals above and below the MLA. We found that being below the MLA was associated with 34% reduction in cannabis-related hospitalization rates relative to those above the MLA compared with expected rates based on prelegalization trends. The protective effect against increases in cannabis-related hospitalizations was consistently observed over a range of MLAs in all regions across Canada and in individuals aged 18 to 20 years in Quebec following an increase in the MLA from 18 to 21 years.

A large body of literature has found that higher MLAs for alcohol and tobacco purchase are associated with reductions in vehicle crashes, youth alcohol or tobacco initiation, or prevalence of use. A review of studies from the United States estimated that lowering the MLA for alcohol from 21 to 18 years increased fatal and nonfatal car crashes by 10%, while raising it from 18 to 21 years reduced crashes by 12%.[18] Raising the MLA from 18 to 21 years for alcohol purchase has been similarly associated with lower levels of alcohol use and alcohol-related injuries in individuals aged younger than 21 years.[19–21] Evidence from the United States suggests declines in the uptake and prevalence of youth smoking after increasing the MLA from 18 to 21 years for tobacco purchases.[22,23]

There is less evidence on the effectiveness of MLAs for cannabis purchase. One study found that increasing the MLA from 18 to 21 years in Quebec was associated with reduced self-reported cannabis use in individuals aged 18 to 20 years but was limited by a small sample size (1005 respondents) and examined past-3-month cannabis use, which has lower clinical relevance.[24] Two studies using health administrative data from Ontario, Canada, found that emergency department visits for cannabis-induced psychosis and cannabis hyperemesis syndrome increased following legalization for individuals above (aged ≥ 19 years) but not below the MLA (aged 15–18 years).[25,26] One study from the United States found that state-level nonmedical legalization was associated with increases in self-reported frequent cannabis use for individuals above the MLA (aged 21–23 years) but not individuals below the MLA (aged 18–20 years).[27] Another study found that the legal cannabis retail stores opening in Washington State was associated with increases in the prevalence of monthly cannabis use for individuals above the MLA (aged 21–25 years) but not in those below (aged 18–20 years).[28]

Adding to the literature, our findings suggest that being below the MLA after legalization was associated with preventing further increases in cannabis-related hospitalizations across multiple regions in Canada. These findings are consistent with available survey data suggesting no increases in past-year cannabis use in youths in Canada after legalization.[29,30] This protective association occurred for MLAs up to 21 years and was consistent both during early periods of legalization with market restrictions and later when the market expanded with more stores and high-potency cannabis products (e.g., vape pens, concentrates). We found that raising the MLA in Quebec from 18 to 21 years in January 2020 may have had a protective effect for individuals aged 18 to 20 years. Reductions in cannabis-related hospitalizations in youths below the MLA may be explained by a decline in their ability to access and obtain cannabis. Mechanistically, this could have occurred through a combination of declines in the size of the illicit market (which is estimated to have contracted by 51% between the start of legalization and the end of our observation period) along with MLA policies and related implementation measures that effectively prevented youths from accessing the legal market that was replacing the illicit market.[31]

Our findings have policy implications. First, while these findings reduce concerns that legalization will result in increased cannabis-related harm in youths, cannabis-related hospitalizations remain high in this age group, and additional evidence-based policy measures are indicated. Second, MLAs were associated with preventing increases in cannabis-related hospitalizations for those below the MLA during both periods of market restrictions and periods of commercialization, which suggests that MLAs work across the spectrum of nonmedical legalization policies and may be a key intervention regardless of the regulatory framework adopted. Third, MLAs were associated with protective effects at least until age 21 years, which suggests that setting a higher MLA in countries pursuing legalization could prevent increases in cannabis-related hospitalizations after legalization for a larger number of youths and young adults.

In contrast to youths aged below the MLA, hospitalizations for individuals above the MLA continued to increase after legalization in Canada. Daily or near-daily cannabis use in Canadian adults and the potency (THC content) of cannabis products in Canada, both predictors of cannabis-related harms, have increased since legalization.[32,33] Rising cannabis-related hospitalizations may reflect increasing overall access to cannabis and align with studies showing that commercialization of cannabis markets increases cannabis use and associated cannabis use disorders and harms.[34–36]

## Limitations

Our study has limitations. First, part of the increases over time in cannabis-related hospitalizations may reflect increasing awareness of, or willingness to document, cannabis use by health care providers. Importantly, these biases would not be expected to have differential impacts based on MLA status. Second, changes in cannabis-related hospitalizations may be partially explained by the willingness of individuals to disclose cannabis use after legalization. This bias may explain some of the ongoing increases in hospitalizations after legalization for individuals above the MLA. However, it is unlikely to explain the observed declines in rates of cannabis-related hospitalizations in individuals below the MLA in whom cannabis possession and use switched from being illegal to decriminalized and consequently would also have been more likely to disclose cannabis use. Finally, these findings may not capture the long-term impacts of a mature legal market (e.g., greater legal access and lower illicit access), and ongoing monitoring is needed.

## Public Health Implications

This population-level study found that MLAs were associated with a protective effect against increases in cannabis-related hospitalizations after legalization for individuals below the MLA compared with those above the MLA. These findings should reduce concerns that legalization will result in increases in cannabis-related harm in youths below the MLA. In contrast, ongoing increases in cannabis-related hospitalizations in young adults aged above the MLA suggest potential harms arising from legalization and highlight the need for additional policy interventions, which could include setting a higher MLA. AJPH

## ABOUT THE AUTHORS

Daniel T. Myran is with the Department of Family Medicine, Faculty of Medicine at the University of Ottawa, Ontario. Robert Talarico is with ICES uOttawa, at the Ottawa Hospital Research Institute. Rosalie Liccardo Pacula is with the Sol Price School of Public Policy and Schaeffer Center for Health Policy and Economics, University of Southern California, Los Angeles. Jennifer Xiao and Lauren Konikoff were with the Clinical Epidemiological Program at the Ottawa Hospital Research Institute at the time of this study. Doug Manuel is with the Clinical Epidemiological Program and ICES uOttawa at the Ottawa Hospital Research Institute, Ottawa. Erin Hobin is with the Dalla Lana School of Public Health, University of Toronto, Ontario. Peter Tanuseputro is with the University of Hong Kong, Department of Family Medicine and Primary Care, Hong Kong. Monica Taljaard is with the Clinical Epidemiology Program at the Ottawa Hospital Research Institute.

## CORRESPONDENCE

Correspondence should be sent to Daniel T. Myran, MD, MPH, CCFP, FRCPC, Ottawa Hospital Research Institute, 1053 Carling Ave, Box 693, Ottawa, Ontario, K1Y 4E9, Canada (e-mail: dmyran@ohri.ca). Reprints can be ordered at https://www.ajph.org by clicking the "Reprints" link.

## PUBLICATION INFORMATION

Full Citation: Myran DT, Talarico R, Pacula RL, et al. Minimum legal age of nonmedical cannabis purchase laws and cannabis-related hospitalizations in Canada, 2015 to 2022. *Am J Public Health*. 2025;115(7):1166–1174.

Acceptance Date: February 19, 2025.

DOI: https://doi.org/10.2105/AJPH.2025.308090

ORCID iDs:

Daniel T. Myran https://orcid.org/0000-0002-8038-300X

Rosalie Liccardo Pacula https://orcid.org/0000-0002-6145-9865

Doug Manuel https://orcid.org/0000-0003-0912-0845

Lauren Konikoff https://orcid.org/0009-0006-2786-7933

## CONTRIBUTORS

D. T. Myran (primary author), R. L. Pacula, P. Tanuseputro, and M. Taljaard generated the idea for the study. D. T. Myran, M. Taljaard, R. Talarico, R. L. Pacula, E. Hobin, P. Tanuseputro, and D. Manuel developed the methodological approach. D. T. Myran and P. Tanuseputro sourced the data for the study, and R. Talarico undertook the statistical analyses. J. Xiao and L. Konikoff provided research support and project coordination. D. T. Myran drafted the article, and all authors provided critical input into the interpretation of the results, revisions, and approval of the final submission. D. T. Myran and R. Talarico accessed and verified the data. D. T. Myran and R. Talarico had full access to all the data in the study. All authors had final responsibility for the decision to submit for publication.

## ACKNOWLEDGMENTS

D. T. Myran was supported by a Canada Research Chair at the University of Ottawa Department of Family Medicine. P. Tanuseputro was supported by a PSI Graham Farquharson Knowledge Translation Fellowship. This study was supported by the University of Ottawa site of ICES, which is funded by an annual grant from the Ontario Ministry of Health and Ministry of Long-Term Care. This study also received funding from the Canadian Institutes of Health Research (grant 200272).

This study used data adapted from the Statistics Canada Postal Code Conversion File, which is based on data licensed from Canada Post Corporation, or from the Ontario Ministry of Health Postal Code Conversion File, which contains data copied under license from Canada Post Corporation and Statistics Canada. Parts of this material are based on data and/or information compiled and provided by the Canadian Institute for Health Information and the Ontario Ministry of Health. Part of the data set from this study is held securely in coded form at ICES. While legal data-sharing agreements between ICES and data providers (e.g., health care organizations and government) prohibit ICES from making the data set publicly available, access may be granted to those who meet prespecified criteria for confidential access, available at https://www.ices.on.ca/DAS (e-mail: das@ices.on.ca). The full data set creation plan and underlying analytic code are available from the authors upon request, with the understanding that the computer programs may rely upon coding templates or macros that are unique to ICES and are therefore either inaccessible or may require modification.

**Note.** The analyses, conclusions, opinions, and statements expressed herein are solely those of the authors and do not reflect those of the funding or data sources; no endorsement is intended or should be inferred.

## CONFLICTS OF INTEREST

The authors declare no conflicts of interest.

## HUMAN PARTICIPANT PROTECTION

The use of the data in this study was approved by the Ottawa Hospital Research Institute Research Ethics Board. Because the study used de-identified aggregate health information, no informed consent was required.

## REFERENCES

1. Parliament of Canada. Bill C-45, The Cannabis Act. 2018. Available at: https://laws-lois.justice.gc.ca/eng/acts/c-24.5. Accessed September 6, 2024.
2. Centre for Addiction and Mental Health. Cannabis Policy Framework. October 2014. Available at: https://www.camh.ca/-/media/files/pdfs—public-policy-submissions/camhcannabispolicyframework-pdf.pdf. Accessed September 6, 2024.
3. Spithoff S, Emerson B, Spithoff A. Cannabis legalization: adhering to public health best practice. *CMAJ*. 2015;187(16):1211–1216. https://doi.org/10.1503/cmaj.150657
4. Murray RM, Hall W. Will legalization and commercialization of cannabis use increase the incidence and prevalence of psychosis? *JAMA Psychiatry*. 2020;77(8):777–778. https://doi.org/10.1001/jamapsychiatry.2020.0339
5. Myran DT, Harrison LD, Pugliese M, et al. Transition to schizophrenia spectrum disorder following emergency department visits due to substance use with and without psychosis. *JAMA Psychiatry*. 2023;80(11):1169–1174. https://doi.org/10.1001/jamapsychiatry.2023.3582
6. Myran DT, Harrison LD, Pugliese M, et al. Development of an anxiety disorder following an emergency department visit due to cannabis use: a population-based cohort study. *EClinicalMedicine*. 2024;69:102455. https://doi.org/10.1016/j.eclinm.2024.102455
7. Harding FM, Hingson RW, Klitzner M, et al. Underage drinking: a review of trends and prevention strategies. *Am J Prev Med*. 2016;51(4):S148–S157. https://doi.org/10.1016/j.amepre.2016.05.020
8. Richardson L, Hemsing N, Greaves L, et al. Preventing smoking in young people: a systematic review of the impact of access interventions. *Int J Environ Res Public Health*. 2009;6(4):1485–1514. https://doi.org/10.3390/ijerph6041485
9. Babor TF, Casswell S, Graham K, et al. *Alcohol: No Ordinary Commodity*—a summary of the third edition. *Addiction*. 2022;117(12):3024–3036. https://doi.org/10.1111/add.16003
10. Mahamad S, Wadsworth E, Rynard V, Goodman S, Hammond D. Availability, retail price and potency of legal and illegal cannabis in Canada after recreational cannabis legalisation. *Drug Alcohol Rev*. 2020;39(4):337–346. https://doi.org/10.1111/dar.13069
11. Shingler, B. Quebec passes cannabis law that will raise legal age to 21. *CBC News*. Available at: https://www.cbc.ca/news/canada/montreal/quebec-cannabis-law-1.5339477. October 30, 2019. Accessed April 3, 2025.
12. Alliance for Healthier Communities. Non-insured clients. Available at: https://www.allianceon.org/Non-Insured-Clients. Accessed July 18, 2024.
13. Statistics Canada. Population estimates on July 1st, by age and sex. Available at: https://www150.statcan.gc.ca/t1/tbl1/en/tv.action?pid=1710000501. Accessed November 29, 2023.
14. Government of Canada. Regulations Amending the Cannabis Regulations (New Classes of Cannabis): SOR/2019-206. *Canada Gazette*. 2019;153(13). https://gazette.gc.ca/rp-pr/p2/

2019/2019-06-26/html/sor-dors206-eng.html. Accessed April9, 2025.

15. Myran DT, Friesen EL, Dickson S, Konikoff L, Arora G, Tanuseputro P. Access to legal cannabis market in Canada over the four years following non-medical cannabis legalisation. *Drug Alcohol Rev.* 2023;42(5):1114–1119. https://doi.org/10.1111/dar.13650
16. Myran DT, Gaudreault A, Konikoff L, Talarico R, Pacula RL. Changes in cannabis-attributable hospitalizations following nonmedical cannabis legalization in Canada. *JAMA Netw Open.* 2023;6(10):e2336113. https://doi.org/10.1001/jamanetworkopen.2023.36113
17. Turner SL, Karahalios A, Forbes AB, Taljaard M, Grimshaw JM, McKenzie JE. Comparison of six statistical methods for interrupted time series studies: empirical evaluation of 190 published series. *BMC Med Res Methodol.* 2021;21(1):134. https://doi.org/10.1186/s12874-021-01306-w
18. Shults RA, Elder RW, Sleet DA, et al. Reviews of evidence regarding interventions to reduce alcohol-impaired driving. *Am J Prev Med.* 2001;21(4):66–88. https://doi.org/10.1016/S0749-3797(01)00381-6
19. DeJong W, Blanchette J. Case closed: research evidence on the positive public health impact of the age 21 minimum legal drinking age in the United States. *J Stud Alcohol Drugs Suppl.* 2014;(17):108–115. https://doi.org/1015288/jsads2014.s17108
20. Toomey TL, Nelson TF, Lenk KM. The age-21 minimum legal drinking age: a case study linking past and current debates. *Addiction.* 2009;104(12):1958–1965. https://doi.org/10.1111/j.1360-0443.2009.02742.x
21. Toomey TL, Rosenfeld C, Wagenaar AC. The minimum legal drinking age: history, effectiveness, and ongoing debate. *Alcohol Health Res World.* 1996;20(4):213–218.
22. Ertan Yörük C, Yörük BK. Do minimum legal tobacco purchase age laws work? *Contemp Econ Policy.* 2016;34(3):415–429. https://doi.org/10.1111/coep.12153
23. Kessel Schneider S, Buka SL, Dash K, Winickoff JP, Donnell LO. Community reductions in youth smoking after raising the minimum tobacco sales age to 21. *Tob Control.* 2016;25(3):355–359. https://doi.org/10.1136/tobaccocontrol-2014-052207
24. Nguyen HV, Mital S. Changes in youth cannabis use after an increase in cannabis minimum legal age in Quebec, Canada. *JAMA Netw Open.* 2022;5(6):e2217648. https://doi.org/10.1001/jamanetworkopen.2022.17648
25. Myran DT, Roberts R, Pugliese M, Taljaard M, Tanuseputro P, Pacula RL. Changes in emergency department visits for cannabis hyperemesis syndrome following recreational cannabis legalization and subsequent commercialization in Ontario, Canada. *JAMA Netw Open.* 2022;5(9):e2231937. https://doi.org/10.1001/jamanetworkopen.2022.31937
26. Myran DT, Pugliese M, Roberts RL, et al. Association between non-medical cannabis legalization and emergency department visits for cannabis-induced psychosis. *Mol Psychiatry.* 2023;28(10):4251–4260. https://doi.org/10.1038/s41380-023-02185-x
27. Kerr DCR, Levy NS, Bae H, Boustead AE, Martins SS. Cannabis and alcohol use by US young adults, 2008–2019: changes in prevalence after recreational cannabis legalization. *Am J Prev Med.* 2023;65(6):983–992. https://doi.org/10.1016/j.amepre.2023.06.009
28. Kilmer JR, Rhew IC, Guttmannova K, et al. Cannabis use among young adults in Washington State after legalization of nonmedical cannabis. *Am J Public Health.* 2022;112(4):638–645. https://doi.org/10.2105/AJPH.2021.306641
29. Statistics Canada. Research to insights: cannabis in Canada. 2023. Available at: https://www150.statcan.gc.ca/n1/pub/11-631-x/11-631-x2023006-eng.htm. Accessed July 12, 2024.
30. Statistics Canada. Prevalence of cannabis use in the past three months, by time relative to legalization and quarter, and selected demographics, household population aged 15 and older, Canada (provinces only), first quarters of 2018 and 2019, and fourth quarter of 2020. 2021. Available at: https://www150.statcan.gc.ca/n1/pub/82-003-x/2021004/article/00001/tbl/tbl01-eng.htm. Accessed June 23, 2024.
31. Health Canada. Canadian Cannabis Survey 2022: summary. Available at: https://www.canada.ca/en/health-canada/services/drugs-medication/cannabis/research-data/canadian-cannabis-survey-2022-summary.html. Accessed October 18, 2023.
32. Naimi T, Vallance K, Churchill S, Callaghan R, Stockwell T, Farrell-Low A. *Sales and Revenue From Regulated Cannabis Products: British Columbia, October 2018–December 2020.* University of Victoria, Canadian Institute for Substance Use Research. June 2021. Available at: https://www.uvic.ca/research/centres/cisur/assets/docs/report-sales-and-revenue-from-regulated-cannabis-products-bc.pdf. Accessed June 16, 2024.
33. Goodman S, Dann MJ, Fataar F, Abramovici H. How have cannabis use and related indicators changed since legalization of cannabis for non-medical purposes? Results of the Canadian Cannabis Survey 2018–2022. *Int J Drug Policy.* 2024;127:104385. https://doi.org/10.1016/j.drugpo.2024.104385
34. Hall W, Stjepanović D, Caulkins J, et al. Public health implications of legalising the production and sale of cannabis for medicinal and recreational use. *Lancet.* 2019;394(10208):1580–1590. https://doi.org/10.1016/S0140-6736(19)31789-1
35. Cantor N, Silverman M, Gaudreault A, et al. The association between physical availability of cannabis retail outlets and frequent cannabis use and related health harms: a systematic review. *Lancet Reg Health Am.* 2024:32:100708. https://doi.org/10.1016/j.lana.2024.100708
36. Myran DT, Imtiaz S, Konikoff L, Douglas L, Elton-Marshall T. Changes in health harms due to cannabis following legalisation of non-medical cannabis in Canada in context of cannabis commercialisation: a scoping review. *Drug Alcohol Rev.* 2023;42(2):277–298. https://doi.org/10.1111/dar.13546

# "Whiteness" and the Opioid Epidemic: A Construct in Need of Elaboration

Akshay Pendyal, MD, MHS

**ABOUT THE AUTHOR**

*Akshay Pendyal is with the School of Medicine, Duke University, Durham, NC.*

Cooper at al. are to be commended for their timely survey-based study of White people who use drugs (PWUD) in 22 rural Appalachian counties.[1] Their study is particularly relevant given the scale and severity of the opioid epidemic. Unsurprisingly, they identify a high prevalence of unmet needs in this population. In their model fully adjusted for relevant sociodemographic covariates, unmet need was not associated with being stopped by law enforcement.

In explaining this finding, the authors unfortunately make claims that extend beyond their own data. Specifically, they note that "Whiteness"—which remains undefined throughout their article—may confer psychological benefits among PWUD in Appalachia, protecting them from policing in a way that is markedly different from predominantly Black jurisdictions. But given the absence of a similarly situated comparator population in their study, a conclusion like this, while provocative, remains conjectural.

The authors write that a "hallmark of Appalachian Whiteness has been freedom from . . . persistent criminal–legal control."[1(p1093)] From this, they infer that because "Whiteness has protected local social networks through sovereignty over home and community,"[1(p1095)] in the case of the participants they sampled, "White Appalachian networks [may] provide essential support—emotional and otherwise—that buffers the effects of criminal–legal encounters,"[1(p1094)] thereby explaining the lack of a statistically significant association between unmet needs and police stops in their data set.

But why invoke Whiteness—a construct that, despite its widespread deployment in the academy, has achieved minimal semantic clarity[2]—to explain this lack of association in the first place? The potted history they sketch over a few paragraphs, which ranges from "White colonists' rage" during the American Revolution to the War on Drugs, does little to bolster their argument. It serves mainly to reify Whiteness as a transhistorical motive force that relegates Blacks to an abject status and Whites to a privileged one (to say nothing of its essentializing effect on racial categories writ large).

The stark baseline prevalence of material deprivation in their study—whether in the form of lack of insurance, homelessness, or unemployment—should put paid to any notion of Whiteness as a salutary phenomenon. If there is any "benefit" to residing in an immiserated geographic region, it seems likely that it would be mediated not through race but rather through other forms of social capital.[3] On this point I agree with the authors that further research, especially involving qualitative methods, is needed to answer central questions about the residents of Appalachia. AJPH



## CORRESPONDENCE

Correspondence should be sent to Akshay Pendyal, MD, MHS, Duke University School of Medicine, Box 90780, Durham, NC 27708-0780 (e-mail: akshay.pendyal@duke.edu). Reprints can be ordered at https://www.ajph.org by clicking the "Reprints" link.

## PUBLICATION INFORMATION

Full Citation: Pendyal A. "Whiteness" and the opioid epidemic: a construct in need of elaboration. *Am J Public Health*. 2025;115(7):1175–1176.

Acceptance Date: January 17, 2025.

DOI: https://doi.org/10.2105/AJPH.2025.308034

ORCID iD:
Akshay Pendyal https://orcid.org/0000-0002-4191-2976

## CONFLICTS OF INTEREST

No conflicts of interest, financial or other, exist with regard to this letter.

## REFERENCES


1. Cooper HLF, Livingston MD, Crawford ND, et al. The War on Drugs, racialized capitalism, and health care utilization among White people who use drugs in 22 rural Appalachian counties. *Am J Public Health*. 2024;114(10):1086–1096. https://doi.org/10.2105/AJPH.2024.307744
2. Arnesen E. Whiteness and the historians' imagination. *Int Labor Working Class Hist*. 2001;60:3–32. https://doi.org/10.1017/S0147547901004380
3. Jonas AB, Young AM, Oser CB, Leukefeld CG, Havens JR. OxyContin as currency: OxyContin use and increased social capital among rural Appalachian drug users. *Soc Sci Med*. 2012;74(10):1602–1609. https://doi.org/10.1016/j.socscimed.2011.12.053

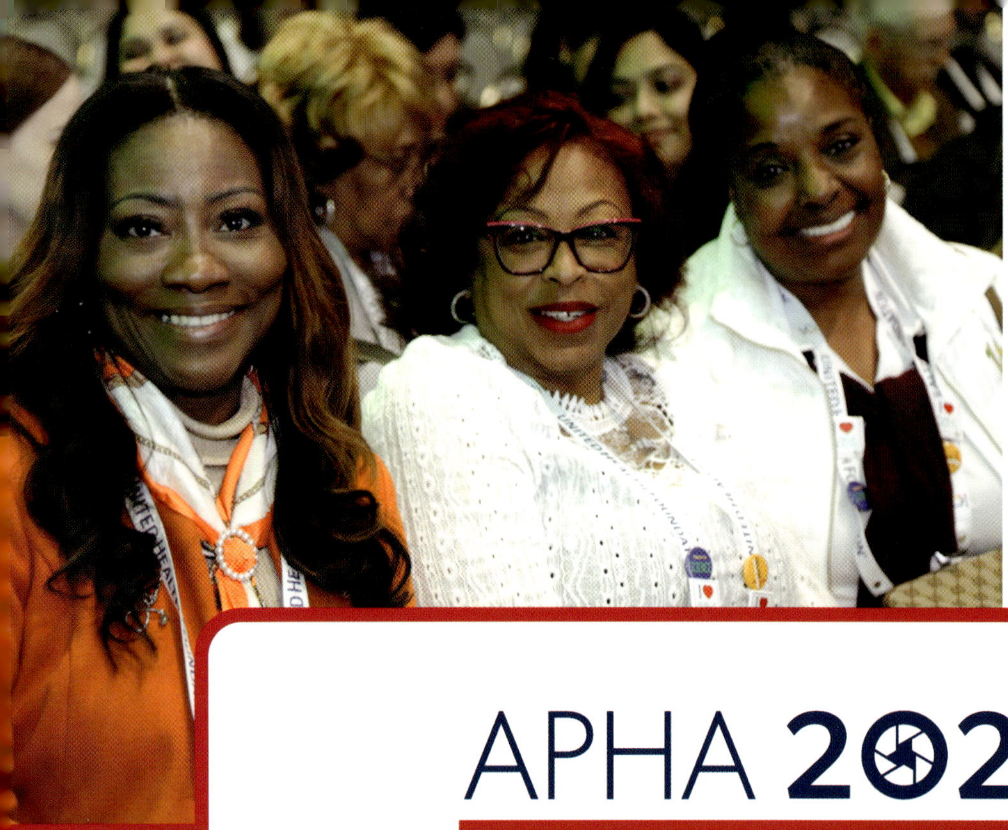

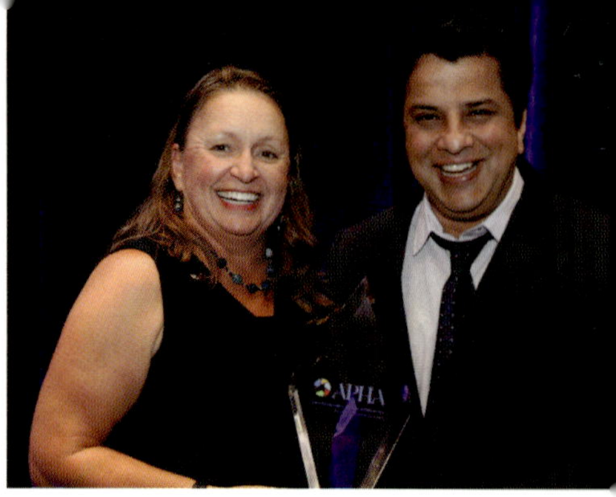

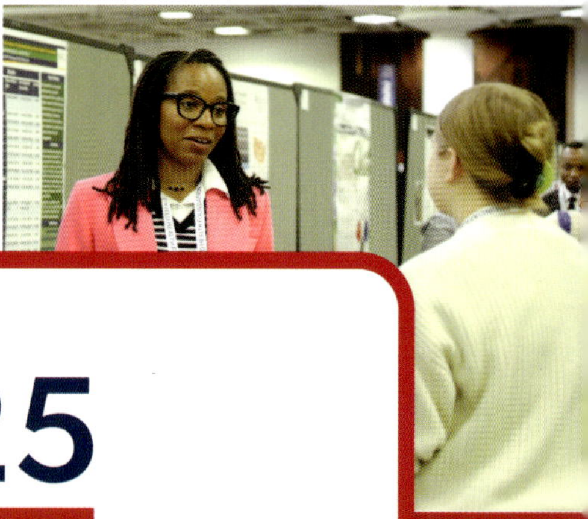